Glutamate as a Neurotransmitter

Advances in Biochemical Psychopharmacology
Volume 27

Advances in Biochemical Psychopharmacology

Series Editors

E. Costa, M.D.
Chief, Laboratory of Preclinical Pharmacology
National Institute of Mental Health
Washington, D.C.

Paul Greengard, Ph.D.
Professor of Pharmacology
Yale University School of Medicine
New Haven, Connecticut

Glutamate as a Neurotransmitter

Advances in Biochemical Psychopharmacology
Volume 27

Editors

Gaetano Di Chiara, M.D.
G. L. Gessa, M.D.

Institute of Pharmacology
University of Cagliari School of Medicine
Cagliari, Italy

Raven Press ■ New York

Raven Press, 1140 Avenue of the Americas, New York, New York 10036

Made in the United States of America

Great care has been taken to maintain the accuracy of the information contained in the volume. However, Raven Press cannot be held responsible for errors or for any consequences arising from the use of the information contained herein.

Materials appearing in this book prepared by individuals as part of their official duties as U.S. Government employees are not covered by the above-mentioned copyright.

Library of Congress Cataloging in Publication Data
Main entry under title:

Glutamate as a neurotransmitter.

(Advances in biochemical psychopharmacology ; v. 27)
"Based on a symposium ... held in Porto Cervo, Sardinia, Italy, in May 1980."
Includes bibliographical references and index.
1. Glutamate—Physiological effect—Congresses.
2. Neurotransmitters—Congresses. I. Di Chiara, Gaetano. II. Gessa, G. L. III. Series.
RM315.A4   vol. 27 [QP562.G5] 615'.78s   80-26264

ISBN 0-89004-420-1   [591.1'88]

Preface

Glutamic acid is an abundant, ubiquitous substance that, in addition to being an intermediary of many metabolic pathways, serves the function, necessarily specific, localized, and phasic, of a neurotransmitter. These characteristics, although demonstrating the importance of compartmentalization in the central nervous system, have limited tremendously the appraisal of glutamate as a neurotransmitter. In fact, the widespread action of glutamate was probably among the factors that led electrophysiologists to consider its powerful excitatory actions on central neurons nonspecific; ubiquity also hampered visual demonstration of glutamate synapses and the study of the synthesis and release of neurotransmitter glutamate. In spite of these difficulties, glutamate, at least in certain systems, now meets most if not all the criteria for being considered a neurotransmitter.

This book is the first specifically dedicated to glutamate and related excitatory amino acids; it is hoped that it will help glutamate along the long, hard road to acquiring its freedom and becoming recognized, not as a by-product of intermediary metabolism, a precursor of GABA, or an oriental flavoring, but at last as a neurotransmitter.

This volume is a comprehensive and systematic review of the anatomy, biochemistry, electrophysiology, and pharmacology of glutamate synapses and receptors and of the role of glutamate analogs, particularly kainic acid, in neuropathology. It will be of interest to anatomists, neurochemists, electrophysiologists, pharmacologists, toxicologists, and pathologists, as well as neurologists.

The Editors

Acknowledgments

This volume is based on a symposium entitled "GABA and Glutamate as Transmitters" held in Porto Cervo, Sardinia, Italy, in May 1980. All symposium participants will testify to its success in providing an enormous amount of new information, stimulating discussions and new ideas, and promoting new collaborations and friendships.

Such a success should be attributed largely to the assembling of the best people in the field, which in turn was made possible by the generous support of FIDIA Research Laboratories, Abano Terme (PD), Italy, which entirely sponsored the symposium.

We particularly acknowledge the contribution made to the organization of the symposium by Dr. Cristina Schirato of FIDIA Research Laboratories and by Miss Francesca Verhagen of our institute, who also acted as secretary in the editing of this book.

Contents

Membrane Changes by Amino Acids

Receptors for Glutamate and Related Excitatory Amino Acids

Kainic Acid, Glutamic Acid, and Neuropathologs

Contributors

R. Balazs
*MRC Developmental Neurobiology
 Unit
Institute of Neurology
London WC1N 2NS, England*

J. L. Barker
*Laboratory of Neurophysiology
NINCDS
Bethesda, Maryland 20205*

A. Beaudet
*Brain Research Institute
University of Zurich
CH-8029 Zurich, Switzerland*

Y. Ben-Ari
*Laboratoire de Physiologie Nerveuse
Département de Neurophysiologie
 Appliquée
C.N.R.S. 91190 Gifs/Yvette, France*

Nathan K. Blank
*Neurology Research
Veterans Administration Medical
 Center
Departments of Neurology, Pathology,
 and Biochemistry
University of Oregon Health Sciences
 Center
Portland, Oregon 97201*

Ch. Bührle
*I. Physiologisches Institut der
 Universität
Im Neuenheimer Feld 326
D-6900 Heidelberg, Federal Republic of
 Germany*

V. Canzek
*Brain Research Institute
University of Zurich
CH-8029 Zurich, Switzerland*

F. Casamenti
*Department of Pharmacology
University of Florence
50134 Florence, Italy*

D. L. Cheney
*Laboratory of Preclinical Pharmacology
National Institute of Mental Health
Saint Elizabeths Hospital
Washington, D.C. 20032*

G. G. S. Collins
*Department of Pharmacology
University of Sheffield
Sheffield S10 2TN, United Kingdom*

J. Collins
*Department of Chemistry
City of London Polytechnic
London EC3N 2EY, England*

J. Constantinidis
*Psychiatric Clinic
University of Geneva
1225 Chêne-Bourg, Switzerland*

R. Corradetti
*Department of Pharmacology
University of Florence
50134 Florence, Italy*

E. Costa
*Laboratory of Preclinical
 Pharmacology
National Institute of Mental Health
Saint Elizabeths Hospital
Washington, D.C. 20032*

C. W. Cotman
*Department of Psychobiology
University of California
Irvine, California 92717*

J. T. Coyle
Departments of Pharmacology and
  Experimental Therapeutics, and
  Psychiatry and the Behavioral
  Sciences
Johns Hopkins University School of
  Medicine
Baltimore, Maryland 21205

M. Cuénod
Brain Research Institute
University of Zurich
CH-8029 Zurich, Switzerland

D. R. Curtis
Department of Pharmacology
The Australian National University
Canberra City, A.C.T. 2601, Australia

J. Davies
Department of Pharmacology
The School of Pharmacy
University of London
London WC1N 1AX, England

Michael Dekin
Department of Physiology
Temple University School of Medicine
Philadelphia, Pennsylvania 19140

G. Di Chiara
Institute of Pharmacology
University of Cagliari
09100 Cagliari, Italy

I. Engberg
Institute of Physiology
University of Aarhus
DK-8000 Aarhus C, Denmark

R. H. Evans
Department of Pharmacology
The Medical School
Bristol BS8 1TD, England

G. Faa
Institute of Pathological Anatomy
University of Cagliari
09100 Cagliari, Italy

J. A. Flatman
Institute of Physiology
University of Aarhus
DK-8000 Aarhus C, Denmark

F. Fonnum
Norwegian Defence Research
  Establishment
Division for Toxicology
N-2007 Kjeller, Norway

M. Fossarello
Institute of Clinical Ophthalmology
University of Cagliari
09100 Cagliari, Italy

A. Foster
Department of Psychobiology
University of California
Irvine, California 92717

A. A. Francis
Department of Pharmacology
The Medical School
Bristol BS8 1TD, England

Alan R. Freeman
Department of Physiology
Temple University School of Medicine
Philadelphia, Pennsylvania 19140

Vittorio Gallo
Laboratorio di Biologia Cellulare
00196 Rome, Italy

J. Garthwaite
MRC Developmental Neurobiology
  Unit
Institute of Neurology
London WC1N 2NS, England

A. Hamberger
Institute of Neurobiology
University of Göteborg
S-400 33 Göteborg, Sweden

J. J. Hansen
Royal Danish School of Pharmacy
Department of Chemistry BC
DK-2100 Copenhagen, Denmark

L. Hertz
Department of Pharmacology
University of Saskatchewan
Saskatoon, Saskatchewan, S7N 0W0,
  Canada

T. Honoré
Royal Danish School of Pharmacy
Department of Chemistry BC
DK-2100 Copenhagen, Denmark

A. Imperato
Institute of Pharmacology
University of Cagliari
09100 Cagliari, Italy

Michiko Ishida
The Tokyo Metropolitan Institute
Bunkyo-ku
Tokyo 113, Japan

I. Jacobsson
Institute of Neurobiology
University of Göteborg
S-400 33 Göteborg, Sweden

A. W. Jones
Department of Pharmacology
The Medical School
Bristol BS8 1TD, England

John Kephart
Department of Physiology
Temple University School of Medicine
Philadelphia, Pennsylvania 19140

Christer Köhler
Research Laboratories
Astra Läkemedel AB
S-15185 Södertälje, Sweden

P. Krogsgaard-Larsen
Royal Danish School of Pharmacy
Department of Chemistry BC
DK-2100 Copenhagen, Denmark

J. Kvale
Norwegian Defence Research
  Establishment
Division for Toxicology
N-2007 Kjeller, Norway

N. Lake
Department of Research in Anaesthesia
McGill University
Montreal, Quebec, H3G 1Y6, Canada

J. D. C. Lambert
Institute of Physiology
University of Aarhus
DK-8000 Aarhus C, Denmark

T. Lanthorn
Department of Psychobiology
University of California
Irvine, California 92717

Arnold L. Leiman
Department of Psychology
University of California
Berkeley, California 94720

Giulio Levi
Laboratorio di Biologia Cellulare
00196 Rome, Italy

D. Lodge
Department of Pharmacology
The Australian National University
Canberra City, A.C.T. 2601, Australia

J. F. MacDonald
Helen Scott Playfair Neuroscience Unit
Toronto Western Hospital
Toronto M5T 2S8, Canada

Richard M. Mangano
Neuroscience Program
Maryland Psychiatric Research Center
Baltimore, Maryland 21228

H. McLennan
Department of Physiology
University of British Columbia
Vancouver, British Columbia, V6T
  1W5, Canada

S.-O. Molin
Institute of Neurobiology
University of Göteborg
S-400 33 Göteborg, Sweden

G. Moneti
Department of Pharmacology
University of Florence
50134 Florence, Italy

M. Morelli
Institute of Pharmacology
University of Cagliari
09100 Cagliari, Italy

F. Moroni
Department of Pharmacology
University of Florence
50134 Florence, Italy

J. Victor Nadler
Department of Pharmacology
Duke University Medical Center
Durham, North Carolina 27710

A. N. Neophytides
Department of Neurology
Veterans Administration Hospital
New York, New York 10010

A. Nistri
Department of Pharmacology
St. Bartholomew's Hospital Medical
College
London EC1M 6BQ, England

B. Nyström
Institute of Neurobiology
University of Göteborg
S-400 33 Göteborg, Sweden

John W. Olney
Department of Psychiatry
Washington University School of
Medicine
St. Louis, Missouri 63110

G. Pepeu
Department of Pharmacology
University of Florence
50134 Florence, Italy

M. L. Porceddu
Institute of Pharmacology
University of Cagliari
09100 Cagliari, Italy

S. J. Potashner
Department of Anatomy
University of Connecticut Health Center
Farmington, Connecticut 06032

Madelon T. Price
Department of Psychiatry
Washington University School of
Medicine
St. Louis, Missouri 63110

Maurizio Raiteri
Istituto di Farmacologia e
Farmacognosia
Facoltà di Farmacia
University of Genova, Italy

Dianna A. Redburn
Department of Neurobiology and
Anatomy
University of Texas Medical School
Houston, Texas 77025

J. C. Reubi
Brain Research Institute
University of Zurich
CH-8029 Zurich, Switzerland

A. V. Revuelta
Laboratory of Preclinical
Pharmacology
National Institute of Mental Health
Saint Elizabeths Hospital
Washington, D.C. 20032

E. Roberts
City of Hope Research Institute
Duarte, California 91010

P. J. Roberts
Department of Physiology and
Pharmacology
School of Biochemical and
Physiological Sciences
University of Southampton
Southampton S09 3TU, United
Kingdom

M. Sandberg
Institute of Neurobiology
University of Göteborg
S-400 33 Göteborg, Sweden

A. Schousboe
Department of Biochemistry A
The Panum Institute
University of Copenhagen
DK-2200 Copenhagen, Denmark

Robert Schwarcz
Neuroscience Program
Maryland Psychiatric Research Center
Baltimore, Maryland 21228

Menahem Segal
Isotope Department
The Weizmann Institute of Science
Rehovot, Israel

Fredrick J. Seil
Neurology Research
Veterans Administration Medical
Center
Departments of Neurology, Pathology,
and Biochemistry
University of Oregon Health Sciences
Center
Portland, Oregon 97201

Richard P. Shank
Department of Physiology
Temple University School of Medicine
Philadelphia, Pennsylvania 19140

N. A. Sharif
Department of Physiology and
Pharmacology
School of Biochemical and
Physiological Sciences
University of Southampton
Southampton S09 3TU, United
Kingdom

H. Shinozaki
The Tokyo Metropolitan Institute
Bunkyo-ku
Tokyo 113, Japan

J. Slevin
Departments of Pharmacology and
Experimental Therapeutics, and
Psychiatry and the Behavioral
Sciences
Johns Hopkins University School of
Medicine
Baltimore, Maryland 21205

U. Sonnhof
I. Physiologisches Institut der
Universität
Im Neuenheimer Feld 326
D-6900 Heidelberg, Federal Republic of
Germany

A. Søreide
Norwegian Defence Research
Establishment
Division for Toxicology
N-2007 Kjeller, Norway

Jon Storm-Mathisen
Anatomical Institute
University of Oslo
Oslo 1, Norway

P. Streit
Brain Research Institute
University of Zurich
CH-8029 Zurich, Switzerland

R. Tissot
Psychiatric Clinic
University of Geneva
1225 Chène-Bourg, Switzerland

P. N. R. Usherwood
Department of Zoology
University of Nottingham
Nottingham NG7 2RD, England

Froylan Vargas
Laboratory of Preclinical
Pharmacology
National Institute of Mental Health
Saint Elizabeths Hospital
Washington, D.C. 20032

I. Walaas
Norwegian Defence Research
Establishment
Division for Toxicology
N-2007 Kjeller, Norway

J. Walker
Norwegian Defence Research
Establishment
Division for Toxicology
N-2007 Kjeller, Norway

Michael Wang
Department of Physiology
Temple University School of Medicine
Philadelphia, Pennsylvania 19140

J. C. Watkins
Department of Physiology
The Medical School
Bristol BS8 1TD, England

R. J. Wenthold
Laboratory of Neuro-otolaryngology
National Institute of Neurological and
Communicative Disorders and Stroke
National Institutes of Health
Bethesda, Maryland 20205

William R. Woodward
Neurology Research
Veterans Administration Medical
Center
Departments of Neurology, Pathology,
and Biochemistry
University of Oregon Health Sciences
Center
Portland, Oregon 97201

R. Zaczek
Departments of Pharmacology and
Experimental Therapeutics, and
Psychiatry and the Behavioral
Sciences
Johns Hopkins University School of
Medicine
Baltimore, Maryland 21205

Glutamate as a Neurotransmitter,
edited by G. Di Chiara and G. L. Gessa
Raven Press, New York © 1981.

An Overview of Glutamate as a Neurotransmitter

C. W. Cotman, A. Foster, and T. Lanthorn

Department of Psychobiology, University of California, Irvine, California 92717

Most transmitters which have been identified have inhibitory actions, e.g. GABA, DA, NE, 5-HT, enkephalins, etc. Yet in the C.N.S. excitatory synapses far outnumber inhibitory ones and play an obvious key role particularly in projection pathways. Many have argued that glutamate and perhaps aspartate are the major excitatory transmitters in the C.N.S. All at least would agree these amino acids are the major candidates for this position of supremacy.

The notion that glutamate may be a major excitatory transmitter came into focus in the 1960's, a few years after GABA gained its status as the candidate for the major inhibitory transmitter. Earlier, in the fifties, it was recognized that glutamic acid concentrations in the brain exceeded those in all other tissues (151). This pointed towards an important role but most felt that glutamate was either a key molecule in cerebral metabolism or it acted to compensate for the brain's anionic deficit (152). It was thus of critical importance when in the early sixties Curtis, Watkins, Krnjevic (29,72) and others demonstrated that glutamate had a powerful excitatory action when applied externally to most central neurons. These studies pointed towards a major neurotransmitter role, a notion still very much alive but difficult to establish rigorously.

The purpose of this paper will be to examine critically the status of glutamate and aspartate as neurotransmitter candidates. We shall focus on their role in the mammalian C.N.S. but also examine their properties in the peripheral nervous system of invertebrates. We will start this survey with a brief look at the possible relationship of glutamate and/or aspartate to specific behaviors and neurological disorders where correlations have been made. In our survey we shall attempt to at least touch upon the major findings and new directions which make this field an active and exciting one. Because of space considerations, and admittedly some bias, we regret we are unable to cite all the relevant studies. Several recent reviews have appeared (28,43,62,64,119,147).

1

BEHAVIORAL CORRELATES AND DISORDERS

One of the principle goals of Neurobiology is to understand the physical and chemical nature of the processes which underlie animal and human behavior, and to apply that knowledge in the treatment of abnormal and disease states. In the search for C.N.S. transmitters and their pathways, correlations with specific behaviors, or with pathological changes, have provided a great stimulus for research. If one considers the dopaminergic system, it can be appreciated how much impetus was provided to workers in this field by the original observations of Hornykiewicz (60) that dopamine (DA) levels are decreased in the caudate nuclei of Parkinsonian patients, thus establishing a link between DA neurons and Parkinson's Disease. A further stimulus was the subsequent development of the rat turning model by Ungerstedt (146) as an animal behavior correlated to the disease. It has only been in recent years that a link between the putative acidic amino acid transmitters and specific behaviors or pathological alterations has been noted.

Several studies have made use of powerful glutamate agonists to study relationships between behavior and acidic amino acid receptors. The glutamate analogue kainic acid (KA) is a potent neurotoxin when injected in vivo (23,88), and anomalous behaviors have been observed after application of this compound in some areas of the C.N.S. (23,35,88,96). Both short term and long term behavioral effects have been seen, and it is difficult to correlate these with any physiological effect on receptors, rather than a consequence of the neurotoxic action. However, it has been shown that unilateral injections of KA into the substantia nigra (especially pars reticulata) produce ipsilateral turning in rats, at doses not associated with neuronal toxicity (103,104). In contrast, ibotenic acid induces contralateral turning when applied in the same manner. This effect is not blocked by picrotoxin, and therefore is not due to the conversion of ibotenate to muscimol (112). The pathways mediating these effects are not known but they do not seem to involve DA neurons (103,104). This difference in turning behavior between the two glutamate analogues is especially interesting in view of the proposal that ibotenate and kainate act at separate excitatory receptors (see Table 3 and Watkins, this volume).

Lanthorn and Isaacson (74) found that intraventricular KA at subtoxic doses produces, in rats, a behavior called the wet dog shakes. This seems to involve the action of KA on the CA3 area of the hippocampus. Such behaviors are produced naturally when animals are placed in situations where a behavioral sequence is blocked, ie. response conflict resulting in displacement behavior. KA-induced wet dog shakes may be similar to shuddering in man associated with extreme anxiety. It is indeed interesting that ingestion of monosodium glutamate has been reported to produce shuddering in some children (117).

Polc and Haefely (111) have demonstrated that spinal reflexes are affected by acidic amino acids. Thus, KA preferentially enhances monosynaptic reflexes, while N-methyl-D-aspartate (NMDA) enhances polysynaptic reflexes. Linking these findings with the earlier neurochemical (32,48) and electrophysiological (37,87) evidence, it was suggested that the IA afferents may use glutamate (or a KA-like molecule) as a transmitter, and spinal interneurones may use aspartate (or a NMDA-like molecule). In connection with this, it may be significant that the powerful anti-spastic agent baclofen, which blocks spinal reflexes (110), has been shown to cause inhibition of the release of acidic amino acids (113).

There are indications that certain neurological disorders may be the result of abnormalities in glutamate or glutamate-like neurotransmission. The pathological changes which are seen in the basal ganglia of patients with Huntington's chorea can be reproduced in similar areas of the rat brain after injection of KA into the striatum (23,88). Thus, striatal KA injections destroy intrinsic neurons, while sparing afferents and axons of passage (22), resulting in an atrophy similar to that which occurs during the disease state. Concurrently, the changes in markers for GABAergic, cholinergic, dopaminergic and serotonergic neurons are similar in the disease state and the rat model (21). In view of the evidence that the corticostriatal pathway uses glutamate as a transmitter (34,70,89, 118,135), and the involvement of this pathway in the neurotoxic action of KA in the striatum (5,90), it has been proposed that the primary cause of Huntington's chorea may be some abnormality in this proposed glutamate-using system (88,91,108).

When KA is injected into the ventricles under carefully controlled conditions, a selective hippocampal lesion is produced in the rat (97). The pyramidal cells in areas CA3, CA4 and CA1 are most susceptible, whereas CA2 and dentate granule cells are extremely resistant. This pattern of cell loss is similar to that produced by status epilepticus, hippocampal stroke and senile dementia in humans, and thus acidic amino acid receptors have been implicated in these neurological disorders (109).

Another way in which acidic amino acids can modify behavior and induce pathological states is through their action on the release of gonadotrophic hormones. Glutamate, KA, NMDA and DL-homo-cysteate, administered subcutaneously at subtoxic doses, all elevate serum levels of testosterone and lutenizing hormone (LH) (107,114,116). At higher doses, convulsions are induced and neurons are destroyed by these agents, resulting in a multifaceted neuroendocrine deficiency including gonadal hypoplasia, impaired reproductive capacity and decreased serum levels of LH (59,101). The potency of a number of excitatory amino acids in causing the convulsive behaviors and neurotoxicity parallels the neuro-excitatory potency of these compounds (63,106).

As a footnote to this section, it is worth mentioning that glutamate and it's neuroexcitatory analogues are strongly

associated with the sensation of taste. There is no evidence
to suggest that glutamate is a transmitter in the taste buds,
but it certainly activates taste receptors, or the nerve endings
associated with them. This is evident from the widespread use
of monosodium glutamate as a flavorant. A number of glutamate
analogues (ibotenate, domoate, tricholomate) reportedly have
similar effects (140), and a derivative of aspartate, phenyl-
alanylaspartate, is used as an artificial sweetener (105). It
would seem that further investigation of acidic amino acid
responses in these sensory organs would give useful information
about the type(s) of receptor involved with, perhaps, less of
the restrictions imposed upon such a study in the C.N.S.
    It is clear that further investigation of the relationship
between acidic amino acids, specific behaviors and pathological
alterations will yield much useful information concerning the
role of these putative transmitters in the C.N.S. Most of the
studies described above are very recent, thus demonstrating the
beginning of a rapidly developing area.

IDENTIFICATION OF GLUTAMATE PATHWAYS

    Progress on the role of glutamate neurons in nervous system
function would be greatly facilitated by advances in two major
areas: 1) the identification of the pathways which use glutamate
as a transmitter and 2) the discovery of specific and powerful
antagonists which block the action of glutamate. Accordingly,
we shall now look at the pathways which appear to use glutamate
and aspartate as transmitters.
    One of the first approaches used in an attempt to identify
excitatory amino acid pathways was to map the distribution of
endogenous glutamate and aspartate levels in the C.N.S. and to
measure the changes induced by a lesion of specific nerve tracts.
However, unlike GABA, the catecholamines and other putative
transmitters, glutamate is a ubiquitous metabolite and there is
no compelling evidence that it even exists in greatly enriched
concentrations in glutamate neurons. Therefore, a high endogenous
level of glutamate or aspartate, or a reduction in levels after
lesioning is not sufficient evidence alone to indicate a
transmitter role. Similarly, no unique enzyme or other molecular
marker associated with a transmitter pool of glutamate has been
found (see also E. Roberts, this volume).
    High-affinity transport has also been proposed as a marker for
glutamate neurons. On the basis of this, several authors have
suggested that the reduction in uptake which occurs after a lesion
of one nerve terminal population is indicative of a transmitter
role (see Table 1).
    However, glutamate uptake is not a specific marker for
"glutamate-using" neurons. Glutamate and aspartate share the same
high-affinity uptake process (78), suggesting that the same uptake
sites are present on both "glutamate-using" and "aspartate-using"
neurons. Also, high-affinity uptake has been demonstrated in

TABLE 1. Pathways in the mammalian C.N.S. which show a reduction in glu/asp uptake after various treatments

Pathway	Treatment	Reference
CEREBELLAR PARALLEL FIBERS	X-radiation	120
	Pre virus	163
	Mutation	61
PERFORANT PATH	Surgical Lesion	97,138
HIPPOCAMPAL COMMISSURAL/ASSOCIATIONAL	Surgical Lesion	97,138
HIPPOCAMPAL-SEPTAL AND MAMMILLARY BODIES	Surgical Lesion	139
CORTICO-STRIATAL PATHWAY	Surgical Lesion	34,91

glial preparations (56), and autoradiography suggests that glial uptake may predominate in vivo (69,92). The existence of any net transport of glutamate by high-affinity systems has also been challenged as being an exchange of external for internal glutamate (75). Such homoexchange mechanisms, however, are only observed in subcellular fractions probably because of the uncoupling of transport during tissue preparation. For these reasons there are problems involved in using glutamate uptake as a marker for "glutamate-using" neurons.

Several studies have attempted to assess the ability of uptake systems to regulate neuronal responses to acidic amino acids. A number of compounds which interfere with glutamate transport systems have been shown to prolong responses to iontophoretically applied amino acids in vivo. Threo-3-hydroxy-aspartate and dihydrokainic acid both block high-affinity glutamate uptake in vitro (1,66), and enhance responses to L-glutamate, L-aspartate and quisqualic acid but not to NMDA and kainic acid which are not transported (67,76,77). However, low-affinity uptake systems also seem to be important. D-glutamate and L-homocysteate are taken up by low-affinity systems only, but have the same onset and cessation of action as L-glutamate and L-aspartate, whereas D-homocysteate (which does not appear to be taken up by any system) has a prolonged action (20). Also, histidine, which competes only for low affinity uptake, is able to prolong L-glutamate and L-aspartate responses (76). It would appear, therefore, that low-affinity transport is a major influence on responses to these exogenously applied amino acids, which casts doubt on the necessity for a high-affinity system. However, it has yet to be established whether responses to synaptically released glutamate are affected by uptake blockers.

PROPERTIES OF GLUTAMATE RELEASE

It is now well established that transmitter release in the mammalian C.N.S. is Ca^{2+}-dependent and stimulated by depolarization (71,122). Thus, glutamate may serve as a transmitter in an area of the brain or spinal cord if it is shown to be released in this manner. Such a demonstration of Ca^{2+}-dependent release is, at present, the best marker for glutamate-using pathways.

Release has now been studied from several specific pathways (Table 2). We will describe glutamate release from hippocampus in order to illustrate the experimental approach and characteristics of the process (see also 17,18).

TABLE 2. Pathways which show the release of acidic amino acids upon stimulation.

Pathway	Amino Acid	Reduction with Lesions[a]	Ref.
AUDITORY NERVE COCHLEAR NUCLEUS	GLU (end., ex.)[b] ASP (end.)	YES	12,155
CORTICO-STRIATAL PATH	GLU (end.)	YES	118,121
CEREBELLAR PARALLEL FIBERS	GLU (end., ex.)	YES	123
LATERAL OLFACTORY TRACT	ASP (end.) (rat) GLU (end.) (guinea pig)	YES ---	16 19
PERFORANT PATH	GLU (end., ex.) ASP (end., ex.)	YES	99
HIPPOCAMPAL COMMISSURAL FIBERS	ASP (end., ex.) GLU (end., ex.) ASP (end., ex.)	YES	99
SCHAEFFER COLLATERALS	GLU (ex.) D-ASP (ex.)	---	83,160
HIPPOCAMPAL SEPTAL PATH	D-ASP (ex.)	---	84

[a]Destruction of the input causes a reduction in release from the terminal field.
[b]end., endogenous
ex., exogenous

   The laminar organization of the hippocampus lends itself
particularly well to the analysis of release from specific
terminal fields. In the dentate gyrus of the hippocampus, the
major cell type (the granule cells) is found in a layer. The zone
which contains the granule cell dendrites and its inputs is called
the molecular layer. Granule cells receive only two major inputs:
one from the entorhinal cortex and another from hippocampal CA4
neurons. The projection from the entorhinal cortex terminates in
the outer 3/4 of the dendritic field; the one from CA4 neurons
terminates in the inner 1/4 of the dendritic field nearest the
granule cell bodies. The entorhinal input accounts for about 60%
of the total input to the granule cells, and is known to be
excitatory. The molecular layer is sufficiently large so that it
can be readily dissected from fresh slices thereby providing
tissue where the main afferent is of entorhinal origin.

   In 1976, Cotman and coworkers (97) provided the first evidence
that entorhinal fibers secrete glutamate in a Ca^{2+} dependent
manner which is stimulated by depolarization. Release has now
been extensively studied in a number of preparations with a number
of different types of depolarizing agents. Slices of the
molecular layer (or fascia dentata) or synaptosomes isolated from
the hippocampus have been employed to analyze the characteristics
of endogenous and exogenous glutamate, aspartate and GABA release.

   Electrical field stimulation released glutamate from slices of
the dentate. Release was Ca^{2+} dependent since in the absence of
Ca^{2+} and in the presence of Mg^{2+} it was greatly reduced (159).
Alternatively, depolarization by 56mM K^+ ions or veratridine in
the presence of Ca^{2+} provoked release. Release was stimulated by
depolarization alone, probably due to reversal of the carrier,
but it was 2-3 times greater in the presence of Ca^{2+}. Other
divalent ions such as Ba^{2+} could substitute for Ca^{2+} and Mg^{2+}
inhibited release (99,100). The release of newly synthesized
glutamate from glutamine or glucose showed similar characteristics
to that of endogenously loaded glutamate (54).

   Subcellular fractionation studies have shown that glutamate
release appears to originate from synaptic boutons. Isolated
synaptosomes prepared from whole hippocampus or dentate gyrus
show an increase in Ca^{2+} dependent release relative to less
homogenous fractions. In fact, fractions which do not contain
synaptosomes fail completely to release glutamate. Potassium
evoked, Ca^{2+} independent efflux appears to decrease upon
purification of synaptosomes. In the presence of the Ca^{2+}
ionophore A23187 and Ca^{2+}, glutamate was released from
synaptosomes in the absence of depolarization (123). Therefore,
in agreement with known properties of other transmitters, the
entry of Ca^{2+} is a necessary and sufficient condition to evoke
release. In all respects GABA release shows the same
characteristics as glutamate release (17, 124). It is not known
whether release originates from synaptic vesicles and a direct
demonstration of this would strengthen the case further.
Nonetheless, the present evidence strongly favors the view that

glutamate, and probably aspartate, are neurotransmitters in the
hippocampus. Data on the postsynaptic action of these acidic
amino acids will be described in a later section.

Calcium dependent glutamate release appeared to come from
entorhinal boutons since it decreased after the entorhinal cortex
was removed (54,97,98). Release, either endogenous or newly
synthesized from glutamine, decreased by 4 days after the lesion
and was reduced for at least 14 days, the longest time period
studied. The effect was selective to glutamate since GABA and
aspartate both increased significantly. The elevation in
aspartate release is probably a result of axon sprouting. CA4
neurons are known to grow new boutons which partially replace the
lost entorhinal fibers (18). The increase in GABA release is
probably an adaptive response by local interneurons to the lesion
but whether new synapses form or existing ones increase the
efficiency of their release is unknown (100).

Table 2 summarizes data on other systems where lesions have
been employed along with release studies in order to identify
the source of the fibers that employ glutamate as a transmitter
candidate. Experiments which employ exogenously loaded amino
acids must be considered with some caution, as these are subject
to the limitations noted previously for high-affinity uptake.

Several toxins or drugs have been identified which appear to
act more or less selectively on glutamate release. Fraction E of
black widow spider venom appears to potentiate both excitatory
and inhibitory postsynaptic potentials at lobster neuromuscular
junction (46), thus probably affecting release of glutamate and
GABA. This fraction does not increase release of ACh (frog) (46)
or GABA from mouse brain slices (145). A fungal toxin,
Verruculogen, increases the spontaneous release of endogenous
glutamate and aspartate, but not GABA from cerebral cortex
synaptosomes (102); curiously, it does not act on synaptosomes
isolated from spinal cord or medulla (102). This toxin also
increases the frequency (but not amplitude) of mepps at the locust
neuromuscular junction, a known glutamate system (102). Penitrem
A, another fungal toxin, increases release of glutamate, aspartate
and GABA from cortical synaptosomes. It also has no effect on
spinal cord or medulla synaptosomes (102). Wasp venom
(Habrobracon) has been reported to decrease excitatory junction
potentials at the locust neuromuscular junction without changing
postsynaptic sensitivity to glutamate (153). Therefore, it causes
presynaptic block. Other wasp venoms have similar effects.
Baclofen (Lioresal) appears to alter glutamate release without
affecting GABA release (112) (see Potashner, this volume).

SYNTHESIS OF GLUTAMATE

As with any neurotransmitter, it must be replenished. Glucose
or glutamine are the two potential precursors of glutamate which
are present in the highest amount in brain. Glutamate can be
synthesized by hydrolysis of glutamine, a reaction catalyzed by

the enzyme(s) glutaminase, or it can be synthesized from glucose
by oxidative metabolism and transamination of the oxoglutarate.
Bradford and Ward (10) showed that nerve terminals contain large
quantities of glutaminase and suggested that this enzyme plays
the major role in the production of transmitter glutamate.
Previous studies on glutamate biosynthesis had revealed a complex
compartmentation (149,152). Studies are needed on a system where
glutamate is strongly expected to serve as a neurotransmitter.

Cotman and coworkers employed dentate gyrus slices in order to
evaluate the relative role of glucose and glutamine as precursors
for the readily releasable glutamate pool (see 17). The
difference in release of endogenous glutamate between slices
incubated in the presence of glucose alone and in the presence
of glucose and glutamine together clearly illustrates the
importance of glutamine for glutamate biosynthesis (53). Slices
exposed to glutamine release much more glutamate than those
incubated with glucose alone. Addition of 2mM free Ca^{2+} to a
K^+ enriched medium evokes a larger efflux of glutamate than
56mM K^+ in the absence of Ca^{2+}, amounting to a total of over
300 nmol/mg protein in 20 min. Thus during incubation with
glutamine, elevated K^+ and Ca^{2+}, approximately 10% of the total
slice content of glutamate is released per minute. Nevertheless
tissue levels of glutamate remain essentially constant. It
follows that the total production of glutamate must have increased
markedly when the slices were stimulated in the presence of
glutamine. In contrast, in the presence of glucose alone little
or no net synthesis of glutamate occurs. Glutamate is released
into the medium at the expense of tissue stores. It thus appears
that extracellular glutamine greatly facilitates the production
of releasable glutamate.

Whereas studies of the release of endogenous glutamate shows
that glutamine better supports the biosynthesis of the releasable
glutamate store than glucose, it was not possible to determine how
much glutamine and glucose was actually converted to releasable
glutamate. For this purpose, studies with radiolabeled precursors
were carried out. In addition, it is important to determine
whether newly synthesized glutamate is preferentially released
and the means by which the biosynthesis of glutamate from
glutamine is controlled.

One way of evaluating the relative contributions of
extracellular glucose and glutamine to the biosynthesis of
releasable glutamate is to compare the specific radioactivity
of glutamate released into the medium to that of its precursors.
Glutamate that appeared in the medium during incubation with
elevated K^+, Ca^{2+} and [^{14}C] glutamine had a specific radioactivity
66% that of the precursor. This result suggests that about two-
thirds of the glutamate released from the slices under these
conditions originated from extracellular glutamine. In contrast,
when [^{14}C] glucose was the precursor, the specific radioactivity
of glutamate released into the medium was only 16% that of the
added glucose. Removal of the entorhinal cortex markedly

decreased the quantity of both newly synthesized and endogenous glutamate released. Thus more than 80% of the glutamate released from perforant path boutons under these conditions was derived from extracellular glucose and glutamine, with about two-thirds of the total originating from glutamine (54,55). Bradford, et al. (11) have reported that about 80% of glutamate released from synaptosomes by elevated K^+ is derived from glutamine, in close agreement with our results. Most of the rest of the radioactive glutamate was derived from glucose. It was possible to demonstrate that most of the glutamate derived from glutamine is available for release, whereas most of the glutamate synthesized from glucose serves a different function, presumably metabolic. Thus, glutamate released by perforant path boutons appears to be derived primarily from glutamine, at least when elevated K^+ is employed as the depolarizing agent. Studies in other systems have also shown that glutamine is a suitable precursor for providing release of glutamate (see Table 2 and Cuenod, this volume).

Glutamine appears to be synthesized primarily in glial cells, rather than in neurons (3,85,149). These data, therefore, imply a dynamic interaction between glutamate boutons and their associated glial cells (Fig. 1). Upon release of glutamate, its biosynthesis is stimulated by an increase in both terminal uptake

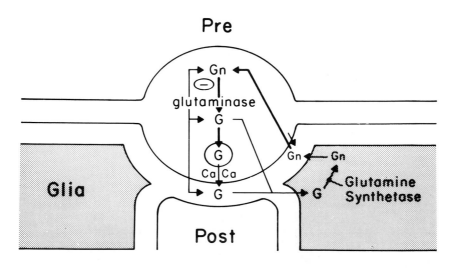

FIG. 1. Pathways in the biosynthesis of the transmitter pool of glutamate (G) with glutamine (Gn) as a precursor (55).

of glutamine and glutaminase activity. Glutamate that is released can be recaptured by the bouton or enter glial cells, where it is converted to glutamine. Glutamine is then released from glia and is available to refuel the releasable glutamate stores in synaptic boutons. Thus glutamate-releasing boutons and associated glial cells appear to have a symbiotic relationship. It appears that glutamine is the major precursor; however, other metabolic pathways may yet prove to play an important, if not unique, role (see E. Roberts, this volume). Hopefully one of these will prove to be present only in glutamate neurons.

IDENTIFICATION OF EXCITATORY AMINO ACID RECEPTORS

The identification of glutamate-using pathways would be greatly facilitated by the discovery of a specific antagonist of glutamate responses. Much of the rapid progress in the field of opiate research can be attributed to the availability of the opiate antagonist, naloxone. Only in recent years have compounds which selectively antagonize acidic amino acid responses been found. With the use of these compounds it has become clear that several types of receptors for amino acids are present in the mammalian C.N.S. (see Watkins, this volume). Multiple receptors for glutamate are known to exist in the invertebrate C.N.S. (for review see 147), and it is interesting to consider these receptor types in relation to those found in mammals.

Glutamate is the primary candidate for neurotransmitter at the crustacean and insect neuromuscular junctions (see Usherwood, this volume). One of the most convincing pieces of evidence in favor of this proposal is the analysis of glutamate noise at the crab neuromuscular junction. Crawford and McBurney (25) analyzed the power spectra of postsynaptic noise caused by the application of glutamate, aspartate and cysteate at the neuromuscular junction. They found that these compounds caused an elementary event, the the response to activation of the postsynaptic membrane by one molecule of agonist, which had the same amplitude (thus opening the same ionic channels), but different average lifetimes, the faster frequency components appearing with application of aspartate and cysteate. The mean lifetime of this event is given by the half frequency, and for glutamate is about 1.5 msec. For aspartate and cysteate, however, the duration is half of that for glutamate, about 0.7 msec. This difference allows one to select which is the best transmitter candidate: if the decay of a response to a quantum of transmitter (the mepp) is controlled by closure of membrane channels, and not by the decline in transmitter concentration at the junction, then the time constant for decay of the mepps should correspond to the average duration of the elementary event, as has been shown at the cholinergic neuromuscular junction (68). At the crab neuromuscular junction, the time course of mepps corresponds to that of glutamate, not aspartate (24). This argues strongly in favor of glutamate as the neurotransmitter.

Glutamate receptors, other than those mediating neurotransmission, have also been found in invertebrates. At the locust
muscle, glutamate applied to extrajunctional regions produces
a biphasic response (depolarizing-hyperpolarizing). The glutamate
analogue ibotenate causes only a hyperpolarization at extrajunctional sites, which is mediated by chloride channels (148),
indicating that the D and H responses are mediated by separate
receptors for glutamate. Glutamate applied at junctional sites
gives only a depolarization, and in general the junctional sites
are more sensitive to glutamate, because they contain a greater
density of glutamate receptors (26). Additionally, more
than one type of junctional receptor for glutamate is present.
Ibotenate causes a depolarization at approximately 20% of the
junctions, and L-aspartate at a further 20% (49). Another feature
of these receptors is that the rapid desensitization of the
junctional and extrajunctional D receptors to glutamate
application is blocked by Concanavalin A (Con A), whereas H
receptor desensitization is not (86). Therefore, at least five
different glutamate receptors have been identified in locust
muscle (Fig. 2; and Usherwood, this volume).

FIG. 2. Receptor types at the locust neuromuscular junction.

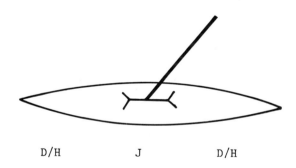

D/H   J   D/H

			Desensitization	Blocked by Con A
H	GLUTAMATE (IBOTENATE)	Cl$^-$	X	
D	GLUTAMATE (NOT IBOTENATE)	cation(s)	X	X
J	GLUTAMATE (≈20% L-ASP, ≈20% IBOTENATE)	cation(s)	X	X

Extrajunctional receptors have also been found in the crayfish, although these appear to be different than those of the locust. Glutamate is the primary candidate as the excitatory transmitter at the crayfish neuromuscular junction (141,143). Kainic acid causes a potentiation of the response to bath-applied glutamate, through an activation of extrajunctional receptors (131,142). The mechanism of this effect is unknown but the kainate analogue domoic acid has the same action (132). The junctional glutamate receptors are activated by quisqualic acid, and cross desensitization experiments between glutamate, quisqualate and the natural transmitter indicate that a common receptor is involved (130,143). Recently, however, Shinozaki and Ishida (129) have shown that Con A will block the desensitization of responses to glutamate applied at the junction but not that of the natural transmitter. The meaning of this observation is not clear at present, but illustrates that even in this relatively simple preparation it has proved difficult to equate excitatory amino acid receptors with those that accept the natural transmitter.

Due to the complexity of the tissue, and the technical difficulties involved, it has not been possible to directly assess the contribution of extrajunctional receptors to glutamate responses in the mammalian C.N.S. However, there are indications that such receptors are present. In their early work on cat spinal neurons, Curtis, et al. (29-31) proposed a non-specific action for acidic amino acids, due in part to the near universality of their action. This contrasted with acetylcholine (ACh) which would only act on certain cells. In fact, it is difficult to find neurons in the C.N.S. which do not respond to glutamate (28), and while it may be that a large percentage of C.N.S. neurons receive a glutamate input, a more plausible explanation might be an activation of extrasynaptic receptors. In agreement with this possibility, it has been shown that the iontophoretic application of glutamate to the cell body layer will excite hippocampal pyramidal neurons, even though no excitatory synapses have been identified there. The maximal action of glutamate, however, is on the dendrites, the locus where most putative glutamate synapses are found (36,125). It is interesting to note that in the cerebellum, responses to glutamate can be hyperpolarizing or depolarizing (161). The hyperpolarization is not mediated through inhibitory transmitters and appears to be a direct response to glutamate. Perhaps these glutamate receptors are analogous to the H extrajunctional receptors of locust muscle.

The clearest pharmacological classification of glutamate receptors has been performed on spinal neurons. Three classes have been identified, based primarily on the sensitivity to the antagonists D-α-aminoadipate (D-α-AA) and glutamate diethyl ester (GDEE) (Table 3). The n-methyl-D-aspartate (NMDA) class is preferentially antagonized by D-α-AA and related compounds, and Mg^{2+} (see Watkins, this volume), and the quisqualic acid class is more sensitive to GDEE (33,93). NMDA and quisqualate are the agonists of highest selectivity for these two receptor

classes. However, other agonists have affinities for both
receptors types, and these can be placed in a ranked order of
sensitivity to the two antagonists (57,93). L-glutamate and
L-aspartate are among these intermediary compounds, although
L-aspartate responses are more sensitive to D-α-AA, and
L-glutamate responses to GDEE (4,50,52,93). On this basis, NMDA
sites have been proposed as aspartate-preferring, and quisqualate
sites as glutamate-preferring receptors (33,65,93,154). In
relation to this classification, Krogsgaard-Larsen, et al. (73)
have shown that ibotenate can be converted from a D-α-AA sensitive
agonist to a GDEE sensitive agonist by rearrangement of the
molecule. Thus, bromohomoibotenate and (RS)-α-amino-3-hydroxy-5-
methyl-4-isoxazole propionic acid (AMPA) are more potent excitants
that ibotenate, but they are relatively insensitive to D-α-AA, and
more so to GDEE.

TABLE 3.   <u>Classes of acidic amino acids receptors in the
mammalian C.N.S.</u>

Agonist	D-α-AA[a]	GDEE[b]
I. N-METHYL-D-ASPARTATE	+	−
IBOTENIC ACID		
II. GLUTAMATE	−	+
AMPA[c]		
QUISQUALATE	−	+
III. KAINATE	−	−

[a] D-α-aminoadipate
[b] glutamate diethyl ester
[c] (RS)-α-amino-3-hydroxy-5-methyl-4-isoxazolepropionic acid

    The third class of receptors are those activated by kainic
acid, the responses of which are relatively insensitive to both
D-α-AA and GDEE. It has been shown that kainate receptors are
distinct from most other acidic amino acid receptors (64), based
on neurophysiological evidence (51,154) and binding data (44,79).
    These three classes of receptors nicely account for most of the
existing data and serve as a useful framework for an otherwise
disarrayed body of information. It is unlikely, however, that
this scheme is the final one which will account for all systems.
    Direct conductance measurements also support the existence of
distinct classes of acidic amino acid receptors. Working on cat
spinal neurons, Engberg, Flatman and Lambert (38,39) showed that
D-homocysteate and NMDA cause a conductance decrease, possibly
by closing K^+ channels, whereas L-glutamate, L-aspartate and
L-homocysteate cause a conductance increase, which rises

continually. The conductance change induced by the application
of kainic acid is qualitatively similar to that of L-glutamate
but is of a much greater size. These data suggest that the
distinction between glutamate and aspartate-preferring receptors
is not as clear as the three class scheme indicates. It may be
that natural ligands other than glutamate or aspartate exist
which use diverse receptors and generate unexpected responses.
Once identified and associated with specific pathways it is
likely that the pharmacological and functional characteristics
of receptors will fall into a unitary scheme.

Do the different classes of acidic amino acid receptors play
a part in synaptic transmission? Evans et al., (40) reported a
striking correlation between the amplitude of the ventral root
potential to dorsal root stimulation, and the sensitivity of
NMDA depolarizations to antagonism by a series of mono- and
diaminodicarboxylic amino acid derivatives. D-α-aminosuberate
and α,ϵ-diaminopimelate were the most potent antagonists of
motorneuron responses. Most significantly, it was found that
synaptic activity and NMDA responses were depressed in parallel
by this series of compounds. This is, at present, the best
correlation between a synaptic response and excitatory amino acid
pharmacology. Thus, it would appear that an NMDA-like molecule
acts naturally in this response, at least in the low Mg^{2+} medium
used.

GDEE has been shown to antagonize synaptic excitation in
several areas of the brain: thalamus (50); striatum (135);
pyramidal tract targets (136,137) and hippocampus (58,127,156).
Although the specificity of this compound has been questioned in
that ACh responses can also be depressed (15), it would appear
that quisqualate-type receptors may be mediating synaptic
transmission in these areas.

In the hippocampus, a distinction can be made between the
synaptic responses to the excitatory pathways by use of acidic
amino acid antagonists. The glutamate analogue 2-amino-4-
phosphonobutyrate (2-APB) has been shown to act as an antagonist
at the invertebrate neuromuscular junction (27). 2-APB
selectively blocks synaptic excitation of the dentate granule
cells evoked by perforant path stimulation, whereas the aspartate
analogue 2-amino-3-phosphonopropionic acid (2-APP) is ineffective
(157). Neither compound will antagonize the response to mossy
fiber stimulation. These results, taken with the neurochemical
evidence described above, favor glutamate as transmitter of the
perforant path fibers. In support of our results, Wheal and
Miller (156) and Hicks and McLennan (58) have shown that
iontophoretically applied GDEE will also block perforant path
synaptic excitation of the dentate granule cells. D-α-AA is
relatively ineffective on perforant path synapses but does block
the dentate commissural response (58). Therefore, it appears
that at least two types of excitatory amino acid receptors are
present on these hippocampal cells (see also McLennan, this
volume).

Binding studies with acidic amino acids have revealed high-affinity receptor sites for L-glutamate, kainate and NMDA in the mammalian C.N.S. (2,6,44,80,95,133,134). The pharmacology of this binding is in broad agreement with electrophysiology experiments. L-glutamate binding is displaced by the potent excitatory compounds quisqualate, DL-homocysteate and ibotenate, but not by kainic acid (2,44,133). Kainic acid binding is displaced by glutamate and quisqualate, but this action may be indirect (79). The density of glutamate binding sites is at least one order of magnitude greater than those for kainic acid. In a preliminary report NMDA binding sites have recently been found which have a lower density than the kainate sites and which are distinct from them (134). The NMDA sites show the same characteristics as NMDA receptors identified in electrophysiological experiments, being potently displaced by D-α-AA and Mg^{2+}. They may be the same sites as those reported to be labeled by D-aspartate (64).

Recently, we have attempted to evaluate the relative importance of junctional and non-junctional receptors for excitatory amino acids. Use has been made of subcellular fractionation techniques to isolate synaptic junctions from rat brain (19), and the binding of L-[^{3}H]-glutamate, L-[^{3}H]-aspartate and [^{3}H]-kainate has been studied. The binding of all three ligands is enriched several fold in synaptic junctions (Table 4), suggesting that acidic amino acid receptors are more concentrated there. Approximately 11 and 26% of the glutamate and aspartate sites in synaptic membranes, respectively, are recovered in the junctions. In contrast, greater than 70% of the kainate binding sites are retained in the junctional membranes (Table 4). This suggests that binding sites for glutamate and aspartate are mainly extrajunctional in nature. Kainate binding sites appear to be predominantly junctional.

These findings with kainic acid are further supported by our experiments using an in vitro autoradiographical technique to localize kainate binding sites in slices of rat brain, as described for opiate and benzodiazepine receptors by Young and Kuhar (164,165). We have found that the kainate binding sites in the hippocampus are enriched in the CA3 region, and appear to be localized in the terminal field of the mossy fibers (Fig. 3). A postsynaptic localization of these receptors could be inferred from the findings that the CA3 pyramidal cells are the most sensitive to the neurotoxic action of kainic acid (96). These data support the possibility that the brain contains endogenous kainate type molecules which may serve as transmitters.

PLASTICITY PROCESSES AT GLUTAMATE PATHWAYS

The study of plasticity processes is one of the important frontiers for future work on acidic amino acids. Many of the pathways, in fact, which display plasticity are expected to use acidic amino acids or their derivatives as transmitters.

Habituation and long term potentiation (LTP) are two elementary forms of plasticity which have attracted great interest in recent

TABLE 4. Specific binding of GLU, ASP and KA to subcellular fractions from rat whole brain.[a]

Fraction	Specific Binding Relative to Homogenate		
	GLU	ASP	KA
WHOLE PARTICULATE	1	1	1
CRUDE MITOCHONDRIAL PELLET (P_2)	1.15+0.07	1.14+0.57	0.73+0.34
SYNAPTIC PLASMA MEMBRANES (SPM)	6.86+3.07	5.20+1.47	2.08+0.41
SYNAPTIC JUNCTIONS (SJ)	4.08+1.39	18.09+6.47	22.37+5.79

[a]Subcellular fractions were prepared by the method of Cotman and Taylor (19), and analyzed for L-3H-GLU, L-3H-ASP and 3H-KA binding using a microfuge assay; at a final concentration of 100nM for labelled L-glutamate and L-aspartate, and 40nM for KA. Specific binding was determined as that which could be displaced by a 100nM concentration of the respective unlabelled ligand. The values were taken from 3-4 separate preparations and are means +S.E.M.

years. Habituation is generally defined as a decrement in response to an initially novel stimulus when it is given repeatedly. A cellular analogue of behavioral habituation can be produced at certain monosynaptic pathways including the hippocampal perforant path. Upon slow repetitive stimulation of the perforant path a decrement in response occurs which fullfils the major criteria for habituation and offers an appropriate brain model of this plasticity (144). Perforant path synapses also exhibit LTP. Tetanic supra-threshold stimulation augments the amplitude of subsequent synaptic potentials. There is a large immediate facilitation that decays rapidly (post-tetanic potentiation (PTP)) and an enhancement of the efficacy of transmission that persists for hours, even days (LTP). LTP can be produced by stimulus parameters well within the physiological range and thus it appears that LTP may underlie certain types of learning or behavioral plasticity.

The mechanisms of habituation and LTP in the brain are largely unknown. However, in the Aplysia abdominal ganglion and frog spinal cord, habituation involves presynaptic changes (13,14,47), while in the hippocampus, postsynaptic changes are implicated in LTP (42,81,82,94,150). A specific postsynaptic antagonist should

aid in the dissection of presynaptic vs postsynaptic events at
hippocampal synapses.

At a concentration of 2.5 mM, 2-APB abolished LTP without
affecting PTP (Fig. 4). Identical results were obtained when
2-APB was removed from the medium within 1 min after tetanization.
The effect of 2-APB was completely reversible, since LTP could be
generated after 2-APB was removed from the medium. Because 2-APB
reduced the amplitude of the population spike and LTP usually
cannot be demonstrated at low response amplitudes, another series
of experiments were conducted in which the stimulus intensity was
increased to yield a population spike of the same amplitude that
had been obtained in the absence of 2-APB. This procedure did not
alter the outcome; 2-APB still abolished LTP without affecting
PTP. In contrast to LTP, habituation was not affected by the
presence of 2-APB (158).

These results demonstrate that habituation and LTP can be
pharmacologically dissociated and thus must be generated by
different processes. Habituation at this synaptic site appears
to be generated presynaptically, in accordance with evidence of
a presynaptic mechanism at other synapses. Our results also
support the prevailing view that LTP is generated post-
synaptically. It has been demonstrated previously that some
minimum number of synapses must be activated for LTP to occur
(7,8,94,126). However, increasing the stimulus intensity to bring
more pyramidal cells to threshold did not overcome the supres-
sion of LTP by APB. This result suggests that the production
of LTP depends not only on the number of synapses that are
activated on each cell, but also on the number of transmitter-
receptor interactions or, more correctly, the number of ionophores
opened at each synapse.

It is important to discover the molecular processes which may
modulate transmission at glutamate synapses. Modulation of
synaptic responses in many transmitter systems seems to be
mediated by cAMP or cGMP. Aspartate and glutamate and their
analogues have been found to increase the amount of cAMP(128) or
cGMP (41) in nervous system tissue. The results of these
increases to subsequent transmission are presently unknown.
However, as the efficacy of excitatory amino acid analogues to
increase or decrease cyclic nucleotide concentrations is similar
to their excitatory potency (see P.J. Roberts, this volume), it is
very likely that such effects will be important to our understanding of excitatory amino acid transmission.

At lobster walking limb muscles, glutamate induces depolari-
zation-mediated contractions, whereas aspartate by itself has
little effect. However, the presence of l-aspartate potentiates
the response to l-glutamate. This potentiation is not correlated
to inhibition of reuptake mechanisms and may be the result of an
increase in the affinity for glutamate. The ratio of aspartate
to glutamate concentrations which gives the maximum potentiation
is about 3:1. The same ratio is found inside the excitatory
axons, and in the superfusate following stimulation of these

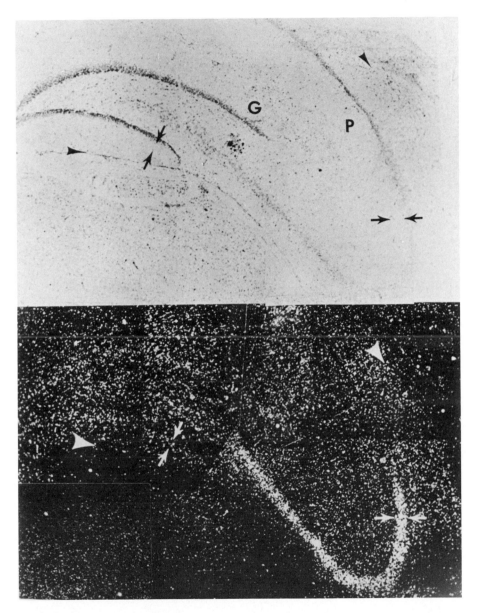

FIG. 3. Autoradiographic localization of kainate receptor sites in the hippocampus (Foster, Mena, Monaghan and Cotman, submitted). TOP: Cresyl violet stain (G) granule cells, (P) pyramidal cells. Paired arrows indicate location of high grain density. Single arrows indicate hippocampal formation border. BOTTOM: Darkfield montage of autoradiograph.

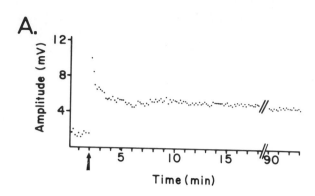

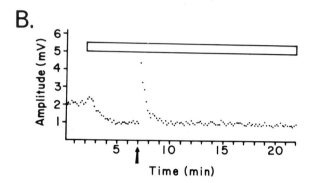

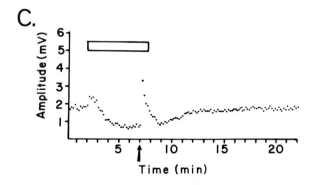

FIG. 4.   Selective inhibition of LTP by 2-APB at the Schaeffer collateral-commissural regio superior pyramidal cell synapse.   Dots
represent the amplitude of the population spike recorded in the
pyramidal cell layer.   APB was present in the perfusion medium
during the period denoted by the open bar.   Arrow indicates the
time at which the conditioning train (100 Hz for 2 sec, 0.05 msec
pulse width) was delivered.

fibers (45). This suggests that aspartate normally modulates glutamate transmission in this preparation.

Curiously, the response of taste mechanisms in the tongue to monosodium glutamate is markedly enhanced by 5'-ribonucleotides, e.g. 5'-AMP and 5'-GMP. The enhancement of glutamate effects by 5'-ribonucleotides has also been observed in a crayfish muscle preparation. The synergistic effects of the 5'-ribonucleotides appear to be on a receptor distinct from the glutamate receptor suggesting a receptor complex (162). The relevance of this modulatory influence to normal transmission has not been examined, though the 5'-ribonucleotides are known to be behaviorally active flavor enhancers. Some type of modulation process is implied.

CONCLUSION

Since the 1960's when glutamate was singled out as a candidate for the major excitatory transmitter in the C.N.S. evidence in support of this hypothesis has grown. Glutamate release, uptake and receptor characteristics are all compatible with a neuro-transmitter role. Moreover, these properties can now be associated with specific central pathways. Some of these pathways display various forms of plasticity and can be related, albeit indirectly at present, to specific behaviors. Moreover, glutamate analogues such as kainic acid produce animal models of such disorders as Huntington's chorea and epilepsy. All these discoveries, many of which are very recent, pave the way for rapid progress in the future.

REFERENCES

1. Balcar, V.J. and Johnston, G.A.R. (1972): J. Neurochem., 19: 2657-2666.
2. Baudry, M. and Lynch, G. (1979): Eur. J. Pharmac., 57:283-285.
3. Benjamin, A.M. and Quastel, J.M. (1972): Biochem J., 128: 631-646.
4. Biscoe, T.J., Evans, R.H., Francis, A.A., Martin, M.R., Watkins, J.C., Davies, J. and Dray, A. (1977): Nature, 270: 743-745.
5. Biziere, K. and Coyle, J.T. (1978): Neurosci. Letters, 8: 303-310.
6. Biziere, K., Thompson, H. and Coyle, J.T. (1980): Brain Res. 183:421-423.
7. Bliss, T.V.P. and Gardner-Medwin, A.R. (1973): J. Physiol. Lond.), 232:357-374.
8. Bliss, T.V.P. and Lømo, T. (1973): J. Physiol. (Lond.), 232: 331-356.
9. Bradford, H.F. and Richards, C.D. (1976): Brain Res., 105: 168-172.
10. Bradford, H.F. and Ward, H.K. (1976): Brain Res., 110:115-125.

11. Bradford, H.F., Ward, H.K. and Thomas, A.J. (1978): J.Neuro-
    chem., 30:1453-1459.
12. Canzek, V. and Reubi, J.C. (1980): Exp. Br. Res., 38:437-441.
13. Capek, R. and Esplin, B. (1977): J. Neurophysiol., 40:95-105.
14. Castellucci, V. and Kandel, E.R. (1976): Science, 194:1176-
    1178.
15. Clarke, G. and Straughan, D.W. (1977): Neuropharmacology,
    16:391-398.
16. Collins, G.G.S. (1979): Brain Res., 171:552-555.
17. Cotman, C.W. and Hamberger, A. (1978): In: Amino Acids as
    Chemical Transmitters, edited by F. Fonnum, pp. 379-412.
    Plenum Press, New York.
18. Cotman, C.W. and Nadler, J.V. (1980 in press): In: Glutamate
    as a Neurotransmitter, edited by P.J. Roberts, J. Storm-
    Mathisen and G. Johnston, John Wiley Press, NY.
19. Cotman, C.W. and Taylor, D. (1972): J. Cell Biol., 55:696-
    711.
20. Cox, D.W.G., Headley, M.H. and Watkins, J.C. (1977): J.
    Neurochem., 29:579-588.
21. Coyle, J.T., McGeer, E.G., McGeer, P.L. and Schwarcz, R.
    (1978): In: Kainic Acid as a Tool in Neurobiology, edited by
    E.G. McGeer, J.W. Olney and P.L. McGeer, pp. 139-160. Raven
    Press, New York.
22. Coyle, J.T., Molliver, M.E. and Kuhar, M.J. (1978): J. Comp.
    Neurol., 180:301-324.
23. Coyle, J.T. and Schwarcz, R. (1977): Nature, 263:244-246.
24. Crawford, A.C. and McBurney, R.N. (1976): J. Physiol. (Lond.)
    254:47P.
25. Crawford, A.C. and McBurney, R.N. (1976): Proc. R. Soc. Lond.
    B 192:481-489.
26. Cull-Candy, S.G. (1978): J. Physiol. (Lond.), 276:165-181.
27. Cull-Candy, S.G., Donnellan, J.F., James, R.W. and Lunt, G.G.
    (1976): Nature, 262:408.
28. Curtis, D.R. and Johnston, G.A.R. (1974): Rev. Physiol.
    Pharmac., 69:97-188.
29. Curtis, D.R., Phillis, J.W. and Watkins, J.C. (1960): J.
    Physiol. (Lond.), 150:656-682.
30. Curtis, D.R. and Watkins, J.C. (1960): J.Neurochem., 6:117-
    141.
31. Curtis, D.R. and Watkins, J.C. (1963): J. Physiol. (Lond.),
    166:1-14.
32. Davidoff, R.A., Graham, L.T., Shank, R.P. and Aprison, M.H.
    (1967): J. Neurochem., 14:1025-1031.
33. Davies, J. and Watkins, J.C. (1979): J. Physiol. (Lond.),
    297:621-635.
34. Divac, I., Fonnum, F. and Storm-Mathisen, J. (1977): Nature,
    266:377-378.
35. Divac, I., Markowitsch, H.J. and Pritzel, M. (1978): Brain
    Res., 151:523-532.
36. Dudar, J.D. (1974): Neuropharmacology, 13:1083-1089.
37. Duggan, A. (1974): Exp. Br. Res., 19:522-525.

38. Engberg, I., Flatman, J.A. and Lambert, J.D.C. (1978): Brit. J. Pharmac., 64:384-385P.

39. Engberg, I., Flatman, J.A. and Lambert, J.D.C. (1979): J. Physiol. (Lond.), 288:227-261.

40. Evans, R.H., Francis, A.A., Hunt, K., Oakes, D.J. and Watkins, J.C. (1979): Br. J. Pharmac., 67:591-603.

41. Ferrendelli, J.A., Chang, M.M. and Kinscherf, D.A. (1974): J. Neurochem., 22:535-540.

42. Fifkova, E. and Van Harreveld, A. (1977): J. Neurocytol., 6:211-230.

43. Fonnum, F., editor (1978): Amino Acids as Chemical Transmitters, Plenum Press, New York.

44. Foster, A.C. and Roberts, P.J. (1978): J. Neurochem., 31: 1467-1477.

45. Freeman, A.R., Shank, R.P., Kephart, J., Dekin, M. and Wang, M. (1979): J. Physiol. (Paris), 75:605-610.

46. Fritz, L.C., Tzeng, M-C. and Mauro, A. (1980): Nature, 283: 485-487.

47. Glanzman, D. and Thompson, R.F. (1980): Brain Res., 189:377- 390.

48. Graham, L.T., Shank, R.P., Werman, R. and Aprison, M.H. (1967): J. Neurochem., 14:465-472.

49. Gration, K.A.F., Clark, R.B. and Usherwood, P.N.R. (1979): Brain Res., 171:360-364.

50. Haldman, S. and McLennan, H. (1972): Brain Res., 45:393-400.

51. Hall, J.G., Hicks, T.P. and McLennan, H. (1978): Neurosci. Letters, 8:171-175.

52. Hall, J.G., Hicks, T.P., McLennan, H., Richardson, T.L. and Wheal, H.V. (1979): J. Physiol. (Lond.), 286:29-39.

53. Hamberger, A., Chiang, G., Nylen, E.S., Scheff, S.W. and Cotman, C.W. (1978): Brain Res., 143:549-555.

54. Hamberger, A.C., Chiang, G.H., Nylen, E.S., Scheff, S.W. and Cotman, C.W. (1979): Brain Res., 168:513-530.

55. Hamberger, A., Chiang, G.H., Sandoval, M.E. and Cotman, C.W. (1979): Brain Res., 168:531-541.

56. Hertz, L. (1979): Prog. in Neurobiol., 13:277-323.

57. Hicks, T.P., Hall, J.G. and McLennan, H. (1978): Can. J. Physiol. Pharmac., 56:901-906.

58. Hicks, T.P. and McLennan, H. (1979): Can. J. Physiol. Pharmac., 57:973-978.

59. Holzworth-McBride, M.A., Hurst, E.M. and Knigge, K.M. (1976): Anatomical Record, 186:185-196.

60. Hornykiewicz, O. (1962): Deutsch Med. Wschr., 87:1807-1810.

61. Hudson, D.B., Valcana, T., Bean, G., and Timiras, P.S. (1976): Neurochem. Res., 1:83-92.

62. Johnson, J.L. (1978): Prog. in Neurobiol., 10:155-202.

63. Johnston, G.A.R. (1972): Biochem. Pharmac., 22:137-140.

64. Johnston, G.A.R. (1979): In: Glutamic Acid: Advances in Biochemistry and Physiology, edited by L.J. Filer, S. Garattini, M.R. Kare, W.A. Reynolds and R.J. Wurtman, pp. 177-185. Raven Press, New York.

65. Johnston, G.A.R., Curtis, D.R., Davies, J. and McCulloch, R.M. (1974): Nature, 248:804-805.
66. Johnston, G.A.R., Kennedy, S.M.E. and Twitchin, B. (1979): J. Neurochem., 32:121-127.
67. Johnston, G.A.R., Lodge, D., Bornstein, J.C. and Curtis, D.R. (1980): J.Neurochem., 34:241-243.
68. Katz, B. and Miledi, R. (1972): J. Physiol. (Lond.), 224:665-699.
69. Kelly, J.S. and Dick, F. (1976): Cold Spring Harbour Symposia on Quantitative Biology, XL: 93-106.
70. Kim, J.S., Hassler, R., Hang, P. and Paik, K-S. (1977): Brain Res., 132:370-374.
71. Krnjevic, K. (1974): Physiological Reviews, 54:418-540.
72. Krnjevic, K. and Phillis, J.W. (1963): J. Physiol. (Lond.), 165:274-304.
73. Krogsgaard-Larsen, P., Honore, T., Hansen, J.J., Curtis, D.R. and Lodge, D. (1980): Nature, 284:64-66.
74. Lanthorn, T. and Isaacson, R.L. (1978): Life Sci., 22:171-178.
75. Levi, G. and Raiteri, M. (1974): Nature, 250:735-737.
76. Lodge, D. (1979): Neurosci. Letters, 14:343-348.
77. Lodge, D., Curtis, D.R., Johnston, G.A.R. and Bornstein, J.C. (1980): Brain Res., 182:491-495.
78. Logan, W.J. and Snyder, S.H. (1972): Brain Res., 42:413-431.
79. London, E.D. and Coyle, J.T. (1979): Eur. J. Pharmac., 56:287-290.
80. London, E.D. and Coyle, J.T. (1979): Mol. Pharmac., 15:492-505.
81. Lynch, G., Dunwiddie, T. and Gribkoff, V. (1977): Nature, 266:737-739.
82. Lynch, G.S., Gribkoff, V.K. and Deadwyler, S.A. (1976): Nature, 263:151-153.
83. Malthe-Sørenssen, D., Skrede, K.K. and Fonnum, F. (1979): Neuroscience, 4:1255-1263.
84. Malthe-Sørenssen, D., Skrede, K.K. and Fonnum, F. (1980): Neuroscience, 5:127-133.
85. Martinez-Hernandez, A., Bell, K.P. and Norenberg, M.D. (1977): Science, 195:1356-1358.
86. Mathers, D.A. and Usherwood, P.N.R. (1976): Nature, 259:409-411.
87. McCulloch, R.M., Johnston, G.A.R., Game, C.J.A. and Curtis, D.R. (1974): Exp. Br. Res., 21:515-518.
88. McGeer, E.G. and McGeer, P.L. (1977): Nature, 263:517-518.
89. McGeer, E.G. and McGeer, P.L. (1979): J. Neurochem., 32:1071-1075.
90. McGeer, E.G., McGeer, P.L. and Singh, K. (1978): Brain Res., 139:381-383.
91. McGeer, P.L., McGeer, E.G., Scheherer, U. and Singh, K. (1977): Brain Res., 128:369-373.
92. McLennan, H. (1976): Brain Res., 115:139-144.
93. McLennan, H. and Lodge, D. (1979): Brain Res., 169:83-90.

94. McNaughton, B.L., Douglas, R.M., and Goddard, G.V. (1978): Brain Res., 157:277-293.
95. Michaelis, E.K., Michaelis, M.L. and Boyarsky, L.L. (1974): Biochim. Biophys. Acta., 367:338-348.
96. Nadler, J.V., Perry, B.W. and Cotman, C.W. (1978): In: Kainic Acid as a Tool in Neurobiology, edited by E.G. McGeer, J.W. Olney and P.L. McGeer, pp. 219-238. Raven Press New York.
97. Nadler, J.V., Vaca, K.W., White, W.F., Lynch, G.S., and Cotman, C.W. (1976): Nature, 260:538-540.
98. Nadler, J.V., White, W.F., Vaca, K.W. and Cotman, C.W. (1978): Nature, 271:676-677.
99. Nadler, J.V., White, W.F., Vaca, K.W., Perry, B.W. and Cotman, C.W. (1978): J. Neurochem., 31:147-155.
100. Nadler, J.V., White, W.F., Vaca, K.W., Redburn, D.A. and Cotman, C.W. (1977): J. Neurochem., 29:279-290.
101. Nemeroff, C.B., Konkol, R.J., Bissette, G., Youngblood, W., Martin, J.B., Brazeau, P., Rone, M.S., Prange Jr., A.J., Breese, G.R. and Kizer, J.S. (1977): Endocrinology, 101:613-622.
102. Norris, P.J., Smith, C.C.T., DeBelleroche, J., Bradford, H.F., Mantle, P.G., Thomas, A.J. and Penny, R.H.C. (1980): J. Neurochem., 34:33-42.
103. Olianas, M.C., DeMontis, G.M., Concu, A., Tagliamonte, A. and DeChiara, G. (1978): Eur. J. Pharmac., 49:223-232.
104. Olianas, M.C. DeMontis, G.M., Mulas, G. and Tagliamonte, A. (1978): Eur. J. Pharmac., 49:233-241.
105. Olney, J.W. (1976): Adv. Exp. Med. Biol., 69:497-505.
106. Olney, J.W., Lan Ho, O. and Rhee, V. (1971): Exp. Br. Res., 14:61-76.
107. Olney, J.W., Cicero, T.J., Meyer, E.R. and DeGubareff, T.S. (1976): Brain Res., 112:420-424.
108. Olney, J.W. and DeGubareff, T. (1978): Nature, 271:557-559.
109. Olney, J.W., Fuller, T. and DeGubareff, T. (1979): Brain Res., 176:91-100.
110. Pinto, O.D.S., Polikar, M. and Debono, G. (1972): Postgrad. Med. J., 48 Supplement, 18-23.
111. Polc, P. and Haefely, W. (1977): Naunyn-Schmiedeberg's Arch. Pharmac., 300:199-203.
112. Porceddu, M.L., Piacente, B., Morelli, M. and DiChiara, G. (1979): Neurosci. Letters, 15:271-276.
113. Potashner, S.J. (1978): Can. J. Physiol. Pharmac., 56:150-154.
114. Price, M.T., Olney, J.W., Anglim, M. and Buchsbaum, S. (1979): Brain Res., 176:165-168.
115. Price, M.T., Olney, J.W. and Cicero, T.J. (1978): Neuroendocrinology, 26:352-358.
116. Price, M.T., Olney, J.W., Mitchell, M.V., Fuller, T. and Cicero, T.J. (1978): Brain Res., 158:461-465.
117. Reif-Lehrer, L. and Stemmermann, M.G. (1975): N. Engl. J. Med., 293:1204-1205.

118. Reubi, J.C. and Cuenod, M. (1979): Brain Res., 176:185-188.
119. Roberts, P.J., Storm-Mathisen, J., Johnston, G. editors (1980 in press): Glutamate as a Transmitter, John Wiley Press, New York.
120. Rohde, B.H., Rea, M.A., Simon, J.R. and McBride, W.J. (1979): J. Neurochem., 32:1431-1435.
121. Rowlands, G.J. and Roberts, P.J. (1980): Exp. Br. Res., 39: 239-240.
122. Rubin, R.P. (1970): Pharmacological Reviews, 22:389-428.
123. Sandoval, M.E. and Cotman, C.W. (1978): Neuroscience, 3:199-206.
124. Sandoval, M.E., Horch, P. and Cotman, C.W. (1978): Brain Res., 142:285-300.
125. Schwartzkroin, P.A. and Andersen, P. (1975): In: Advances in Neurology Vol. 12, edited by G.W. Kreutzberg, pp. 45-51. Raven Press, New York.
126. Schwartzkroin, P.A. and Wester, K. (1975): Brain Res., 89: 107-119.
127. Segal, M. (1976): Br. J. Pharmac., 58:341-345.
128. Shimizu, H., Ichishita, H., Tateishi, M. and Umeda, I. (1975): Mol. Pharmacol., 11:223-231.
129. Shinozaki, H. and Ishida, M. (1979): Brain Res., 161:493-501.
130. Shinozaki, H. and Shibuya, I. (1974): Neuropharmacology, 13: 665-672.
131. Shinozaki, H. and Shibuya, I. (1974): Neuropharmacology, 13: 1057-1065.
132. Shinozaki, H. and Shibuya, I. (1976): Neuropharmacology, 15: 145-147.
133. Simon, J.R., Contrera, J.F. and Kuhar, M.J. (1976): J. Neurochem., 26:141-147.
134. Snodgrass, S.R. (1979): Abs. Soc. Neurosci., 5:1943.
135. Spencer, H.J. (1976): Brain Res., 102:91-101.
136. Stone, T.W. (1973): J. Physiol. (Lond.), 233:211-225.
137. Stone, T.W. (1976): J. Physiol. (Lond.), 257:187-198.
138. Storm-Mathisen, J. (1977): Brain Res., 120:379-386.
139. Storm-Mathisen, J. and Woxen-Opsahl, M. (1978): Neurosci. Letters, 9:65-70.
140. Takemoto, T. (1978): In: Kainic Acid as a Tool in Neurobiology, edited by E.G. McGeer, J.W. Olney and P.L.McGeer, pp. 1-16. Raven Press, New York.
141. Takeuchi, A. and Onodera, K. (1973): Nature New Biol., 242: 124-126.
142. Takeuchi, A. and Onodera, K. (1975): Neuropharmacology, 14: 619-625.
143. Takeuchi, A. and Takeuchi, N. (1964): J. Physiol. (Lond.), 170:296-317.
144. Teyler, T.J. and Alger, B.E. (1976): Brain Res., 115:413-425.
145. Tzeng, M-C, Cohen, R.S. and Siekevitz, P. (1978): Proc. Natl. Acad. Sci. U.S.A., 75:4016-4020.
146. Ungerstedt, V. (1973): Neurosci. Res., 5:73-96.

147. Usherwood, P.N.R. (1978): Adv. Comp. Physiol. Biochem., 7: 227-309.
148. Usherwood, P.N.R., Clark, R.B., Gration, K.A., Ozeki, M. and Patlak, J. (1979): J. Physiol. (Paris), 75:615-621.
149. Van den Berg, D.J. and Garfinkel, D. (1971): Biochem. J., 123: 211-218.
150. Van Harreveld, A. and Fifkova, E. (1975): Exp. Neurol., 49: 736-749.
151. Waelsch, H. (1951): Adv. Protein Chem., 6:301.
152. Waelsch, H. (1962): In: Neurochemistry: The Chemistry of Brain and Nerve, edited by K.A.C. Elliot, I.H. Page and J.H. Quastel, pp. 288-320. Charles C. Thomas, Springfield, Illinois, U.S.A.
153. Walther, U.C. and Rathmayer, W. (1974): J. Comp. Physiol., 89:23-38.
154. Watkins, J.C. (1978): In: Kainic Acid as a Tool in Neuro- biology, edited by E.G. McGeer, J.W. Olney and P.L. McGeer, pp. 37-69. Raven Press.
155. Wenthold, R.J. (1979): Brain Res., 162:338-343.
156. Wheal, H.V. and Miller, J.J. (1980): Brain Res., 182:145-155.
157. White, W.F., Nadler, J.V. and Cotman, C.W. (1979): Brain Res., 164:177-194.
158. White, W.F., Nadler, J.V. and Cotman, C.W. (1979): Brain Res., 178:41-53.
159. White, W.F., Nadler, J.V., Hamberger, A., Cotman, C.W., and Cummins, J.T. (1977): Nature, 270:356-357.
160. Wieraszko, A. and Lynch, G. (1979): Brain Res., 160:372-376.
161. Yamamoto, C., Yamashita, H. and Chujo, T. (1976): Nature, 262:786-787.
162. Yamashita, S., Ogawa, H. and Sato, M. (1973): Jap. J. Physiol., 23:59-68.
163. Young, A.B., Oster-Granite, M.L., Herndon, R.M. and Snyder, S.H. (1974): Brain Res., 73:1-13.
164. Young, W.S. and Kuhar, M.J. (1979): Brain Res., 179:255-270.
165. Young, W.S. and Kuhar, M.J. (1980): J. Pharmac. Exp. Therap., 212:337-346.

Glutamate as a Neurotransmitter,
edited by G. Di Chiara and G. L. Gessa
Raven Press, New York © 1981.

Glutamate in Cortical Fibers

F. Fonnum, A. Søreide, I. Kvale, J. Walker, and I. Walaas

*Norwegian Defence Research Establishment, Division for Toxicology,
N-2007, Kjeller, Norway*

Studies have accumulated showing that amino acids may constitute the quantitatively most important group of neurotransmitters in mammalian brain (6,7,9,11,17). Both glutamate (GLU) and aspartate (ASP) excites most neurons and are strong candidates for excitatory neurotransmitters. The two amino acids play an important part in brain metabolism and it is therefore a problem to establish methods which enable us to identify the transmitter pool of glutamate and aspartate. Based on the properties of other amino acids and amines that function as neurotransmitters, 3 methods for identifying the neurotransmitter pool of glutamate and aspartate have been suggested (11):

1) High affinity uptake of D-Asp or L-Glu. Evidence is accumulating that the GLU/ASP nerve terminals exhibit a specific uptake activity for both Glu and Asp (11). The uptake can be demonstrated either autoradiographically in slices (Fig 1-4) or biochemically in brain homogenates. The results obtained by the two techniques are similar in that a high uptake activity was found in neocortex, striatum, hippocampus and thalamus, whereas low activities were found in globus pallidus and hypothalamus. A substantial loss in this activity is found after lesion of putative glutamergic terminals (see below). It is, however, well established that injection of labelled GLU into brain give rise to heavy glial labelling (15). The interference from glial cells does not, however, seem to constitute a major problem in our experiments (11). It is possible that the glial cells are labile and lose their uptake activity during preparation of our slices or homogenates. The

29

slices were 400 μ thick and prepared with a Sorvall TC2 tissue chopper.

2) Ca^{++} dependent release of GLU and ASP on depolarization of brain slices or synaptosomes. The release of exogenous or endogenous amino acids can either be studied by specific stimulation of fibers in slices (25,26), or by chemical (K^{+}, veratridine) stimulation of slices or synaptosome preparation (Cotman, Chapter 1). The latter procedure is only of value when combined with lesion experiments.

3) High intraterminal concentration of ASP or GLU. By analogy to the situation in GABA (13), the terminal is expected to contain a very high concentration of its neurotransmitter. Amino acid analysis after lesion of GLU/ASP nerve terminals is therefore expected to give a loss in the endogenous level of amino acid. Since the amino acids have other functions in brain, the loss will not be complete as is the case for GABA.

By studying these 3 parameters in different brain regions, particularly the changes introduced by specific brain lesions, it has been possible to map out several glutamate pathways in brain.

DISTRIBUTION OF GLUTAMERGIC STRUCTURES IN CORTEX

Somatosensory and cingulate cortex

Homogenates of cerebral cortex possess every active HA uptake of D-Asp (12). Autoradiography after uptake of D-Asp into cortical slices shows that the uptake is localized in a laminar pattern which corresponds to the different cortical layers. In the somatosensory cortex the highest uptake is seen in layer I (Fig 2), much higher than in layer II and III. It is particularly interesting to note that the labelling of D-Asp in layer IV confirm to the barrel pattern described by Wolsey and van der Loos (36). The dark stripes correspond to the barrel sides and the lighter areas to the hollows. Thus the barrel sides showed a high uptake of D-Asp whereas the uptake was very low in the barrel hollows, which receive the so called specific thalamocortical fibers (34,35). The barrel sides contain small neurons, large dendrites, synaptic terminals and axons. From high power lm we believe that the activity is localized to the terminals which are derived from cortical neurons outside the somatosensory cortex. The barrel pattern was restricted to the somatosensory part of parietal cortex. The labelling in layer V and VI are very strong.

There are many candidates among efferent fibers which could, in part, be responsible for the cortex staining pattern. The commissural fibers end in layer I, III and Va, other thalamocortical fibers end in layers I and Vb. The small intrinsic corticofugal fibers (30), may well also contribute to the autoradiographic staining pattern.

The autoradiographic distribution of D-Asp was slightly different in the cingulate cortex (Fig 3). The highest activity was localized to layer I, the molecular layer. Since the uptake was restricted to this layer in both cortical areas, we do not think it represents an artifact. In cingulate cortex, layer II is very small or absent. The uptake pattern in the other layers resemble that in somatosensory cortex in that the activity is weak in layer III and IV, but strong in the deeper layers.

Olfactory cortex and tuberculum

Autoradiographic slices also showed a laminar distribution of D-Asp uptake in olfactory cortex (Fig.4). The highest activity was found in the deep part of the plexiform layer (1b), which received a cortical input (15). Conspicuously lower activity was found in the more superficial part of the plexiform layer (1a), which receives an imput from LOT. LOT itself is

FIG 1. Autoradiography of HA uptake of D-ASP in a frontal slice of the mouse brain. A high uptake is seen in cerebral cortex, striatum and thalamus, while the uptake is low in globus pallidus and hypothalamus. Hippocampus shows a laminar pattern and many thalamic nuclei are visualized. ad: anteriodorsal nucleus, F: fornix, av: anteroventral nucleus, VGp: globus pallidus, Hb: habenula, Wi: hippocampus, Ht: hypothalamus, Ic: capsula interna, Id: laterodorsal nucleus, lp: lateroposterior nucleus, r: reticular nucleus, s: ventral complex.

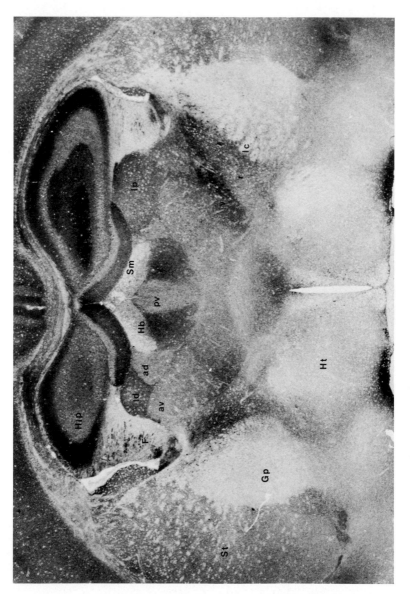

FIG.1. See legend on preceding page

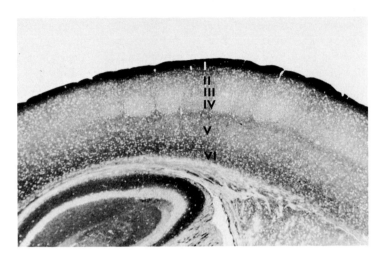

FIG 2. Autoradiography of HA uptake of D-Asp in slices
from somatosensory cortex of mouse cerebrum.
Note the barrel septa in layer IV and the distribution of
grains in distinct layers.

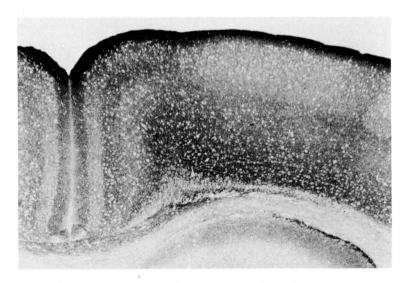

FIG 3. Autoradiography after HA uptake of D-Asp in slices
from mouse cortex. Note that the uptake is distributed in
distinct layers in both cingulate cortex and the parietal
region.

pale. The cells in layer II, as most cells in our radiographic studies, are pale. We do not know to what extent our methods of preparing slices preserve cell perikarya and their ability to take up neurotransmitters. The polyform cell layer III shows intermediate uptake activity.

Cortical ablations, particularly those involving the mediofrontal part, was accompanied by a substantial loss in D-Asp uptake (60%) in the olfactory tubercle. The cortical projection to olfactory tubercle therefore probably contains Asp/Glu as a transmitter.

GLUTAMATE IN NEOCORTICOFUGAL FIBERS

Neostriatum

The ablation of the frontal or entire hemicortex was accompanied by a significant loss of HA-Glu uptake in the whole rostrocaudal extent of neostriatum (52-75%). Most of the uptake could be accounted for by the synaptosome fraction (8,12). In addition a large fall in endogenous Glu (15-40%) was obtained (12,19). A high proportion of the decrease in uptake in neostriatum could be accounted for by a lesion restricted to the frontal cortex (3), in aggreement with anatomical studies that neostriatal fibers from this region predominates (14,18). Further, in aggreement with the anatomical studies (4), there was also a small but significant reduction in uptake (15%) on the contralateral side (12). Several independent biochemical investigations now support the concept that glutamate is the neurotransmitter of the corticostriatal pathway (8,12,15,27). In aggreement the excitatory response to cortical stimulation could be suppressed by iontophoretic application of glutamate diethylester (28).

Nucleus accumbens

Anatomical and neurochemical evidence indicates that nucleus accumbens septi may be regarded as part of the ventral neostriatum (14,33). The ipsilateral frontal neocortex projects to nucleus accumbens (3) and ablation of the frontal cortex was therefore accompanied by 18-25% reduction of Glu uptake in the ipsilateral nl accumbens. A quantitatively more important cortical input was derived from subiculum. Transection of fimbria/fornix was accompanied by 50% decrease of Glu uptake in nl accumbens. It was interesting to see that the medial part of nl accumbens resembled septum and the lateral part of resembled neostriatum in their organization of cortical inputs (33).

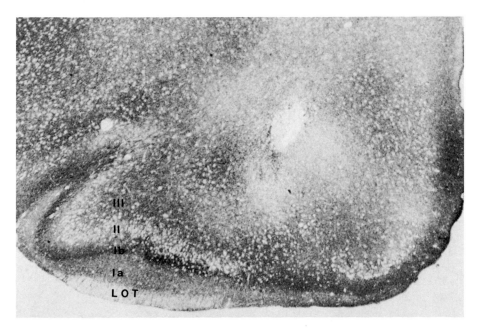

FIG 4. Autoradiography of HA uptake of D-Asp in slices from primary olfactory cortex of mouse. Note the high uptake in the deep part of the plexiform layer (1b).

Substantia nigra

The existence of cortical input to substantia nigra has long been disputed. Recent anatomical studies have, however, provided some evidence for a cortico-nigral projection (1,20). The HA Glu uptake in substantia nigra was only 20 percent of the corresponding uptake in neostriatum. Still ablation of frontal cortex was accompanied by a loss of Glu uptake (20–50%) in substantia nigra and indicates that cortico-nigral fibers may use Glu or Asp as their transmitter. Electropharmacological studies also support such findings (5). When

compared to HA uptake Glu in striatum, the cortico-nigral
proportion can only be a few percent of the density of the
cortico-striatal projection.

Thalamus

Autoradiography of thalamic slices after HA uptake of
D-Asp revealed an interesting pattern which could be correlated to the different thalamic nuclei (Fig 1). Biochemical
studies confirmed the high activity in this region and
showed that the pattern probably was due to corticothalamic
projections. The corticothalamic projection is unilateral and
reciprocal to the thalamocortical projection (35). In aggreement with the anatomical knowledge, hemidecortication was
accompanied by a large reduction (70%) in D-Asp uptake
on the ipsilateral side of the lesion (12). Further studies
have shown that a large part of this reduction was obtained
after removal of pyriform cortex alone. Amino acid analysis
after hemidecortication showed a significant fall in L-Glu
(40%) and a smaller fall in L-Asp (15%) (12). It would be
of interest to study the changes in the autoradiographic
pattern after specific cortical lesion. Such studies are on
the way. Ablation of visual cortex in adult alone, lead to
a substantial fall in L-Glu (75%) uptakes and endogenous
glutamate (30%) in lateral geniculate body (24), in aggreement with the view that cortico-thalamic fibers are glutamergic. The postnatal development of HA Glu uptake in lateral
geniculate body was also correlated with the formation of
corticofugal nerve terminals (20). When the visual cortex
on one side was removed in the young animal, there was
a reduction in Glu uptake in lateral geniculate body on both
sides in adult animal (35-50%) (21). This indicates that the
neonatal lesion has induced changes in the remaining cortico-
thalamic projection (21).

Superior colliculus

The HA Glu uptake in superior colliculus was less than
half of that in lateral geniculate body. Still the uptake
was reduced by 50% and the endogenous glutamate by 30%
after removal of the visual cortex in the adult animal (24).
The finding is thus in aggreement with the concept that glutamate is the neurotransmitter of the corticofugal fibers

from visual cortex.

When visual cortex was removed on one side in the neonatal animal, the Glu uptake was reduced by 50% in both
superior colliculi in the adult animal. When the remaining
visual cortex was removed, the uptake was reduced by a
further 25% on both sides. These results are in agreement
with the recent morphological and electrophysiological studies which show that neonatal lesion of visual cortex induces an aberrant crossing of the visual cortex projection and
that these fibers also use Glu as their transmitter (21).

Amygdala

Amygdala receives fibers from both medio-frontal, pyriform and enthorinalis cortex (15). Lesions in the pyriform
cortex, which will also disrupt fibers from the enthorinalis
cortex, reduced Glu uptake in amygdala by more than 50%.
Lesions in the mediofrontal cortex was not accompanied by
significant changes in Glu uptake. This does not exclude
that also these fibers contain glutamate, but it clearly demonstrate that this glutamergic input is at least quantitatively less important.

GLUTAMATE IN ALLOCORTICAL PROJECTIONS

Lateral septum

The pyramidal cells in CA-3 hippocampus project bilaterally through fimbria-fornix to the lateral but not the medial part of septum (2,23,29). When the pyramidal cells were
degenerated by intrahippocampal injection of kainic acid
or when the fimbria-fornix was transected, the Glu uptake
and the endogenous level of Glu was reduced in the lateral
but not medial septum (10). Collaterals of the hippocampal-
septal fibers, the so called Schaffer collaterals, go to the
stratum radiatum in hippocampus CA-1, where L-Glu should
also be a transmitter candidate. By electrical stimulation
of the fibers in the hippocampal-septal slice and in the
transverse hippocampal slice, we were able to demonstrate
an evoked release of 3H-D-Asp from both the hippocampal
septal terminals and the Schaffer collateral terminals (25,
26). The release was Ca^{++} dependent and did not occur with

L-leucine or GABA under similar conditions. Together, these experiments strongly suggest that at least some of the fornix fibers use Glu as their chemical transmitter.

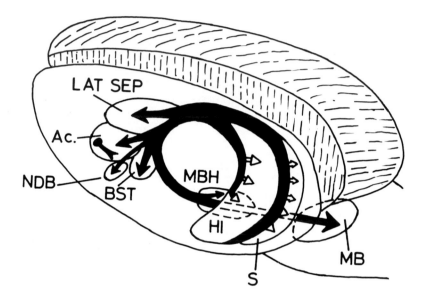

FIG 5.   Distribution of fornix/fimbria fibers from hippocampus-subiculum. Lat sep, lateral septum; Ac, nucleus accumbens; NDB, nucleus of diagonal band; MBH, mediobasal hypothalamus; MB, mammillary body; S, subiculum; HI, hippocampus. The fibers to lat sep and NDB come mainly from hippocampus, whereas the other fibers come mainly from subiculum.

We (23) have therefore also investigated whether L-Glu could be the transmitter in other regions of the brain such as nl of the diagonal band, bed nl of stria terminalis, nl accumbens, mediobasal hypothalamus and corpus mammillare, which receive fornix fiber mainly from the pyramidal cells in subiculum (2,29). The results show that in all these nuclei there was a significant decrease in HA-Glu uptake (40-

70%) and in the endogenous level of Glu (15–34%) (33). Only
in the nl of the diagonal band and in the mammillary body
there was also a significant reduction in aspartate, but
not in other amino acids. From these studies it is clear
that the subicular pyramidal cell constitutes an important
center for glutamergic fibers which distribute widely into
the brain.

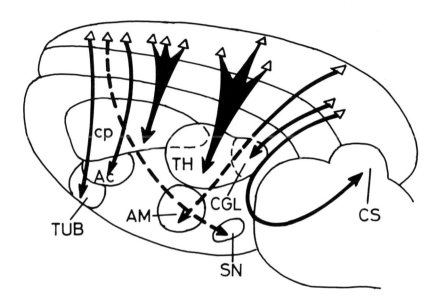

FIG 6.   The origin and distribution of glutamate fibers from
neocortex. Ac, nucleus accumbens; cp, neostriatum; TH, thalamus; CGL, lateral geniculate body; CS, colliculus superior; SN, substantia nigra; AM, amygdala; TUB, olfactory
tubercle. The projections to AC, TUB and cp come mainly
from the frontal part of cortex. The projection to SN is
very small and probably also comes mainly from the frontal part. The projection to TH comes from the entire cortex, but particularly from pyriform cortex. The projection
to AM also passes through the pyriform cortex. The projections to GGL and SC come mainly from visual cortex.

CONCLUSION

Glutamate appears to be a very important transmitter candidate for both intrinsic and afferent fibers in both neocortex and allocortex. Three very important glutamate fiber systems have been identified. In neocorticofugal fiber, glutamate seems in general to be the major transmitter candidate (Fig 6). In allocortico fibers, particularly from the pyramidal cells in subiculum, glutamergic fibers distribute to several parts of the brain (Fig 5). Thirdly, fiber systems in hippocampus proper also seem to use to a large extent glutamate as a neurotransmitter (11,26).

REFERENCES

1. Afifi, A.K., Balruth, N.B., Kaelber, W.W., Mikhael, E. and Nassar, S. (1974):J. Anat., 118:469–476.
2. Andersen, P., Bland, B.H. and Dudar, J.D. (1973):Expl. Brain Res., 17:152–168.
3. Beckstead, R.M. (1979):Neuroscience Letters, 12:59–69.
4. Carman, J.B., Cowan, W.M., Powell, T.S.P. and Webster, K.E. (1965):J. Neurol.Neurosurg.Psychiat., 28: 71–77.
5. Collingridge, G.L. and Davies, J. (1979):Neuropharmacology, 18:193–199.
6. Curtis, D.R. and Johnston, G.A.R. (1974):Ergebn. Physiol., 69:94–188.
7. Curtis, D.R. (1979):In:Glutamic acid Advances in biochemistry and physiology. Edited by L.J. Filler Jr., S. Garrattini, M.K. Kane, W.A. Reynolds and R.J. Wurtman, pp.163–176. Raven Press.
8. Divac, I., Fonnum, F. and Storm-Mathisen, J. (1977): Nature (Lond.), 266:377–378.
9. Fonnum, F. (1978):Amino Acids as Chemical Transmitters Nato Advances Study Series, Series A, Life Sciences, 16, Plenum Press.
10. Fonnum, F. and Walaas, I. (1978):J. Neurochem., 31: 1173–1181.
11. Fonnum, F., Lund-Karlsen, R., Malthe-Sorenssen, D., Skrede, K.K. and Walaas, I. (1979):Prog. Brain Res., 51:167–191.
12. Fonnum, F., Storm-Mathisen, J. and Divac, I. (1980):

Neuroscience, in press.
13. Fonnum, F. and Walberg, F. (1973):Brain Res., 54:115–127.
14. Goldman, P.S. and Nauta, H.J.H. (1977):J. Comp. Neurol., 171:369–385.
15. Heimer, L. (1978):In:The limbic system, edited by K.E. Levingston and O. Hornykiewiz, Plenum Press.
16. Hokfelt, T. and Ljungdahl, A. (1972):Exp. Brain Res., 14:354–362.
17. Iversen, L.L. and Bloom, F.E. (1972):Brain Res., 41: 131–143.
18. Kemp, K.M. and Powell, T.P.S. (1970):Brain, 93:525–546.
19. Kim, J.S., Hassler, R., Haug, P. and Paik, K.S. (1977) Brain Res., 132:370–374.
20. Kunzle, H. (1978):Brain Behav.Evol., 15:185–234.
21. Kvale, I. and Fonnum, F. (1980):Brain Res., In press.
22. Kvale, I. and Fonnum, F. (1981):Brain Res., In press.
23. Lorente de Nò, R. (1934):J. Psychol.Neurol.(Lpz)., 46: 113–177.
24. Lund Karlsen, R. and Fonnum, F. (1978):Brain Res., 151:457–467.
25. Malthe-Sorenssen, D., Skrede, K.K. and Fonnum, F. (1979):Neuroscience, 5:127–133.
26. Malthe-Sorenssen, D., Skrede, K.K. and Fonnum, F. (1979):Neuroscience, 4:1255–1265.
27. McGeer, P.L., McGeer, E.G., Scherer, V. and Singh, K. (1977):Brain Res., 128:369–373.
28. Spencer, H.J. (1976):Brain Res., 102:91–101.
29. Swanson, L.W. and Cowan, W.M. (1977):J. Comp. Neurol. 172:49–84.
30. Szentagothai, J. (1978):Proc.R.Soc., London, B,201: 219–248.
31. Soreide, A. and Fonnum, F. (1980):Brain Res., In press
32. Walaas, I. (1980):Neuroscience. In press.
33. Walaas, I. and Fonnum, F. (1980):Neuroscience.In press
34. White, E.L. (1978):J. Comp. Neurol., 181:627–662.
35. Wise, S.P. and Jones, E.G. (1976):J. Comp. Neurol., 168:313–343.
36. Woolsey, T.A. and Van der Loos, H. (1970):Brain Res., 17:205–242.

Glutamate as a Neurotransmitter,
edited by G. Di Chiara and G. L. Gessa
Raven Press, New York © 1981.

Glutamate in Hippocampal Pathways*

Jon Storm-Mathisen

Anatomical Institute, University of Oslo, Oslo 1, Norway

The hippocampal formation is one of the brain
regions where the transmitter role of glutamate (Glu)
has been most thoroughly studied and documented. In
the present communication I will deal mainly with the
autoradiographic and microbiochemical localization of
Glu uptake sites. Other aspects of Glu as a
transmitter in this region are dealt with elsewhere
in this volume. The use of high affinity membrane
transport of Glu as a possible marker for neurones
using Glu as their transmitter was introduced by
Solomon Snyder's group, who showed that radiolabelled
Glu was taken up preferentially in a subpopulation of
brain nerve ending particles (40) and provided the
first evidence that some of these belong to certain
excitatory neurones (42).

PATHWAYS

The hippocampal formation is ideally suited for
studying the localization of transmitter candidates
in excitatory neurones. The region contains several
excitatory systems which are well characterized and
are organized in distinct laminae (Fig. 1). Thus the
main input to the region is from the entorhinal cortex via the perforant path, which terminates on the
outer 2/3 of the dendrites of the granular cells in
area dentata, with lateral fibres ending in the superficial zone and medial fibres in the middle zone of
the dentate molecular layer (13,29). The terminals
of this pathway constitute a very large proportion
of the total population of nerve endings in their
target area and typically form synaptic contacts
with asymmetric thickenings on spines (21). Fibres
from the entorhinal cortex go also to the molecular

*Supported by grant C. 20.30-40 from the Norwegian
Council for Science and the Humanities.

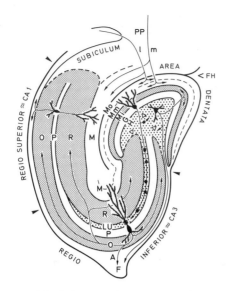

FIG. 1 - Diagram of transverse slice of the rat
hippocampal formation
showing the three-link
chain of excitatory
neurones: perforant path
axons (PP) with lateral
and medial parts (l & m),
granular cell axons (mossy
fibres), and pyramidal
cell axons from regio
inferior (CA3) or hilus
fasciae dentatae (CA4).
The target areas of the
CA3 and CA4 axons are
shown in fine stippling,
that of the mossy fibres
in coarse stippling.
Solid arrowheads show
limits between cortical
subfields. Other symbols: F, fimbria; FH, fissura
hippocampi. A, alveus; O, stratum oriens; P, str.
pyramidale; R, str. radiatum; M, str. moleculare of
hippocampus; Mo, Mm & Mi, outer, middle & inner zones
of str. moleculare of area dentata; G, str. granulare;
H, hilus fasciae denatae; L, str. lucidum (mossy fibre
layer of CA3).

layer of hippocampus (29). The excitation of the dentate granules is brought on to pyramidal cells in
regio inferior (CA3) of the hippocampus and to
modified pyramidal cells in the hilus region (CA4) of
area dentata by means of the mossy fibre system (9,
36, and references therein).
     The target of the pyramidal cells of regio inferior
within the hippocampus is the stratum oriens and stratum radiatum, ipsilaterally and contralaterally. Ipsilateral fibres are more prevalent in radiatum than in
oriens, while commissural fibres are more numerous in
oriens than in radiatum. Altogether boutons of commissural fibres are considerably less numerous than
those of ipsilateral fibres and their proportion
decreases in the dorsal (septal) to ventral (temporal)
direction (7,14,18,36). Ipsilateral fibres to stratum
radiatum of CA1 are known as Schaffer collaterals.
The target of the hilus (CA4) cells is the inner 1/3
of the molecular layer of area dentata (7,15,18,36,43).
Again, the ipsilateral projection is the more abundant. The terminals of the pyramidal cell axons from
CA3 and CA4 form synapses with asymmetric thickenings,

typically on spines. The systems provide a feed-back
excitation of the regio inferior pyramids and of the
granular cells. In addition, the regio inferior pyramids propagate the excitation on to the regio superior
(CA1) as well as out of the region, notably to the
lateral septal nucleus. The boutons in CA1 that are
of CA3 origin constitute a very large proportion of
the total population of boutons in their target areas
(8).

There are several other connections in the hippocampal formation, but in the following I will concentrate on these three classes which are the most
important excitatory projections: the entorhino-dentate
and entorhino-hippocampal axons (perforant path), the
granular cell axons (mossy fibres) and the CA3 and CA4
pyramidal cell axons (including the Schaffer
collaterals).

The pyramidal and granular cells are inhibited by
local neurones. At least some of these contain glutamic acid decarboxylase (GAD), and have their terminals
and axons concentrated on the pyramidal and granular
perikarya, and in addition in a zone adjacent to the
cortical surface (1,28,30). Their distribution is
thus distinct from that of the excitatory system.

PYRAMIDAL CELL AXONS

The initial results were obtained in 1974 when I
brought some slices of rat hippocampus incubated with
[^{3}H]-L-Glu and fixed in glutaraldehyde to Leslie
Iversen's laboratory in Cambridge. The slices were
embedded in plastic, sectioned and processed for
autoradiography (17,34). The uptake was concentrated
in the target zones of the pyramidal cell axons in
hippocampus and area dentata (Fig. 1, fine stippling).

Subsequently, we have developed a technique for
producing autoradiograms of the surface of the slices
exposed to the incubation medium, thus avoiding
problems related to the penetration of [^{3}H]-L-Glu
through the tissue (32,37,38). By this technique the
zonal pattern was very clearly demonstrated (Fig. 2A).
It was the same for [^{3}H]-L-aspartate, [^{3}H]-D-Asp, and
[^{3}H]-L-Glu, as expected from biochemical results
(5,42) which suggest that the uptake systems for these
amino acids are identical or very similar. The uptake
of [^{3}H]GABA shows an entirely different localization
(Fig. 2B), conforming to that of GAD (1,30), with the
highest uptake close to the pyramidal and granular
cell bodies and immediately subjacent to the cortical
surface. The distribution is also different micro-
scopically: GABA is accumulated in relatively coarse

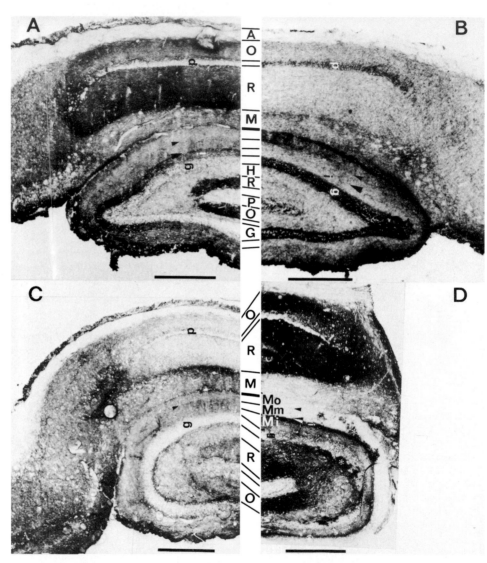

Fig. 2 - Surface autoradiograms of hippocampal slices incubated in 3 uM of [^{3}H]-D-Asp (A,C,D) or [^{3}H]GABA (B) in Krebs' solution and fixed with glutaraldehyde. The regions shown are mainly regio superior of hippocampus (CA1) above and area dentata below. A and B, normal hippocampus. C, 18 days after ipsilateral lesion of regio inferior (CA3) (section between two arrowheads in Fig. 1) plus commissural transection. Note loss of uptake in zones O and R. At more basal

levels even hilus fasciae dentatae (CA4) was damaged,
leading to partial loss of uptake in zone Mi. D, 9
days after ipsilateral transection of perforant path.
Note loss of uptake in zones Mo, Mm and M. (A and B
are from dorsal 1/3 of the hippocampal formation, C
and D from middle 1/3). Symbols: see Fig. 1. Scale
bar, 500 um.

TABLE 1. Summary of results on glutamate and aspar-
        tate uptake in pyramidal and perforant
                  path axons

	Activities in target zones of	
	Pyramidal axons	Perforant path axons
Glu or Asp uptake	3	1
Loss on axotomy	80%	50%
GAD or GABA uptake	0.4	1
Loss on axotomy	None	None

Normal activities in the stratum oriens + radiatum of
CA1 are given relative to those in the perforant path
target zone (Fig. 1, Mo + Mm). Loss on axotomy is
given as % of unoperated controls. (Data from refs.
32,37,38).

axonal and boutonlike structures, while the structures
the acidic amino acids enter are more delicate and
resemble the "dustlike" appearance of the degeneration
products seen in silver impregnated sections after
degeneration of the pyramidal cell axons (14,18).
Electronmicroscopic autoradiography of the target zone
in area dentata (Fig. 1, Mi) showed the highest
labelling intensity over boutons and unmyelinated
axons (34).

The radioactivity accumulated in the slices
was present almost entirely as the unchanged amino
acid (34). The fixation employed (5% distilled glutaraldehyde in Krebs' solution) retained 50% of the
acidic amino acids and 70% of GABA (37).

The uptake activities in the target zones were
assayed biochemically in suspensions of nerve ending
particles prepared by homogenizing samples microdissected from slices. The uptake of $[^3H]$-L-Glu
in the CA1 target zones of pyramidal axons from
CA3 was about 3 times the uptake in the outer

parts of the molecular layer of area dentata, while the ratio for GAD was 0.4 (37) (Table 1). This confirms that the uptake distributions visualized autoradiographically are real and not due to any technical peculiarities of the autoradiographic procedure (e.g., selective loss of [^{3}H]aminoacids from some sites on fixation).

The CA3 axons to CA1 were severed by cutting away the CA3 ipsilaterally and transecting the commissural fibres by a parasagittal cut contralaterally. This resulted in a selective and virtually complete disappearance of [^{3}H]-L-Glu and [^{3}H]-D-Asp uptake from the target zones in CA1, as revealed autoradiographically (Fig. 2C) or biochemically (Table 1). Thus the reduction measured in homogenates of strata oriens plus radiatum dissected from CA1 was by 80% at 4-27 days survival (13 animals) and by 70% at 3 days (3 animals). There was no reduction in [^{3}H]GABA uptake or GAD (38). When the hilus fasciae dentatae (CA4) was damaged a loss of uptake in the target zone of the CA4 axons in the inner part of the dentate molecular layer was observed autoradiographically (38).

These dramatic losses of uptake occur simultaneously with an intense glial proliferation and remain unchanged when the glial reaction subsides (compare ref. 8). Partial lesions produced by ipsilateral parasagittal transections of the hippocampal formation which destroy the numerous longitudinally directed fibres, reduced the uptake of [^{3}H]-D-Asp by up to 50% in strata oriens plus radiatum of CA1 and CA3 (3-14 days survival). The reduction in uptake contralateral to a parasagittal cut was much less than ipsilaterally (about 20% in oriens plus radiatum of CA1 in the dorsal 1/3 of the hippocampal formation), in agreement with the anatomical data (see above).

Kinetic analysis confirmed that the changes induced by lesions were due to reductions in the number of uptake sites (Vmax) and not in the affinity (Km 1.5 uM for [^{3}H]-D-Asp).

The findings outlined above were all obtained in vitro, and it may be argued that some tissue compartment (e.g. glia) could be destroyed under these conditions. Previous results of in vivo injections have suggested that [^{3}H]-L-Glu goes mainly into glia and nonselectively into neurones (16,22). Those studies used high concentrations of aminoacids and/or unphysiological injection medium. We have infused [^{3}H]-D-Asp intraventricularly in rats, mice and hamsters (usually for 1 h) at low concentrations (5 uM) in Krebs' solution (41). D-Asp was chosen for these experiments since it is little metabolized and

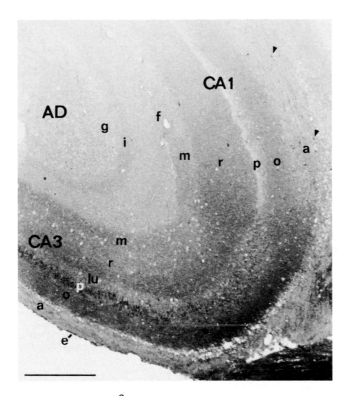

Fig. 3. Uptake of [³H]-D-Asp (5 uM) in vivo infused intraventricularly in Krebs' solution for 50 min, followed by fresh Krebs' solution for 18 min. Fixed by cardiac perfusion with 5% glutaraldehyde. Horizontal kryostat section through dorsal hippocampus. AD, area dentata; CA1, regio superior; CA3, regio inferior; f, fissura hippocampi; i, inner part of dentate molecular layer; e, ependymal cells; ▾, glial cells. Other symbols: see Figs. 1 and 2. (Dark artifact in lower right corner.) Scale bar, 500 um.

not expected to be incorporated into protein (5). The characteristic zonal pattern was clearly revealed in the hippocampal formation (Fig. 3) with the highest labelling intensities in the target zones of the CA3 and CA4 derived axons. Intensely labelled glial and ependymal cells were seen, particularly close to the ventricles. These were much less apparent when the ventricles were flushed for 15-25 min. with Krebs' without [³H]-D-Asp before perfusion-fixing the animal. Interestingly, the pyramidal cell bodies of CA3, but not those of CA1, were conspicuously labelled. This

was never seen in slices, maybe due to poor condition
of the cells. The labelling may represent direct
uptake or retrograde axonal transport from the axon
terminals. The neuropil in the target area of CA3
pyramidal cell axons in the lateral septum also showed
intense uptake activity in vivo, in accordance with
the 70% loss of Glu and Asp uptake in this area after
axotomy (6,35).

In conclusion, the CA3 and CA4 pyramidal cell axon
terminals show high affinity acidic amino acid uptake
in vivo and in vitro. The aminoacid accumulated can
be released on stimulation in a Ca^{++} dependent manner
(19,20,39). The uptake data fit nicely with the evidence for the presence of a greater than average concentration of endogenous L-Asp and L-Glu in these
fibres (6,33), and of a Ca^{++} dependent mechanism
releasing endogenous Asp and Glu, maybe selectively
from commissural and ipsilateral components of the
fibre populations, respectively (4,23, Cotman, this
volume).

PERFORANT PATH AXONS

The target zones of the perforant path contain
uptake sites for [3H]-L-Glu, [3H]-L-Asp and
[3H]-D-Asp, although the density is less than in the
target zones of the pyramidal cell axons (Fig. 2A).
The medial perforant path zone has a somewhat higher
uptake than the lateral. After unilateral transection
of the perforant path there was a selective reduction
in the uptake of acidic aminoacids in its target zones
(Fig. 2D). The reduction in [3H]-L-Glu uptake in
these zones was about 50% when measured biochemically
in microdissected samples (32) (Table 1). The autoradiograms indicated a concomitant widening and increase
in uptake activity in the inner zone of the molecular
layer, in agreement with the well known reactive
synaptogenesis in the CA4 derived fibres after this
type of lesion (3). There was also an increase in
[3H]GABA uptake intensity in the autoradiograms, and
an increase in GAD based on protein. Since there is a
reduction in the tissue volume, it is difficult to be
certain that such observations represent a net
increase in the activities signifying reactive proliferation (31), but there is evidence for increased
GABA release from the dentate area after entorhinal
lesions (24).

Electronmicroscopic autoradiography showed that the
greatest concentrations of silver grains occurred over
nerve endings and axons also in the target zones of
the perforant path in area dentata (34). The middle

part of the dentate molecular layer was analysed by
the hypothetical grain method devised by Blackett and
Parry (2,27). This method corrects for the cross-
firing effects which make it impossible to obtain
accurate results by conventional grain-counts on
complex tissues such as neuropil. While 50% of the
grain centres occurred over axons and boutons, the
analysis indicated that 80% of the radioactivity was
present in these structures, and that they had
radioactive concentrations 3 to 5 times the average
for the tissue. The corresponding figures for glial
profiles were 13% of the radioactivity and 2 times the
average radioactive concentration. The content of
glial cytoplasm in the present material incubated in
vitro was only about 5% of the volume, which is the
same as the value found in the neuropil layers in normal rat hippocampus CA1 perfusion fixed with aldehydes
(S. Laurberg and T.W. Blackstad, personal communication; see also ref. 26). The low content of glial
profiles may be part of the reason for the success in
demonstrating selective neuronal accumulation of
transmitter amino acids in the hippocampal formation.
     The perforant path is probably the best documented
Glu pathway in the brain, according to data on
release, synthesis and pharmacology (4,12,23, Cotman,
this volume). Still, the concentration of uptake
sites in the target zones and the percent reduction on
axotomy suggest that the number of uptake sites per
terminal is considerably smaller in the perforant path
than in the pyramidal cell system.

MOSSY FIBRES

     In autoradiograms of plastic sections through sli-
ces incubated with [^{3}H]-L-Glu the mossy fibre layer in
CA3 and hilus fasciae dentatae (Fig. 1) contained
large clusters of silver grains suggestive of labelled
mossy fibre endings. Electronmicroscopy revealed that
many but not all mossy fibre boutons were labelled
(34). Possibly there are granular cell axons with and
without Glu uptake sites. Perhaps more likely, the
giant mossy fibre endings are less well preserved in
the incubated slices than the smaller nerve endings
(compare above about neuronal perikarya). The damage
would be expected to be worst at the surface of the
slice. In agreement, the mossy fibre layer showed
very little labelling in the surface autoradiograms.
     After in vivo infusion of [^{3}H]-D-Asp the mossy
fibre layer was uniformly labelled, although less
intensely than strata oriens and radiatum (Fig. 3). In
two hamsters where the infusion cannula penetrated

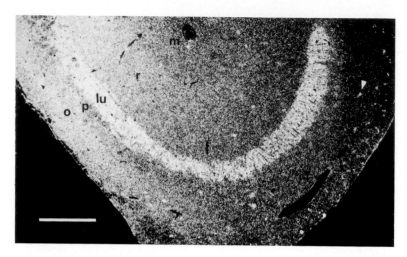

Fig. 4. Orthograde axonal transport of [³H]-D-Asp in
mossy fibres in hippocampus CA3. Intracerebral infusion for 30 min with tip of cannula in hilus fasciae
dentatae, followed immediately by cardiac perfusion
with glutaraldehyde. Dark-field photograph of autora-
diogram of 2 um Araldite section. The stratum lucidum
(lu) is strongly labelled along its whole length.
Note coarse clusters of grains, probably representing
labelled mossy fibre boutons, between poorly labelled
apical dendrites. Symbols: see Fig. 3. Scale bar,
200 um.

into the dentate area the mossy fibre layer was selectively and intensely labelled (Fig. 4). This was presumably due to fast anterograde axonal transport of
[³H]-D-Asp taken up into the granular cells and the
proximal parts of their axons (compare Cuenod,
following paper).
     It thus appears that also the granular cell axons
possess uptake sites for acidic amino acids. The
negative findings on release, uptake and content of
Glu and Asp in this system (25, Cotman, this volume)
may be ascribed to the fact that the mossy fibre layer
constituted only a small proportion of the tissue
samples analysed (whole CA3).
     The mossy fibres are held to contain high con-
centrations of heavy metals, e.g. Zn, but the same is
true of the CA3 and CA4 derived fibres, as well as of
the lateral (but not the medial) perforant path
(10,11). The metals are localized in the terminals.
Although the metal staining pattern bears a certain
resemblance to the pattern of acidic amino acid uptake

there are many differences, and neither Zn^{++} (up to
0.1 mM) nor the complexing agent diethyldithiocar-
bamate (up to 3 mM) added to the incubation medium
affected the uptake of $[^3H]$-L-Glu (2 uM) in hippocampal homogenates (unpublished observations).

SUMMARY

The three consecutive main excitatory neurone projections in the hippocampal formation (the perforant
path, the mossy fibres and the pyramidal cell axons)
all show acidic amino acid uptake in their terminals.
This is in accordance with other data pointing to the
transmitter function of glutamate and/or aspartate in
the perforant path and pyramidal cell axons. In the
mossy fibres the role of these amino acids has so far
not been determined. The localization of glutamate and
aspartate uptake in the excitatory axon systems
contrasts with the localization of GABA uptake in the
axons of the inhibitory basket cells and other short
axon neurones.

REFERENCES

1. Barber, R., and Saito, K. (1976): In: GABA in
   Nervous System Function, Kroc Foundation Series,
   Vol. 5, edited by E. Roberts, T.N. Chase, and
   D.B.Tower, pp. 113-132. Raven Press, New York.
2. Blackett, N.M., and Parry, D.M. (1973): J. Cell
   Biol., 57: 9-15.
3. Cotman, C.W., and Nadler, J.V. (1978): In: Neuronal Plasticity, edited by C.W. Cotman, pp. 227-271.
   Raven Press, New York.
4. Cotman, C.W., and Nadler, J.V. (1980): In: Glutamate: Transmitter in the Central Nervous System
   edited by P.J. Roberts, J.Storm-Mathisen, and
   G.A.R. Johnston, (in press) Wiley.
5. Davies, L.P., and Johnston, G.A.R. (1976):
   J. Neurochem., 26: 1007-1014.
6. Fonnum, F., and Walaas, I. (1978): J. Neurochem.,
   31: 1173-1181.
7. Fricke, R., and Cowan, W.M. (1978): J. comp.
   Neurol., 181: 253-270.
8. Goldowitz, D., Scheff, S.W., and Cotman, C.W.
   (1979): Brain Res., 170: 427-441.
9. Gaarskjaer, F.B. (1978): J. comp. Neurol., 178:
   73-88.
10. Haug, F.-M.Š. (1975): J. Hirnforsch., 16:
    147-158.
11. Haug, F.-M.Š. (1976): Exp. Brain Res., suppl. 1,
    177-178.

12. Hicks, T.P., and McLennan, H. (1979): Can. J. Physiol.Pharmacol., 57: 973-978.
13. Hjorth-Simonsen, A. (1972): J. comp. Neurol.,146: 219-231.
14. Hjorth-Simonsen, A. (1973): J.comp. Neurol., 147: 145-162.
15. Hjorth-Simonsen, A., and Laurberg, S. (1977): J. comp. Neurol.,174: 591-606.
16. Hökfelt, T., and Ljungdahl, Å. (1972): Adv. biochem. Psychopharmacol., 6: 1-36.
17. Iversen, L.L., and Storm-Mathisen, J. (1976): Acta physiol. scand., 96: 22A-23A.
18. Laurberg, S. (1979): J. comp. Neurol., 184: 685-708.
19. Malthe-Sørenssen, D., Skrede, K.K., and Fonnum, F. (1979): Neuroscience, 4: 1255-1263.
20. Malthe-Sørenssen, D., Skrede, K.K., and Fonnum, F. (1980): Neuroscience, 5: 127-133.
21. Matthews, D.A., Cotman, C., and Lynch, G. (1976): Brain Res., 115: 1-21.
22. McLennan, H. (1976): Brain Res., 115: 139-144.
23. Nadler, J.V., Vaca, K.W., White, W.F., Lynch, G.S., and Cotman, C.W. (1976): Nature, (Lond.), 260: 538-540.
24. Nadler, J.V., White, W.F., Vaca, K.W., and Cotman, C.W. (1977): Brain Res., 131: 241-258.
25. Nadler, J.V., White, W.F., Vaca, K.W., Perry, B.W., and Cotman, C.W. (1978):J. Neurochem., 31: 147-155.
26. Nafstad, P.H.J. and Blackstad, T.W. (1966): Z. Zellforsch. mikrosk. Anat., 73: 234-245.
27. Parry, D.M. (1976): J. Microsc. Biol. cell., 27: 185-190.
28. Ribak, C.E., Vaughn, J.E., and Saito, K. (1978): Brain Res., 140: 315-332.
29. Steward, O., and Scoville, S.A. (1976): J. comp. Neurol.,169: 347-370.
30. Storm-Mathisen, J. (1972): Brain Res., 40: 215-235.
31. Storm-Mathisen, J. (1976): In: GABA in Nervous System Function, Kroc Foundation Series, Vol. 5, edited by E. Roberts, T.N.Chase, and D.B.Tower, pp. 149-168. Raven Press, New York.
32. Storm-Mathisen, J. (1977): Brain Res., 120: 379-386.
33. Storm-Mathisen, J. (1978): In: Functions of the Septo-Hippocampal System, Ciba Foundation Symposium, 58, pp. 49-86.
34. Storm-Mathisen, J., and Iversen, L.L. (1979): Neuroscience, 4: 1237-1253.

35. Storm-Mathisen, J., and Woxen Opsahl, M. (1978): Neurosci. Lett., 9: 65-70.
36. Swanson, L.W., Wyss, J.M., and Cowan, W.M. (1978): J. comp. Neurol., 181: 681-716.
37. Taxt, T., and Storm-Mathisen, J. (1979): J. Physiol.(Paris), 75: 677-684.
38. Taxt, T., and Storm-Mathisen, J. (1980): (To be submitted to Neuroscience).
39. Wieraszko, A., and Lynch, G. (1979): Brain Res., 160: 372-376.
40. Wofsey, A.R., Kuhar, M.J., and Snyder, S.H.(1971): Proc. nat. Acad. Sci. (U.S.A.), 68: 1102-1106.
41. Wold, J.E., and Storm-Mathisen, J. (1980): (in preparation).
42. Young, A.B., Oster-Granite, M.L., Herndon, R.M., and Snyder, S.H. (1974): Brain Res. 73: 1-13.
43. Zimmer, J. (1971): J. comp. Neurol., 142: 393-416.

Glutamate as a Neurotransmitter,
edited by G. Di Chiara and G. L. Gessa
Raven Press, New York © 1981.

Glutamatergic Pathways in the Pigeon and the Rat Brain

M. Cuénod, A. Beaudet, V. Canzek, P. Streit, and J. C. Reubi

Brain Research Institute, University of Zurich, CH-8029 Zurich, Switzerland

Glutamate or possibly glutamate-like substances have gained considerable credibility as excitatory neuro-transmitters in the vertebrate central nervous system over the recent years. Work done in perforant pathway of the hippocampus (13,14) in the cortico-striate pathway (6,12) as well as in other cortico-fugal pathways (Fonnum, this symposium) or in the parallel fibers of the cerebellum (27) support in these neurons the trans-mitter role of glutamate by most, if not all, criteria presently available. These criteria are based on two categories of observations: (a) Effects induced by the activation of a pathway on its presynaptic or postsynap-tic side, with or without specific receptor blockers (which are not yet well established for glutamate) and (b) effects induced by the degeneration of a pathway on presynaptic parameters such as transmitter pool, synthe-tising enzymes, high affinity uptake or in vitro release. As this battery of criteria is often very difficult to complete for one given pathway, a tendency has developed to consider one or two criteria as very suggestive if not conclusive evidence that it uses glutamate as trans-mitter. This paper should once more point to the risks of such generalisation.

It should also provide indications that selective labeling of pathways might be used to detect a chemical specificity possibly related to the neurotransmitter.

GLUTAMATE IN THE PIGEON RETINO-TECTAL NEURONS

In the retino-tectal neurons of the pigeon, Henke and Fonnum (7) observed a 50% decrease of glutamate and a 40% decrease of aspartate in the optic tectum following degeneration of the optic nerve. This decrease was restricted to the tectal layers containing optic nerve fibers and terminals, and was not observed for control substances such as glutamine. In the same pathway, the high affinity uptake of glutamate in tectal synaptosomes was decreased by 40-50% after optic nerve degeneration (8). More recently, following up the model described in the rat neostriatum, Streit et al. (25) described histotoxic effects of kainic acid injections in the pigeon optic tectum: while a general cell loss was observed within a sphere of about 1 mm around the injection, at more distant sites, the lesion was restricted to one layer of the tectum (5b), rich in terminals of retinal origin, and consisted in a large number of small vesicular profiles (Fig. 4b). At the electronmicroscopic level, they appeared as ballooning dendrites, surrounded by normal presynaptic boutons partly identified as originating from the retina. These ultrastructural alterations were very similar to those observed by Olney (15) in other CNS regions treated with kainic acid. Following retinal ablation and at least two weeks of optic nerve degeneration, identical kainic acid injections in the tectum remained practically without histotoxic effects. This suggests that some cooperation between kainic acid and a population of optic fibers or terminals is required in order to induce the histotoxic effects (25), an observation similar to that made by McGeer et al. (12) in the striatum, where the kainic acid induced histotoxicity is dependent upon the presence of cortico-striate elements.

IN VITRO GLUTAMATE AND GABA RELEASE
IN RAT AND PIGEON CNS

Reubi et al. (19) devised a technique to measure in brain slices the Ca^{++}-dependent K^+-induced release of glutamate and GABA newly synthetized from radioactive glutamine. Using this technique, Reubi and collaborators (5,16,17,19) determined the glutamate and GABA release in various central nervous system structures of the rat and pigeon brain. The release of glutamate was high in the rat striatum, medium in the rat and pigeon hippocampus and low in the rat cerebellum, sub-

stantia nigra and cochlear nucleus as well as in the
pigeon paleostriatum, cerebellum and optic tectum. The
release of GABA was high in the rat hippocampus and substantia nigra, medium in the rat striatum and cochlear
nucleus and low in the rat cerebellum and in all pigeon
structures analysed. This distribution is in general
agreement with the established localisation of glutamate and GABA neurons and projections in the rat CNS.
Thus, the glutamate release would be expected to be
relatively high in the rat striatum and hippocampus
and the GABA release in the substantia nigra and the
hippocampus. It is, however, surprising that the cerebellum, whose very abundant parallel fibers are supposed to use glutamate as transmitter, show in both
rat and pigeon a relatively moderate release of glutamate. This might indicate either that a subpopulation
of granule cells only is releasing glutamate, or that
the release observed is not everywhere similarly related to the density of terminals: such differences
could be due to alternative synthetic pathways or to
more or less effective reuptake mechanisms in various
structures. Furthermore, the variability among various
structures of the ratio of glutamate versus GABA release, synthetized from glutamine, suggests a segre-
gation of the two respective compartments.

Using this approach unilateral fronto-parietal decortication in the rat led to a massive decrease of glutamate release in striatal slices incubated with $[^3H]$-glu-
tamine, while the GABA release remained unaffected, thus
confirming the transmitter role of glutamate in cortico-
striate neurons (17). Furthermore, after incubation of
striatal slices in $[^3H]$-asparagine, high K^+ concentration
induced a release of $[^3H]$-aspartate, a phenomenon which
is also drastically reduced after decortication (18).
This suggests that aspartate may play a transmitter role
in cortico-striate neurons. This, however, requires further investigations to make sure that one is not dealing
with a false transmitter, using the metabolic machinery
of the physiological one. In the auditory system, Canzek
and Reubi (5) obtained evidence for a transmitter role
of glutamate by showing a decrease of glutamate release
in slices of the cochlear nucleus after section of the
acoustic nerve in the cat, thus confirming the finding
of Wenthold (26).

In the pigeon retino-tectal pathway however, where
evidence reviewed above suggests a special role of glutamate, degeneration of the retina did not alter the
glutamate release in the tectum (16). This observation

could indicate that glutamate, while specially related to retino-tectal fibers, might not be massively released by these neurons.

TRANSMITTER RELATED LABELING OF NEURAL PATHWAYS

The hypothesis has been proposed, that the chemospecificity of neural pathways in the central nervous system could be established by transmitter related retrograde tracing (9,22,23,24). Basically, selective labeling of the perikarya would be observed after injection, in the area of terminals, of the radioactive transmitter used by these neurons. Radioautographic observations compatible with this interpretation have been made for the following transmitters in various pathways of two species: GABA in the rat striato-nigral pathway and in the pigeon anterior Ipc-tectal neurons, glycine in the pigeon central Ipc-tectal neurons, dopamine in the rat nigro-striate pathway, serotonin in the projections from the nucleus raphe dorsalis to substantia nigra, to the striatum (10,22,23), and to the cortex (3,22). However, evidence has been as yet obtained only for amino acids and amines. Furthermore, the selectivity seems to be relative rather than absolute, particularly among amines. The mechanisms involved in this retrograde transport have been recently investigated: In the rapheostriatal serotonergic pathway, the retrograde migration of $[^3H]$-5-HT is prevented by administration of either a 5-HT uptake inhibitor or colchicin, suggesting that it involves uptake and active retrograde transport of the radioactive transmitter(3).

FIG. 1. Radioautographic retrograde perikaryal labeling with $[^3H]$-D-aspartate. (a) Tangential section of the pigeon retina (foveal region) 6 h after injection of $[^3H]$-D-aspartate (25 µl) in the superficial layers of the contralateral optic tectum. Numerous labeled ganglion cell bodies are detected among unreactive perikarya. Note in the upper part of the micrograph the presence of their efferent labeled axons. Scale bar = 50 µm.
(b) Perikaryal labeling in layer V of rat dorso-lateral cortex following injection of $[^3H]$-D-aspartate (14 µCi) into the ipsilateral striatum. Scale bar = 0.5 mm.

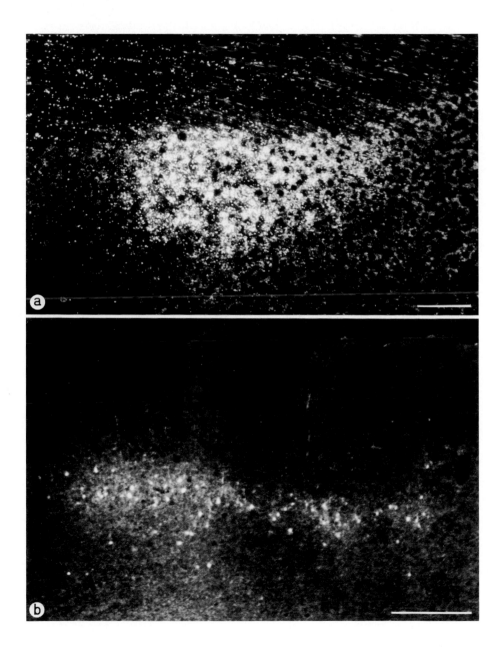

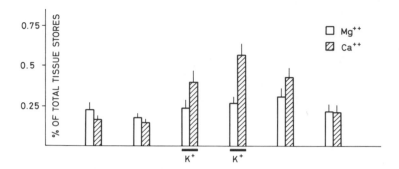

FIG. 2. Ca[++]-dependent release of [^{3}H]-D-aspartate from
rat frontal cortex slices, induced by 47 mM K+ (black
bars) 24 h after [^{3}H]-D-aspartate injection (75 μCi) in
contralateral frontal cortex. Double columns correspond
to consecutive collections over periods of 2.5 min.
Incubation in Krebs solution containing 0.1 mM Ca++,
12 mM Mg++ (white columns) or 12 mM Ca++ (hatched
columns). Mean ± S.E.M. (N=5).

FIG. 3. Superficial layers of the pigeon optic tectum.
(a) Drawing of Golgi-stained optic nerve fibers (layer 1)
and terminal arborisations (layers 2,3,4,5 and 7) modified from Cajal and van Gehuchten. (b) Corresponding
tectal layers after kainic acid injection (2 μg in 0.5
μl) performed two days before sacrifice at a site distant
from 1.5 mm. Note the presence of small and large (arrow)
vacuoles in the lower part of layer 5. These cytotoxic
effects are prevented after optic nerve degeneration.
(c) Dark field radioautograph from the same region 48 h
after contralateral intraocular injection of [^{3}H]-D-
aspartate (500 μCi). Silver grains are visible over
layer 1,2,4 and 5, but not 7, suggesting a differential
labeling of the optic nerve terminal fields. Note the
correlation in layer 5 between the zone of maximal
aspartate labeling and the optic nerve dependent kainate
toxicity illustrated in (b). (d) Radioautoradiograph of
the tectum 24 h after intraocular injection of [^{3}H]-pro-
line (25 μCi). All layers containing optic nerve fibers
and terminals are labeled. Comparison of the density
patterns between c and d indicates that radiolabeled
proteins reach terminal areas more rapidly than unme-
tabolized, soluble D-aspartate. Scale bar = 50 μm.

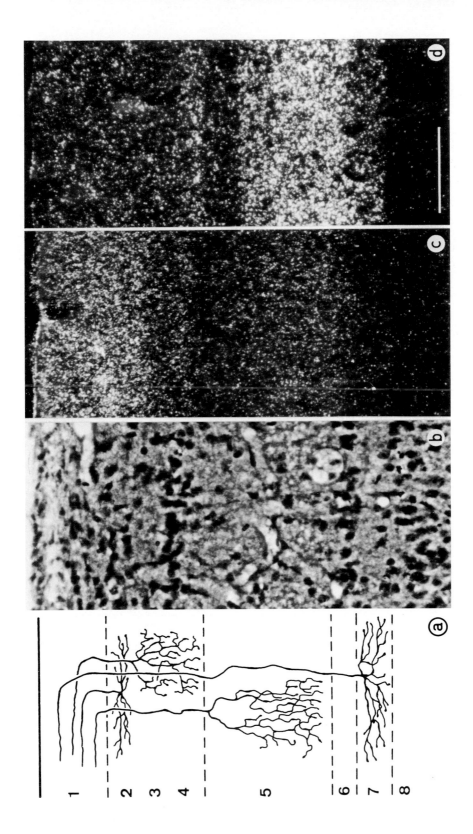

The selective labeling of CNS neurons using glutamate or aspartate as transmitter would be of great interest. Injections of [3H]-L-glutamate in the rat striatum led only to diffuse labeling at the injection site, presumably because the amino acid is to a large extent taken into a metabolic pool. D-aspartate has been proposed as an analog which is taken up as the L-form, but practically not metabolised (1,11,21). After micro-injections of [3H]-D-aspartate in the rat striatum, labeled cell bodies were observed by radioautography in the cortex (fig. 1b) and the thalamus but not, for instance, in substantia nigra or nucleus raphe dorsalis (22). In cortex, the labeled perikarya were scattered in layer V within an area known to project to the striatal injected zone. Glutamate and/or aspartate are well established transmitters in this pathway. However, labeled somata were also observed in the nucleus parafascicularis of the thalamus, whose projection to the striatum has been suggested to use acetylcholine rather than glutamate as transmitter (20). At the moment, it is unclear whether this reflects a poor selectivity of the labeling or indicates the presence of glutamate or aspartate neurons in the thalamo-striate connections.

Conversely, after injection of [3H]-D-aspartate (75 µCi) in the rat frontal cortex, anterograde labeling could be observed in the ipsilateral striatum and the contralateral cortex. Interestingly, 24 h after such intra-cortical injections, the radioactivity could be released in vitro from both these regions by 47 mM K^+, in a Ca^{++}-dependent manner (fig. 2) (4). In keeping with these results, Fonnum (pers. communication) recently observed a decrease in the uptake of D-aspartate in the frontal cortex following contralateral decortication.

In the pigeon retino-tectal pathway, both retrograde and anterograde migration of radioactivity were also observed, following injection of [3H]-D-aspartate (2). Six hours after intra-tectal instillation of 25 µCi of [3H]-D-aspartate, light microscope radioautographs of the optic tectum exhibited an intense labeling of incoming retinal fibers, within layer I. The labeled axons could be traced back along the optic tract and through the optic nerve, up to their parent perikarya in the ganglion cell layer of the retina (fig. 1a).

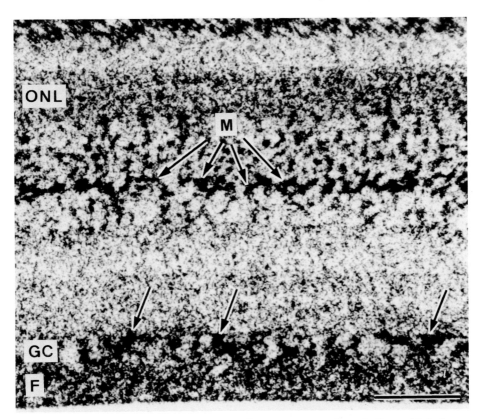

FIG. 4. Light microscope radioautograph of 1 μ-thick, epon embedded cross-section of the pigeon retina 6 h after intraocular injection of [^{3}H]-D-aspartate (500 μCi). Note the preferential labeling of Müller cells (M) and of scattered perikarya (arrows) in the ganglion cell layer (GC). Both the outer nuclear layers (ONL) and fiber layer (F) are the site of an intense and diffuse labeling. Scale bar = 50 μm.

Conversely, after intra-vitreous administration of 500 µCi of [^{3}H]-D-aspartate, heavily labeled optic fibers were found to emerge from the retinal fiber layer, and could be traced up to layer V in the contra-lateral tectum (fig. 3c). These labeled fibers presumably originate from intensely reactive cell bodies, heterogeneously distributed in the ganglion cell layer of the retina (fig. 4). These neuronal perikarya were small, intermingled with unlabeled ganglion cells, and particularly numerous in the postero-superior quadrant of the retina which is known to project to the ventral aspect of the tectum. In keeping with these results, radioactivity measurements in the tectum indicated that 48 h after intra-ocular [^{3}H]-D-aspartate injections, a major proportion of the transported radioactivity (95% in TCA-soluble form) was indeed accumulated in the ventral quadrant of the tectum.

It was thus concluded that [^{3}H]-D-aspartate could be selectively taken up and transported, both retrogradely and anterogradely, within a sub-population of retino-tectal neurons.

In this system too, the radioactivity which has migrated to the tectum 48 h after an intra-ocular injection of [^{3}H]-D-aspartate can be released by high potassium in a Ca^{++}-dependent manner (2).

It thus seems that with D-aspartate, selective tracing of neurons can be obtained, both in anterograde and in retrograde directions, that the material transported from the cell body to the terminals is still TCA-soluble and belongs to a pool which can be released by potassium depolarisation in a calcium-dependent manner. It is tempting to speculate that D-aspartate functions here as false transmitter mimicking L-glutamate, L-aspartate or an unknown similar transmitter.

ACKNOWLEDGEMENTS

The excellent technical assistance of D. Savini and M. Jäckli is gratefully acknowledged. This work has been supported by Grants 3.505.79 and 3.506.79 of the Swiss National Science Foundation, the Dr. Eric Slack-Gyr Foundation, the Roche Research Foundation for Scientifique Exchange and the Medical Research Council of Canada.

REFERENCES

1. Balcar, V.J., and Johnston, G.A.R. (1972): J. Neurochem., 19:2657-2666.
2. Beaudet, A., Burkhalter, A., Reubi, J.C., and Cuénod, M.: unpublished observations.
3. Beaudet, A., Stella, M., and Cuénod, M.: unpublished observations.
4. Canzek, V., Beaudet, A., and Cuénod, M.: unpublished observations.
5. Canzek, V., and Reubi, J.C. (1980): Exp. Brain Res., 38:437-441.
6. Divac, I., Fonnum, F., and Storm-Mathisen, J. (1977): Nature, 266:377-378.
7. Fonnum, F., and Henke, H. (1979): Experientia, 35:919.
8. Henke, H., Schenker, T.M., and Cuénod, M. (1976): J. Neurochem., 26:131-134.
9. Hunt, S.P., Streit, P., Künzle, H., and Cuénod, M. (1977): Brain Res., 129:197-212.
10. Leger, L., Pujol, J.F., Bobillier, P., and Jouvet, M. (1977): C.R. Acad. Sci. (Paris), 285:1179-1182.
11. Lund Karlsen, R., and Fonnum, F. (1978): Brain Res., 151:457-467.
12. McGeer, P.L., McGeer, E.G., Scherer, U., and Singh, K. (1977): Brain Res., 128:369-373.
13. Nadler, J.V., Vaca, K.W., White, W.F., Lynch, G.S., and Cotman, C.W. (1976): Nature, 260:538-540.
14. Nadler, J.V., White, W.F., Vaca, K.W., and Cotman, C.W. (1977), Brain Res., 131:241-258.
15. Olney, J.W. (1978): In: Kainic Acid as a Tool in Neurobiology, edited by E.G. McGeer, J.W. Olney, and P.L. McGeer, pp. 95-121. Raven Press, New York.
16. Reubi, J.C. (1980): Neuroscience (in press).
17. Reubi, J.C., and Cuénod, M. (1979): Brain Res., 176:185-188.
18. Reubi, J.C., Toggenburger, G., and Cuénod M. (1980): J. Neurochem., (in press).
19. Reubi, J.C., Van den Berg, C., and Cuénod, M. (1978): Neurosci. Lett., 10:171-174.
20. Saelens, J.K., Edwards-Neale, S., and Simke, J.P. (1978): J. Neurochem., 32:1093-1094.
21. Storm-Mathisen, J., and Woxen Opsahl, M. (1978): Neurosci. Lett., 9:65-70.
22. Streit, P. (1980): J. comp. Neurol., (in press).
23. Streit, P., Knecht, E., and Cuénod, M. (1979): Science, 205:306-308.

24. Streit, P., Knecht, E., and Cuénod, M. (1980):
    Brain Res., 187:59-67.
25. Streit, P., Stella, M., and Cuénod, M. (1980):
    Brain Res., 187:47-57.
26. Wenthold, R.J. (1979): Brain Res., 162:338-343.
27. Young, A.B., Oster-Granite, M.L., Herndon, R.M.,
    and Snyder, S.H. (1974): Brain Res., 1-13.

Glutamate as a Neurotransmitter,
edited by G. Di Chiara and G. L. Gessa
Raven Press, New York © 1981.

Glutamate and Aspartate as Neurotransmitters for the Auditory Nerve

R. J. Wenthold

Laboratory of Neuro-otolaryngology, National Institute of Neurological and Communicative Disorders and Stroke, National Institutes of Health, Bethesda, Maryland 20205

INTRODUCTION

Although much information has been obtained on the biochemistry, pharmacology and physiology of the putative neurotransmitters, glutamate and aspartate, these substances cannot yet be considered as proven neurotransmitters at any synapse in the mammalian central nervous system. However, over the past several years a number of possible excitatory amino acid pathways have been identified. One of these is the auditory nerve. Evidence supporting this contention falls in three areas: presence of glutamate and aspartate in terminals of the auditory nerve, release of glutamate and aspartate from slices of the cochlear nucleus and pharmacological similarity of the auditory nerve neurotransmitter to glutamate and aspartate.

The cell bodies of the auditory nerve are the spiral ganglion cells located in the modiolus of the cochlea. Morphologically, at least two types of spiral ganglion cells have been described, with one population including 95% of the cells and the other the remaining 5% (51). Functional differences between these two populations of cells are not known. The peripheral processes of the spiral ganglion cells synapse with the sensory cells in the organ of Corti, and central processes, which make up the auditory nerve, terminate in the cochlear nucleus. This input is heaviest throughout the ventral cochlear nucleus except for the granule cell region which receives little innervation (43). The innervation to the dorsal cochlear nucleus is confined mostly to the deeper layers. Several putative neurotransmitters, including GABA (21), acetylcholine (18), glycine (21), catecholamines (18, 20,29), enkephalins (27; R. Altschuler, personal communication) and somatostatin (44; R. Elde, personal communication), are present in the cochlear nucleus and may be associated with distinct groups of neurons, but not with terminals of the auditory nerve.

PRESENCE OF GLUTAMATE AND ASPARTATE IN PRESYNAPTIC
TERMINALS OF THE AUDITORY NERVE

A neurotransmitter must be present in the appropriate presynaptic terminal and this terminal must have the capability of
accumulating and(or) synthesizing the neurotransmitter in adequate amounts. A major difficulty in satisfying this criterion
for amino acids is distinguishing between the neurotransmitter
pool of the amino acid and its metabolic pools. All α amino
acids have metabolic roles in all neurons. Therefore, demonstration of the presence of an amino acid in a population of presynaptic terminals does not rule out an exclusively metabolic
function. However, it seems likely that a neuron which uses an
amino acid in a specialized role, such as a neurotransmitter,
would have properties unlike those of neurons in which amino
acids are used only metabolically. Investigators have used an
unusually high concentration of an amino acid in a specific
region of brain or in a specific population of presynaptic terminals and fibers as an indication of a possible neurotransmitter
role. This has probably been most successfully applied to the
study of glycine in the spinal cord (1,2). This technique is restricted to the analysis of major populations of synapses since
a minor population would not sufficiently affect the total concentration of a substance in a specific region of brain. This is
especially applicable to glutamate and aspartate since both are
found in relatively high concentrations throughout the mammalian
central nervous system.

The first report which indicates that glutamate or aspartate
are concentrated in terminals of the auditory nerve came from
Godfrey et al (21) who measured the levels of glutamate, aspartate, GABA and glycine in regions of the cochlear nucleus and
auditory nerve of the cat. Of these substances only aspartate
somewhat follows the distribution of auditory nerve fibers and
terminals in the cochlear nucleus. The distribution of glutamate is more uniform, generally paralleling that of the nonlipid
fraction of dry weight. While aspartate is lower in the auditory
nerve than in the cochlear nucleus, it is higher in the auditory
nerve than in most other white matter studied. Similar distributions of glutamate and aspartate have also been found in the
cochlear nucleus of the rat (22) and the guinea pig (54).

Evidence which more directly links glutamate and aspartate
with auditory nerve terminals is that both amino acids decrease
in the cochlear nucleus after lesion of the auditory nerve (57).
The time course of decrease of aspartate parallels the morphological degeneration of auditory nerve terminals. Glutamate also
decreases at this time but shows a continued decrease suggesting
additional pools of the amino acid are affected. No other amino
acid or neurotransmitter was found to decrease with the exception
of alanine which decreases slightly and mostly after auditory
nerve terminals had degenerated. The decrease in aspartate and
glutamate in the cochlear nucleus when auditory nerve terminals

degenerate has been confirmed in the waltzing guinea pig (58), a
genetically deaf mutant which exhibits an age dependent decrease
in spiral ganlgion cells and auditory nerve terminals (24).
Decreases in aspartate and glutamate in subdivisions of the
cochlear nucleus after auditory nerve lesions is consistent with
these amino acids being concentrated in auditory nerve terminals
(Table 1) (54). For both whole cochlear nucleus and subdivisions, the magnitude of decrease, expressed as percent of amino
acid in the control, is always greater for aspartate. However,
for early times after lesion, the decrease in actual nmoles is
similar for both amino acids and, since glutamate continues to
decrease, at later times, is greater for glutamate.

TABLE 1.   Glutamate and aspartate in subdivisions of the cochlear
           nucleus two days after auditory nerve lesion

Subdivision	Lesion[a]	Control[a]	Change (nmoles/mg)	Change (% of control)
Glutamate				
Superficial dorsal	73.0± 2.5	67.7± 2.3	+ 5.3	+ 7.8
Deep dorsal	60.8± 1.4	65.3± 3.3	- 4.5	- 6.9
Posteroventral	51.3± 2.6	65.9± 1.7	-14.6	-22.2
Auditory nerve root	35.5± 4.1	48.0± 3.0	-12.5	-26.0
Granule cell region	54.2± 1.3	62.3± 2.6	- 8.1	-13.0
Posterior antero- ventral	42.9± 0.8	65.0± 2.0	-22.1	-34.0
Anterior antero- ventral	46.8± 2.9	62.1± 3.2	-15.3	-24.6
Aspartate				
Superficial dorsal	23.0± 1.2	22.8± 0.6	+ 0.2	+ 0.8
Deep dorsal	20.8± 0.9	24.6± 0.9	- 3.8	-15.4
Posteroventral	15.0± 1.2	25.6± 0.6	-10.6	-41.4
Auditory nerve root	10.7± 1.5	22.8± 2.1	-12.1	-53.1
Granule cell region	18.6± 1.0	23.6± 0.5	- 5.0	-21.2
Posterior antero- ventral	14.2± 0.9	34.5± 0.8	-20.3	-58.8
Anterior antero- ventral	16.5± 2.2	34.2± 2.1	-17.7	-51.8

a Values expressed as nmoles per mg protein
  (From Reference 54)

A neurotransmitter can be supplied to the presynaptic terminal in three ways: axonal transport from the soma to the terminal, uptake into the terminal and enzymatic synthesis in the terminal from available precursor. For the non-peptide neurotransmitters, axonal transport does not appear to be a major route of supply to the terminal. The ability of a presynaptic terminal to concentrate a specific neurotransmitter has been used in attempts to identify some neurotransmitters. However, it is not yet clear if there is substantial uptake of glutamate or aspartate into presynaptic terminals. Autoradiographic analysis reveals most uptake of ^{3}H-glutamate applied in vivo to be associated with glial cells and neuronal cell bodies and little with synaptic terminals (36). On the other hand, studies have shown that synaptosomes take up both glutamate and aspartate (3,4,30). Also, several investigators have reported a decrease in the uptake of glutamate and aspartate with the destruction of specific populations of neurons (19,35,39,46,61).

In the cochlear nucleus there appears to be relatively little high affinity uptake of glutamate or aspartate into terminals of the auditory nerve. After lesion of the auditory nerve, uptake of ^{3}H-glutamate and ^{3}H-aspartate (0.1 - 1 μM) into washed sucrose homogenates of the ventral cochlear nucleus does not decrease, but, rather shows a time-dependent increase with the uptake of both amino acids being about 50% greater two weeks after lesion (unpublished observation). Similar results were seen in studies using slices or synaptosome fractions of the cochlear nucleus. These results are consistent with much of the uptake being associated with glial cells.

The fact that uptake may not be the major means for auditory nerve terminals to acquire neurotransmitter suggests enzymatic routes for the production of glutamate and aspartate. Enzymes involved in the metabolism of the neurotransmitters glutamate and aspartate are probably the same as those involved in the metabolism of these amino acids when they are not acting as neurotransmitters. Therefore, the amount of transmitter-related enzyme localized in a specific glutamate or aspartate pathway is likely to be small compared to the total tissue levels of the enzyme. In the spinal cord there is no correlation between the distribution of glutamate and aspartate and the distribution of enzymes involved in their metabolism (23,28). A number of studies with a variety of neuronal tissues suggest that glutamine may be the immediate precursor of the neurotransmitter glutamate, with the conversion catalyzed by the enzyme glutaminase (8,25,49,50). Glutaminase is also found to be concentrated in synaptosomes (7,53). However, it has been reported that lesioning pathways in the hippocampus and striatum which are suggested to be glutamergic or aspartergic does not cause a decrease in glutaminase, aspartate aminotransferase or glutamate dehydrogenase (34,40). Immunohistochemical localization of glutamine synthetase shows it to be associated with glial cells (33,42).

Four enzymes known to be associated with the metabolism of

glutamate and aspartate, glutaminase, aspartate aminotransferase, glutamate dehydrogenase and glutamine synthetase were measured in the cochlear nucleus after lesion of the auditory nerve (56). Consistent decreases are observed for glutaminase and aspartate aminotransferase in the ventral cochlear nucleus. At 3 and 14 days after lesion the level of glutamate dehydrogenase does change and that of glutamine synthetase increases. Earlier studies have also shown that another glutamate related enzyme, glutamate decarboxylase does not change in the cochlear nucleus after auditory nerve lesion (59). The increase in glutamine synthetase after auditory nerve lesion is consistent with a glial localization for this enzyme. Although the levels of both enzymes are no higher in the cochlear nucleus than in other regions of brain, glutaminase and aspartate aminotransferase are higher in the auditory nerve than in several other nerves analyzed (Table 2).

The presence of glutaminase and aspartate aminotransferase in auditory nerve terminals indicates that both glutamate and aspartate can be synthesized within the terminal and supports the data showing both amino acids are concentrated in the terminals. Although one cannot rule out that the decrease in glutamate and aspartate in the cochlear nucleus after auditory nerve lesion may be a postsynaptic event, this does not appear likely for glutaminase and aspartate aminotransferase. Unlike small molecules such as amino acids, the levels of proteins are less likely to be rapidly changed due to alterations in levels of precursors or products. Furthermore, immunochemical localization of aspartate aminotransferase in the cochlear nucleus confirms that the enzyme

TABLE 2.   Enzymes in the auditory nerve

	Auditory Nerve	Facial Nerve	Trigeminal Nerve	Optic Nerve	Sciatic Nerve
Glutaminase[a]	39.2	7.5	14.4	12.2	—
Aspartate Aminotransferase[a]	325	112	120	142	109
Glutamate Dehydrogenase[a]	49.4	20.9	29.2	78.6	—
Glutamate Decarboxylase[a]	0.08	—	—	—	0.07
Choline Acetyltransferase[b]	1.7	—	—	—	673
Tyrosine Hydroxylase[b]	1.0	—	—	—	17.8

[a] nmoles product formed/min/mg protein

[b] pmoles product formed/min/mg protein.
(From References 18,56).

is present in terminals of the auditory nerve (unpublished observation).

RELEASE OF GLUTAMATE AND ASPARTATE FROM COCHLEAR NUCLEUS SLICES

A neurotransmitter must be released from the appropriate nerve terminals by stimulation of the presynaptic nerve. Although one of the more specific criteria for the identification of a neurotransmitter, demonstration of release in vivo has been limited in the central nervous system. The site of collection is usually relatively far from the point of actual release. Although release of some neurotransmitters can be demonstrated by blocking their inactivation systems, specific blockers have not yet been identified for inactivation systems of glutamate and aspartate, presumably high affinity uptake into glial cells, neurons and synaptic terminals. Therefore, to date, no convincing demonstration of release of glutamate or aspartate from the central nervous system after stimulation of a specific tract has been made.

Release of substances from the central nervous system has been studied in vitro by measuring release of endogenous, or more frequently, preloaded substances from slices or synaptosomes after chemical or electrical stimulation. With this technique the release of several putative neurotransmitters, including glutamate and aspartate, has been demonstrated. It is generally considered that release from presynaptic terminals is calcium-dependent and this criterion is often used to differentiate between specific release of neurotransmitter and non-specific release from other pools (47). However, both calcium-dependent and calcium-independent release of amino acids have been reported to occur from glial cells and neuronal cell bodies as well as from presynaptic terminals (15,16,17,37,38,41,45,48). An additional concern when measuring the release of preloaded substances, is that it is necessary that the substance taken up is at least partially located in the neurotransmitter compartment. Destruction of a specific neuronal pathway has been combined with in vitro release to determine the origin of the substances released (39,55).

Release of glutamate and aspartate from cochlear nucleus slices has been studied by measuring both the release of endogenous amino acids (55) and release of preloaded radioactive amino acids (9). Eighty percent of the endogenous glutamate and 50% of the aspartate released in elevated potassium from cochlear nucleus slices is calcium-dependent. Auditory nerve lesion decreases the calcium-dependent release of endogenous glutamate by 41% and that of aspartate by 26%, while the release of GABA and glycine is not affected. Similar results are obtained by measuring the release of radioactive glutamate and aspartate after incubation of cat cochlear nucleus slices with labeled glutamate or glutamine. In both cases glutamate is the major radioactive substance released and its release is reduced about 75% by prior lesion of the auditory nerve. The release of aspartate, after labeling with glutamate, is reduced about 45% by auditory nerve lesion. Auditory nerve lesion has no effect on the release of GABA, formed from either glutamate or glutamine.

PHARMACOLOGICAL CHARACTERIZATION OF THE AUDITORY NERVE NEUROTRANSMITTER

Lack of specific excitatory amino acid antagonists has frustrated the pharmacological characterization of glutamate and aspartate receptors. However, recently a number of compounds have been reported to selectively antagonize excitatory amino acid responses (5,6,12,13,14). From these studies at least two populations of excitatory amino acid receptors have been differentiated. One (NMDA receptor) is activated by N-methyl-D-aspartate (NMDA) and blocked by D-α-aminoadipate (DαAA), D-α-aminosuberate (DαAS), HA966 and Mg^{++}. The other (non-NMDA receptor) is activated by kainate and quisqualate and is relatively insensitive to the above antagonists. Since DαAA, DαAS and Mg^{++} consistently affect aspartate responses more than glutamate responses, it is suggested that aspartate is the natural neurotransmitter for NMDA receptors. The non-NMDA receptor may be composed of several classes of receptors, some of which may be extrasynaptic.

The pharmacology of auditory nerve neurotransmitter receptors has been studied by Martin and Adams (31) and Martin (32). DαAA, DαAS, HA966 and Mg^{++} reduce the synaptically evoked excitation of the auditory nerve. DαAA was found to depress aspartate responses more than glutamate responses. L-glutamate diethyl ester (GDEE), an amino acid antagonist which has little effect on NMDA responses, depresses glutamate responses more than aspartate responses and does not depress synaptically evoked activity. These data suggest that the auditory nerve receptor in the ventral cochlear nucleus is of the NMDA type. The fact that GDEE reduces amino acid responses but not synaptic responses suggests the presence of additional excitatory amino acid receptors which are unrelated to the function of the auditory nerve.

CONCLUSION

The data obtained on glutamate and aspartate in auditory nerve terminals are consistent in many ways with models presented for a glutamergic neuron (26,50,52). In such models glutamate is synthesized from both glutamine and glucose with glutamine being the major precursor. After release glutamate is taken up into the terminal from which it was released or into glial cells. In the glial cell, which contains glutamine synthetase, glutamate is converted to glutamine which can then be supplied back to the neuron. In the auditory nerve terminal there is a large pool of both glutamate and aspartate as well as the enzymes, glutaminase and aspartate aminotransferase. In vitro glutamine can serve as a precursor for glutamate which is released from auditory nerve terminals, with glutaminase probably catalyzing the conversion. Aspartate aminotransferase catalyzes the reversible reaction converting aspartate to oxaloacetate and α–ketoglutarate to glutamate. Both oxaloacetate and α–ketoglutarate are citric acid cycle intermediates which suggest a role of the citric acid cycle in the synthesis of the neurotransmitters glutamate and aspartate. Therefore, aspartate aminotransferase could be involved in producing either glutamate or aspartate for release or in regulating their relative levels in the presynaptic terminal.

Although all available evidence is consistent with glutamate or aspartate being the neurotransmitter of the auditory nerve, this is not yet proven. Several criteria must be met in order to prove a substance to be a neurotransmitter at a specific synapse (10,11,60). The evidence is strong that glutamate and aspartate are concentrated in the terminals of the auditory nerve and this is supported by the fact that two enzymes capable of synthesizing these amino acids are also present in these terminals. A high affinity uptake system for glutamate and aspartate is present in the cochlear nucleus, but it has not been shown that this system is functional in inactivating the auditory nerve neurotransmitter after it is released. The auditory nerve neurotransmitter is pharmacologically similar to glutamate and aspartate as determined using the currently available antagonists. Release of glutamate and aspartate has been demonstrated in slices of the cochlear nucleus and this release has been shown to be substantially reduced in the absence of auditory nerve terminals. Although supportive of a transmitter role for glutamate and aspartate in the cochlear nucleus, these data cannot be directly related to release which occurs in vivo. Changes in the postsynaptic membrane properties in response to glutamate, aspartate and the auditory nerve neurotransmitter have not been studied in the cochlear nucleus.

ACKNOWLEDGMENTS

I thank Drs. J. C. Adams, J. Fex and M. Martin for helpful comments on this manuscript and M. L. Adams for assistance in preparing this manuscript.

REFERENCES

1. Aprison, M.H., Daly, E.C., Shank, R.P. and McBride, W.J. (1975): In: Metabolic Compartmentation and Neurotransmission: Relation to Brain Structure and Function, edited by S. Berl, D. D. Clarke and D. Schneider, pp. 37-63, Plenum Press, New York.
2. Aprison, M.H. and Werman, R. (1965): Life Sci. 4: 2075-2083.
3. Balcar, V.J. and Johnston, G. A. R. (1973): J. Neurochem. 20: 529-539.
4. Beart, P.M. (1976): Brain Res. 103: 350-355.
5. Biscoe, T.J., Davies, J., Dray, A., Evans, R.H., Francis,

A.A., Martin, M.R. and Watkins, J.C. (1977): Nature (Lond.) 270: 743-745.

6. Biscoe, T.J., Davies, J., Dray, A., Evans, R.H., Martin, M. R. and Watkins, J.C. (1978): Brain Res. 148: 543-548.
7. Bradford, H.F. and Ward, H.K. (1976): Brain Res. 110: 115-125.
8. Bradford, H.F., Ward, H.K. and Thomas, A.J. (1978): J. Neurochem. 30: 1453-1459.
9. Canzek, V. and Reubi, J.C. (1980): Exp. Brain Res. 38, 437-441.
10. Curtis, D.R. (1975): In: Metabolic Compartmentation and Neurotransmission: Relation to Brain Structure and Function, edited by S. Berl, D. D. Clarke and D. Schneider, pp. 11-36, Plenum Press, New York.
11. Curtis, D.R. and Johnston, G.A.R. (1974): Ergebn. Physiol. 69: 97-188.
12. Davies, J., Evans, R.H., Francis, A.A. and Watkins, J.C. (1979): In: Advances in Pharmacology and Therapeutics, Vol. 2, edited by P. Simon, pp. 161-170, Pergamon Press, New York.
13. Davies, J., Evans, R.H., Francis, A.A. and Watkins, J.C. (1979): J. Physiol. (Paris) 75: 641-645.
14. Davies, J. and Watkins, J.C. (1979): J. Physiol. (Lond.) 297: 621-635.
15. Davies, L.P. and Johnston, G. A. R. (1976): J. Neurochem. 26: 1007-1014.
16. Davies, L.P., Johnston, G.A.R. and Stephanson, A.L. (1975): J. Neurochem. 25: 387-392.
17. DeBelleroche, J.S. and Bradford, H.F. (1977): J. Neurochem. 29: 335-343.
18. Fex, J. and Wenthold, R.J. (1976): Brain Res. 109: 575-585.
19. Fonnum, F. and Storm-Mathisen, J. (1977): Nature 266: 377-378.
20. Fuxe, K. (1965): Acta Physiol. Scand. 64: (Suppl. 247) 39-85.
21. Godfrey, A. A., Carter, J.A., Berger, S.J., Lowry, O.H. and Matschinsky, F.M. (1977): J. Histochem. Cytochem. 25: 417-431.
22. Godfrey, D.A., Carter, J.A., Lowry, O.H. and Matschinsky, F.M. (1978): J. Histochem. Cytochem. 26: 118-126.
23. Graham, L.T. and Aprison, M.H. (1969): J. Neurochem. 16: 559-566.
24. Gulley, R.L., Wenthold, R.J. and Neises, G.R. (1978): Brain Res. 158: 279-294.
25. Hamberger, A., Chiang, G., Nylen, E.S., Schaff, S.W. and Cotman, C.W. (1978): Brain Res. 143: 549-555.
26. Hamberger, A.C., Chiang, G.H., Nylen, E.S., Scheff, S.W. and Cotman, C.W. (1979): Brain Res. 168: 513-530.
27. Hokfelt, T., Elde, R., Johansson, O., Terenius, L. and Stein, L. (1977): Neurosci. Letters 5: 25-31.
28. Johnson, J.L. (1972): Brain Res. 45: 205-215.
29. Kromer, L.F. and Moore, R.Y. (1976): Brain Res. 118: 531-537.
30. Logan, W.J. and Snyder, S.H. (1972): Brain Res. 42: 413-431.

31. Martin, M.R. (1980): Neuropharmacology, In press.
32. Martin, M.R. and Adams, J.C. (1979): Neuroscience 4: 1097–1105.
33. Martinez-Hernandez, A., Bell, K.P. and Norenberg, M.D. (1977): Science 195: 1356–1358.
34. McGeer, E.G. and McGeer, P.L. (1979): J. Neurochem. 32: 1071–1975.
35. McGeer, P.L., McGeer, E.G., Scherer, U. and Singh, K. (1977): Brain Res. 128: 369–373.
36. McLennan, H. (1976): Brain Res. 115: 139–144.
37. Minchin, M.C.W. and Iversen, L.L. (1974): J. Neurochem. 23: 533–540.
38. Mulder, A.H. and Snyder, S.H. (1974): Brain Res. 76: 297–308.
39. Nadler, J.V., Vaca, K.W., White, W.F., Lynch, G.S. and Cotman, C.W. (1976): Nature (Lond.) 260: 538–540.
40. Nadler, J.V., White, W.F., Vaca, K.W., Perry, B.W. and Cotman, C.W. (1979): J. Neurochem. 31: 147–155.
41. Nadler, J.V., White, W.F., Vaca, K.W., Redburn, D.A. and Cotman, C.W. (1977): J. Neurochem. 29: 279–290.
42. Norenberg, M.D. and Martinez-Hernandez, A. (1979): Brain Res. 161: 303–310.
43. Osen, K.K. (1970): Arch. ital. Biol. 108: 21–51.
44. Parsons, J.A., Erlandsen, S.L., Hegre, O.D., McEvoy, R.C. and Elde, R.P. (1976): J. Histochem. Cytochem. 24: 872–882.
45. Roberts, P.J. (1974): Brain Res. 74: 327–332.
46. Rohde, B.H., Rea, M.A., Simon, J.R. and McBride, W.J. (1979): J. Neurochem. 32: 1431–1435.
47. Rubin, R.P. (1970): Pharmacol. Rev. 22: 389–428.
48. Sellström, A. and Hamberger, A. (1977): Brain Res. 119: 189–198.
49. Shank, R.P. and Aprison, M.H. (1977): J. Neurochem. 28: 1189–1196.
50. Shank, R.P. and Aprison, M.H. (1979): In Glutamic Acid: Advances in Biochemistry and Physiology, edited by L. J. Filer, S. Garattini, M. R. Kare, W. A. Reynolds and R. J. Wurtman, pp. 139–150, Raven Press, New York.
51. Spoendlin, H. (1973): In: Basic Mechanisms in Hearing, edited by A. R. Moller, pp. 185–234, Academic Press, New York.
52. Watkins, J.C. (1973): Biochem. Soc. Symp. 36: 33–47.
53. Weiler, G.T., Nystrom, B. and Hamberger, A. (1979): Brain Res. 160: 539–543.
54. Wenthold, R.J. (1978): Brain Res. 143: 544–548.
55. Wenthold, R.J. (1979): Brain Res. 162: 338–343.
56. Wenthold, R.J. (1980): Brain Res. In press.
57. Wenthold, R.J. and Gulley, R.L. (1977): Brain Res. 138: 111–123.
58. Wenthold, R.J. and Gulley, R.L. (1978): Brain Res. 158: 279–284.
59. Wenthold, R.J. and Morest, D.K. (1976): Neurosci. Abst. 2: 28.
60. Werman, R. (1972): Ann Rev. Physiol. 34: 337–374.
61. Young, A.B., Oster-Granite, M.L., Herndon, R.M. and Snyder, S.H. (1974): Brain Res. 73: 1–13.

Glutamate as a Neurotransmitter,
edited by G. Di Chiara and G. L. Gessa
Raven Press, New York © 1981.

GABA and Glutamate as Retina Neurotransmitters in Rabbit Retina

Dianna A. Redburn

*Department of Neurobiology and Anatomy, University of Texas Medical School,
Houston, Texas 77025*

Interest in glutamate as a retinal neurotransmitter began to emerge when Potts et al. (21) first demonstrated that glutamate causes potent excitation of retinal neurons and eventually renders them inexcitable, probably due to excessive depolarization. Photoreceptor cells are the only retinal neurons which are not affected. It has also been known for many years (19) that high concentrations of glutamate, particularly in developing retina, causes degeneration of all retinal neurons except photoreceptor cells. Further attempts to define the role of glutamate as a transmitter in retina have been hampered by the uncertainty in general about the specificity of glutamate action. In spite of this uncertainty, a variety of experiments have demonstrated the presence of a glutamate system in retina which exhibits characteristics that meet most of the criteria for a functional neurotransmitter system.

GLUTAMATE AS A TRANSMITTER IN THE INNER PLEXIFORM LAYER

Autoradiography

Perhaps the most convincing data for glutaminergic transmission in retina has been reported for a relatively small population of cells shown by autoradiography to be located in the amacrine and ganglion cell layers with terminals in the inner plexiform layer (5). Autoradiograms of rabbit retina after a 15 min incubation in 5 μM ^{3}H-glutamate show preferential localization of label in Muller (glial) cells (Fig 1A). Some accumulation of label is noted in amacrine cell bodies and within the inner plexiform layer. However, if the tissue is postincubated in label-free medium for 30 min, label in the Muller cell is lost, presumably through metabolism, and the remaining label is concentrated in cells of the amacrine and ganglion cell layer with diffuse banding in the inner plexiform layer (Fig 1B).

It is of interest to note that autoradiographic patterns of aspartate are significantly different from glutamate in that neuronal localization is never observed (5). Autoradiograms of rabbit retina after a 15 min

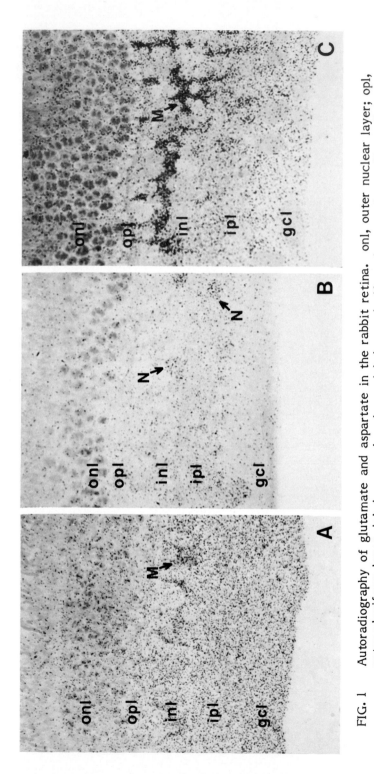

FIG. 1   Autoradiography of glutamate and aspartate in the rabbit retina. onl, outer nuclear layer; opl, outer plexiform layer; inl, inner nuclear layer; ipl, inner plexiform layer; gcl, ganglion cell layer; M, Muller cell; N, neuron. A) Retina incubated in ³H-glutamate for 15 min. B) Same as (A) with addition of a 30 min postincubation in buffer. C) Retina incubated in ³H-aspartate for 15 min. X 480.

incubation of 5 µM ^{3}H-aspartate show that label is limited exclusively to Muller cells. Post-incubation in label-free medium causes a loss of the Muller cell label with no increase in neuronal labeling (Fig 1C).

Uptake Systems

A transport system for glutamate and aspartate has been demonstrated by biochemical studies using a synaptosomal (P_2) fraction containing terminals from the inner plexiform layer (26, 27). The high affinity uptake systems described for a variety of neurotransmitters in brain all have several characteristics in common: saturation kinetics with increasing time and with increasing ligand concentration, and dependency upon external Na^+ and temperature (10). The uptake of ^{14}C-aspartate and ^{14}C-glutamate also demonstrate these characteristics. The amount of ^{14}C-aspartate taken up by retinal fractions increase with time up to 20 min, however, the rate of the increase begins to decline after approximately 15-20 min. Similar results are obtained with ^{14}C-glutamate.

Uptake at $4°C$ is less than 30% of the total uptake at $37°C$ for both ^{14}C-aspartate and ^{14}C-glutamate. Uptake of both ligands in Na^+-free media is inhibited more than 95% as compared to controls at $37°C$.

Uptake kinetics of the two ligands show many similarities (Table 1). The uptake sites for both ligands appear to have high affinities since uptake is saturated with ligand concentrations of less than 5 µM. The rate of maximum uptake/mg protein is highest in the P_2 fraction and is approximately the same for both ligands, 600-700 pmol/mg protein/4 min.

The differences observed in the kinetic analysis of the two ligands are (1) a significantly lower K_m for glutamate uptake than for aspartate uptake in both fractions; (2) a significantly higher (approx 2 fold) V_{max} for ^{14}C-aspartate uptake than for ^{14}C-glutamate uptake in homogenate fractions. See Table 1.

In brain as well as intact retina, both glutamate and aspartate are thought to share the same carrier for uptake and to compete with each other (17). To study this transport phenomenon in retinal synaptosomes, ^{14}C-aspartate or ^{14}C-glutamate (0.5 µM) were incubated in the presence of unlabeled glutamate or aspartate respectively. A 50% inhibition of ^{14}C-aspartate uptake occurred when the two ligands were in approximately equal concentrations, i.e., 0.5 µM ^{14}C-aspartate, 0.55 µM unlabeled glutamate. There was virtually 100% inhibition of ^{14}C-aspartate uptake in the presence of a tenfold excess of unlabeled glutamate. In contrast, ^{14}C-glutamate uptake was inhibited only 80-85% even in the presence of a tenfold excess of aspartate. This aspartate-insensitive glutamate uptake may represent the specific neuronal accumulation of glutamate observed in autoradiograms.

TABLE I

CHARACTERISTICS OF AMINO ACID TRANSPORT
IN RETINAL FRACTIONS

	Vmax (pmol/mg prt./4 min)	Km (µM)
Glutamate		
Retinal Homogenate	104	1.61
P_2 Synaptosomal Fraction	584	0.48
Aspartate		
Retinal Homogenate	293	2.87
P_2 Synaptosomal Fraction	672	1.46
GABA		
Retinal Homogenate	241	3.45
P_2 Synaptosomal Fraction	840	1.86

TABLE II

INHIBITION OF GLUTAMATE RECEPTOR BINDING
BY GLUTAMATE ANALOGUES IN P_2 SYNAPTOSOLMAL FRACTIONS
FROM BOVINE RETINA

	IC_{50}'s (µM)
Cysteic acid	1.4
DL-α-aminoadipic acid	6.0
L-glutamate	6.5
Aspartate	15
Homocystetic acid	17
Glutamic acid diethyl ester	> 1000
Glutamic acid dimethyl ester	> 1000
Kainic acid	> 1000

Effect of Kainic Acid

We have recently described some effects of kainic acid on the morphology of the retina and on the uptake systems of three putative retinal transmitters (5,9). Inasmuch as kainic acid may exert excitotoxic effects preferentially on glutamoreceptive cells (2,6,20), a discussion of these results is presented here.

Retinas incubated at 10^{-5}M kainic acid for 15 or 30 min show minor morphological damage consisting of vacuolation in the cytoplasm of a few cells in the ganglion cell layer. After 15 min in 10^{-4}M kainic acid, more dramatic changes are noted in the inner plexiform layer and associated elements. The layer is filled with vacuoles presumably from swollen neuron terminals or dendrites. Many cells in the ganglion cell layer show signs of necrosis with a "bubbly" appearance in the cytoplasm. At higher concentrations (10^{-3}M) of kainic acid, or longer exposure times (30 min) many cells in the amacrine cell layer show signs of necrosis and degeneration. In contrast, necrotic cells are rarely seen in other portions of the retina, although extreme swelling is noted in horizontal cell bodies and terminals. These experiments demonstrate differential sensitivity of various retinal neurons to the toxic effects of kainic acid. Elements of the inner plexiform layer are clearly affected, and cells of the ganglion cell layer are more sensitive than cells of the amacrine cell layer.

Although the mechanism of action of kainic acid is still unclear, it has been recently reported (8) that kainic acid is an inhibitor of glutamate transport systems in brain synaptosomes. Our autoradiographic studies in retina are consistent with this suggestion (5). When kainic acid (10^{-4}M) is included during a 15 min incubation of rabbit retina in buffer containing 0.5 µM ^{3}H-glutamate, normal autoradiographic patterns are disrupted. While Muller cell accumulation is apparently unaffected, neuronal accumulation is entirely blocked, even after a 30 min postincubation in the absence of kainic acid.

This effect is in contrast to the effect of kainic acid on the autoradiographic patterns of ^{3}H-GABA (Fig 2C). When kainic acid (10^{-4} M) is included during a 15 min incubation of rabbit retina in buffer containing 2 µM ^{3}H-GABA, neuronal accumulation is entirely blocked, with Muller cell accumulation only slightly decreased. However, a 30 min post-incubation in the absence of kainic acid causes a dramatic enhancement in neuronal labeling. One suggestion is that kainic acid causes tonic release of ^{3}H-GABA by depolarization, thus decreasing net accumulation. After removal of kainic acid, the increased accumulation of ^{3}H-GABA may result from a compensatory action of these GABA depleted neurons.

Glutamate receptor binding

A variety of assay techniques have been developed for analysis of specific postsynaptic glutamate receptors. We have modified the assay system developed by Foster and Roberts (4) for cerebellar membranes in order to analyze presumptive glutamate receptors in retina (15). Our results show the presence of very high affinity binding sites in bovine retina with a reasonable degree of pharmacological specificity. Approximately 75% of the total binding of low concentrations of ^{3}H-glutamate was displaced by 1 mM unlabeled glutamate and thus, is designated as specific binding. Scatchard analysis of specific binding using concentrations of 1-100 nM ^{3}H-glutamate revealed a single affinity site with a K_D of 72 nM. Little difference was noted in the K_D of freeze-thawed samples (72 nM) vs. samples which were never frozen (94 nM). However, the Bmax was increased three-fold from 0.46 to 1.5 pmoles/mg prt. after the freeze-thaw procedure due in part to a decrease in nonspecific binding.

Eight glutamate analogues were tested for their ability to displace ^{3}H-glutamate binding (See Table II). The potent excitatory compound, cysteic acid was the most potent displacer with a $1C_{50}$ of 1.4 μM. Aminoadipic acid and glutamate were equipotent; aspartate and homocysteic acid were slightly less effective. Glutamic acid diethyl ester and dimethyl ester as well as kainic acid were very weak displacers of glutamate binding.

GABA AS A TRANSMITTER IN THE INNER PLEXIFORM LAYER

Autoradiography

There is substantial evidence that GABAnergic transmission is important in information processing in the inner plexiform layer (1,5,22). Autoradiograms of rabbit retina after 15 min incubation of 2 μM ^{3}H-GABA show heavy accumulation by Muller cells, cells of the amacrine cell layer, and elements of the inner plexiform layer. Postincubation in label-free medium causes a loss of Muller cell labeling, while neuron cell labeling is enhanced (Fig 2A,B). Three faint bands of label can also be discerned in the inner plexiform layer after postincubation. As in the case of glutamate, GABA is metabolized rapidly by Muller cells while neuronal stores are relatively protected from metabolism.

GABA Uptake

A GABA transport system has been described in a synaptosomal fraction from inner plexiform layer terminals (2). The transport of ^{14}C-GABA by retinal fractions is inhibited 75% by reducing the incubation temperature from 37 to 4°C. Replacement of $NaCl_2$ with choline chloride in the incubation medium also reduces binding approximately 75%. The transport sites demonstrate a very high affinity ($K_D \simeq 1$μM) and are highly concentrated in the P_2 synaptosomal fraction. Retinal ^{14}C-GABA transport thus demonstrates the characteristics which are similar to the high affinity, GABA uptake system previously described in brain (7).

GABA Release

Efflux rates of the previously bound ^{14}C-GABA were determined (22) by immobilizing retinal samples on a filter and washing sequentially, first with Ca^{++}-free, modified Ringer solution (standard buffer), then with

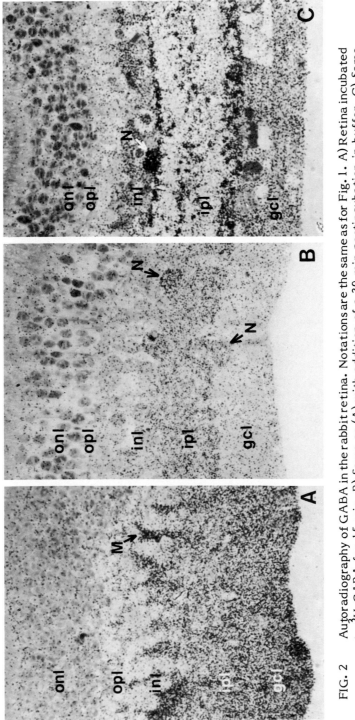

FIG. 2 Autoradiography of GABA in the rabbit retina. Notations are the same as for Fig. 1. A) Retina incubated in ³H-GABA for 15 min. B) Same as (A) with addition of a 30 min postincubation in buffer. C) Same as (B) with addition of 10⁻⁴ M kainic acid during the 15 min incubation in ³H-GABA. X 480.

buffer containing an additional 50 mM KCl (56.2 mM total) and finally with buffer containing 56.2 mM KCl and 6 mM $CaCl_2$. EGTA (1mM) was present in all solutions. The calculated free Ca^{+2} concentration was between 4-5 mM in solutions containing 1 mM-EGTA and 6 mM-$CaCl_2$.

In standard Ca^{++}-free, EGTA buffer, the amount of ^{14}C-GABA released per min declined with each succeeding wash until a relatively stable baseline efflux rate was reached after three or four, 1 min washes. Addition of depolarizing levels of K^+ caused a significant increase in the amount of GABA released per minute. Subsequent addition of 6 mM-Ca^{++} caused an additional increase in the release rate of ^{14}C-GABA from the P_2 fraction to about 4-5% of the available ^{14}C-GABA pool.

GABA Receptor Binding

GABA receptor binding has also been demonstrated to be highly enriched in this fraction in bovine retina (23,24,25). Using ^3H-GABA (3,16) and ^3H-Muscimol (28) binding assays, we have demonstrated two sets of binding sites, one with higher affinity (Site 1); the other with lower affinity (Site 2). See Table III. Pretreatment with concentrations of Triton X-100 between .001 and 0.1% enhanced specific ^3H-GABA binding, with a maximal effect noted at 0.05%. Freezing caused a small but significant enhancement of specific binding at all concentrations of Triton tested. Sodium perchlorate also stimulated specific ^3H-GABA binding with maximum stimulation noted at 100 mM.

Binding curves using a wide range of ligand concentrations revealed a striking difference between the two treatments. In the presence of perchlorate, a Scatchard plot from the P_2 fraction revealed a single high affinity site with a K_D of 14 nM (Site #1). Site #2 was absent. The opposite was seen with Triton treated material with the lower affinity site (K_D 380 nM, Site #2) present but the higher affinity site (K_D 14 nM, Site #1) absent. Both sites exhibit a high degree of pharmacological specificity.

Specific ^3H-muscimol binding in washed bovine retina synaptosomal fractions demonstrated high affinity binding showing two points of saturation similar to Site 1 and Site 2 for ^3H-GABA binding (See Table 2). Muscimol binding in retina demonstrated a high degree of pharmacological specificity with K_i's for agonists and antagonists somewhat higher but in the same rank order seen with ^3H-GABA binding.

INTERACTION OF GABA AND GLUTAMATE
IN THE INNER PLEXIFORM LAYER

There is considerable evidence that GABAnergic transmission in the inner plexiform layer modulates the activity of a well-characterized excitatory cholinergic pathway. Masland (11,12) has demonstrated auto-radiographically and electrophysiologically, that two sets of cholinergic neurons are present in rabbit retina. One population has cell bodies in the amacrine cell layer and a discrete band of terminals in the outer portion of the inner plexiform layer. The second population has cell bodies in the ganglion cell layer, and a discrete band of terminals in the inner portion

TABLE III

CHARACTERISTICS OF GABA RECEPTOR BINDING
IN P_2 SYNAPTOSOMAL FRACTIONS FROM BOVINE RETINA

Constants Derived from Scatchard Analysis

	Site 1		Site 2	
	Bmax (pmoles/mg prt.)	K_D (nM)	Bmax (pmoles/mg prt.)	K_D (nM)
^{3}H-GABA Binding Triton Treated	-	-	10.0	380
Sodium Perchlorate Treated	1.28	14	-	-
^{3}H-Muscimol Binding	0.55	25	1.76	88.4

Inhibitory Constants (K_i, μM) of GABA Agonists and Antagonists

	^{3}H-GABA Binding Triton Treated	^{3}H-GABA Binding Perchlorate Treated	^{3}H-Muscimol Binding
GABA	0.015	-	0.27
Muscimol	0.0035	0.0030	0.06
Imidazole Acetic Acid	0.26	0.41	-
+Bicuculline	2.03	1.75	5.0
THIP	-	0.011	1.17
Diaminobutyric Acid	>1000	-	-
Picrotoxin	> 500	-	-
Nipocotic Acid	-	>1000	-

of the inner plexiform layer. These cholinergic neurons make synaptic contact with on-center ganglion cells, i.e., cells which exhibit a transient burst of firing activity when the light is turned on. Ariel et al.(1) has also demonstrated electrophysiologically the presence of cholinoreceptive on-center ganglion cells. In addition, he has demonstrated that GABA receptor blockers cause a loss of specificity in this pathway so that these ganglion cells now fire both when the lights are turned on and when the lights are turned off. In other words, on-center cells become on-off cells in the presence of bicuculline.

Massey (13,14,18) has monitored the light evoked release of endo-genously synthesized ^{3}H-ACh using an <u>in vivo</u> eye cup preparation in rabbit. This release is Ca^{++} dependent and is maximal in dark adapted retinas exposed to flashes of light at a frequency of 3 Hz. GABA receptor blockers stimulate (disinhibit) the tonic release as well as the light evoked release of ACh. Also, the GABA neuron appears to be stimulated by an excitatory input which uses a transmitter other than ACh. This is demonstrated by the fact that ACh receptor blockers do not alter the inhibitory effect of bicuculline on light evoked ACh release.

In view of the apparent stimulating effect of kainic acid on GABA accumulation, it is tempting to speculate that glutamate may be the excitatory neurotransmitter which impinges on these GABAnergic cells.

SUMMARY

In summary, both glutamate and GABA appear to be functional neurotransmitters in the inner plexiform layer of the rabbit retina. Autoradiograph localization suggests they are both subpopulations of amacrine cells which are found primarily in the amacrine cell layer, although some appear as displaced amacrines in the ganglion cell layer. The characteristics of these two transmitter systems are similar to those described in brain including systems for transport, release and receptor binding. There is considerable evidence that GABAnergic cells may be responsible for the specificity of on-center ganglion cells through inhibi-tory modulation of cholinergic transmission. The role of glutamate is much more speculative at this point, however, it is suggested that the excitatory input to the GABAnergic neurons may be mediated by gluta-minergic transmission.

This work was supported by NEI grant EYO-1655-04 and Research Career Development Award 1 K04 EY 00088-03.

REFERENCES

1.   Ariel, M., Daw, N.W. and Rader, R.K. (1980): Invest. Ophthal. Vis Sci. Supp., p. 132.
2.   Curtis, D.R., Perrin, D.D. and Watkins, J.C. (1960): <u>J. Physiol.</u>, 150: 656-660.
3.   Enna, S.J. and Snyder, S.H. (1977): Molec. Pharmacol., 13: 442-453.

4. Foster, A.C. and Roberts, P.J. (1978): J. Neurochem., 31: 1467-1477.
5. Hampton, C.K. and Redburn, D.A. (1980): Invest. Opthal. Vis. Sci. supp., p. 72.
6. Herndon, R.M. and Coyle, J.T. (1977): Science 198: 71-72.
7. Hutchison, H.T., Werrback, F., Vance, C. and Haber, B. (1974): Brain Res., 66: 265-274.
8. Johns, G.A.R., Kennedy, S.M. E. and Twitchin, B. (1979): J. Neurochem., 32: 121-127.
9. Keiller, C.A. and Redburn, D.A. (1979): Invest. Opthal. Vis. Sci. supp., p. 85.
10. Levi, G. and Raiteri, M. (1973): Brain Res., 57: 165-185.
11. Masland, R.H. and Ames, A. (1976): J. Neurophys., 39: 1327-1329.
12. Masland, R.H. and Mills, J.W. (1979): J. Cell Biol., 83: 159-178.
13. Massey, S.C. and Neal, M.J. (1979): J. Neurochem., 32: 1327-1329.
14. Massey, S.C. and Redburn, D.A. (1980): Invest. Ophthal. Vis. Sci., supp., p. 283.
15. Mitchell, C.K. and Redburn, D.A. (1980): Invest. Opthal. Vis. Sci. Supp. p. 185.
16. Mohler, H. (1980): In: Gaba-Biochemistry and CNS Function, edited by P. Mandel, F.V. DeFeudis, and J. Mark. Pergamon Pres Ltd., New York.
17. Neal, M.J. (1976): Gen. Pharmac., 7: 331-333.
18. Neal, M.J. and Massey, S.C. In: Neurochemistry of the Retina, edited by N.G. Bazan and R.N. Lolley, (in press). Pergamon Press Ltd., New York.
19. Olney, J.W. (1968): J. Neuropathol. Exp. Neurol., 28: 455-474.
20. Olney, J.W., Rhee, V., and Ho, O.L. (1974): Brain Res., 77: 507-512.
21. Potts, A.M., Modrell, R.W., and Kingsbury, C. (1960): Am. J. Ophthal., 50: 900-907.
22. Redburn, D.A. (1977): Exp. Eye Res., 25: 265-275.
23. Redburn, D.A., Kyles, C. and Ferkany, J. (1979): Exp. Eye Res., 28: 525-532.
24. Redburn, D.A. and Mitchell, C.K. Brain Res. Bul., (in press).
25. Redburn, D.A. and Mitchell, C.K. (1980): Life Sci., (in press).
26. Redburn, D.A. and Thomas, T.N. (1979): J. Neurosci. Meth., 1: 235-242.
27. Thomas, T.N. and Redburn, D.A. (1978): J. Neurochem., 31: 63-68.
28. Williams, M. and Resley, E.A. (1979): J. Neurochem., 32: 713-718.

Glutamate as a Neurotransmitter,
edited by G. Di Chiara and G. L. Gessa
Raven Press, New York © 1981.

Strategies for Identifying Sources and Sites of Formation of GABA-Precursor or Transmitter Glutamate in Brain

E. Roberts

City of Hope Research Institute, Duarte, California 91010

INTRODUCTION

Recently, much attention has been devoted to the function of the GABA system because GABAergic neurons are important for the control of activity in all parts of the vertebrate CNS (11,17). Derangements in function of these neurons may be involved in various forms of epilepsy, in Huntington's and Parkinson's diseases, in schizophrenia, and possibly in the genesis of brain stem- and hypothalamus-related "psychosomatic disorders." Many GABA studies have dealt with a) its synthesis from glutamate, b) its release, c) its postsynaptic action, d) its synaptic inactivation by carrier-mediated transport, and e) its metabolic destruction by transamination and oxidation of the carbon chain. The immunocytochemical localization of GABAergic neurons has allowed us to begin to study identified inhibitory local circuit and projection neurons in various parts of the normal vertebrate CNS and to apply our findings to the study of focal epilepsy and related problems (16).

Important controls in regulation of the GABA system may be exerted at points related to the availability of L-glutamic acid, the substrate for GABA synthesis in nerve endings by L-glutamic acid decarboxylase (GAD), which is the terminal enzyme in GABA biosynthesis. Experience with immunocytochemistry of the GABA system suggests that the most likely hope for a definitive resolution of the GABA-precursor question would be to achieve direct visualization, at light and electron microscopic levels, of pertinent substances or enzymes in glutamate biosynthesis that would show specific localization in neurons previously shown to be GABAergic (e.g., Purkinje cells).

An urgent need is to be able to trace the connectivities of the mainline and local circuit excitatory neurons that impinge on inhibitory local circuit and projection neurons and, in turn, whose activities the latter serve to regulate. Glutamate and aspartate, or still undefined derivatives thereof, may be major excitatory transmitters in vertebrate and invertebrate nervous

systems. If this is so, eventually it will be necessary to
identify the relationships of the neurons liberating these substances by techniques similar to those developed for GABAergic
neurons. Currently, knowledge is lacking as to what enzymes may
be rate-limiting in the biosynthesis of these amino acids in the
presynaptic endings of the neurons that may liberate them or,
what may be less likely, in glial cells that may "feed" precursors (e.g., glutamine) to the presynaptic endings of excitatory
neurons. If these enzymes were identified with certainty, their
purification, development of antisera to them, and application of
immunocytochemical procedures to CNS tissue for their visualization probably could be achieved rapidly. The major difficulty
for the biochemist lies in the multiplicity of metabolic pathways
in which these ubiquitously occurring amino acids participate.

It seems to me that in the case of glutamate, for example,
either as precursor for GABA synthesis or possibly as an excitatory transmitter, itself, or as excitatory transmitter precursor,
that quantitatively less important metabolic pathways, such as
arginine$\rightarrow$ornithine$\rightarrow$glutamate and proline$\rightarrow\Delta^1$-pyrroline-5-
carboxylate$\rightarrow$glutamate more likely would be used for transmitter
or transmitter-precursor synthesis than would the more common
aminotransferases (aspartic or alanine), glutaminase, or glutamic
dehydrogenase. This would be in keeping with the need for specificity of control and sequestration that generally seem to be
part of neurotransmitter logistics. Of course, a variant of one
or more of the generally occurring enzymes with unique control
properties also might possess suitable characteristics. At this
point, it seems that a systematic search for such enzymes might
yield rich scientific dividends.

It would be important to have additional biochemical markers
for GABAergic neurons, the only current one being GAD, which
would be useful in studies of development of the GABA system and
in disease states such as Huntington's disease and seizure disorders. In addition, knowledge of specific properties of the
enzymes involved might furnish new pharmacologically active
agents for manipulation of the GABA system or help explain the
action of some old ones. Specific localization of a particular
glutamate-forming enzyme (or enzymes) in the presynaptic endings
of known excitatory neurons, e.g., primary afferents in spinal
cord, would strengthen the possibility that glutamate is, indeed,
an excitatory transmitter and also might give possibilities of
developing specific tools for pharmacologic manipulation of such
glutamatergic neurons. It would then be possible to determine
whether or not the same pathways furnish substrate glutamate for
GABAergic nerve endings and transmitter glutamate for the putative glutamatergic ones or whether different pathways are employed for them, e.g., proline as precursor for the former and
arginine as precursor for the latter. If the latter were the
case, immunocytochemical tools would be at hand for distinguishing the two types of endings and for the development of agents
for the specific manipulation of one system or the other.

Even though it is not feasible at present to work with ultra thin sections to visualize two antigens in the same synaptic terminal or to routinely perform experiments in which two or more antigens can be visualized on the same section, a judicious blending of approaches visualizing one antigen at a time should make the proposed tracing techniques yield valuable information. For example, the somata of neurons in the nucleus interpositus in the rat are literally studded with GABAergic terminals coming from the Purkinje cells of the cerebellar cortex; the terminals, as well as somata and dendrites of Purkinje, stellate, basket, and Golgi II cells in the cerebellar cortex, are GAD-positive after colchicine injection (16). The visualization of other antigens by this technique can be extended to the several neural regions in which GAD already has been studied in order to increase the confidence that the other antigens either are or are not found at the same sites as GAD. Work is in progress in a number of laboratories in which techniques are being sought for the visualization of more than one antigen in a single section. Visualizing different combinations of two enzymes of a series at one time would, of course, make it much easier to determine whether or not the enzymes of a particular metabolic sequence coexist in a particular neural structure.

PERTINENT METABOLIC RELATIONSHIPS IN NERVOUS TISSUE

Quantitatively, the major overall sources of glutamate in neural tissue probably are the pathways by which ammonia is fixed via glutamate dehydrogenase (Fig. 1, reaction 8) and by which ammonia is liberated from glutamine by glutaminase (reaction 6). Although the latter two enzymes probably play major roles in the glutamate and ammonia economy of nervous tissue, from a variety of experiments it does not seem conclusive that the reactions which they catalyze are immediate sources for the glutamate that is the direct substrate for L-glutamate decarboxylase (reaction 5) in presynaptic endings of GABAergic neurons (3,4,25). Other important sources of glutamate nitrogen may be the several amino acids that can undergo α-transaminations in brain, among which are arginine and ornithine (23). The most common nitrogen acceptor is α-ketoglutarate (reaction 9), although transaminations also can occur with pyruvate, oxalacetate, and glyoxylate (not shown in Fig. 1).

An important link between amino acid and carbohydrate metabolism in brain occurs at the level of the ornithine-α-ketoglutarate ω-aminotransferase (reaction 2). The ornithine cycle (illustrated in the upper left-hand portion of Fig. 1), by which urea is formed in liver, is incompletely functional in brain; carbamoyl transferase (reaction 10), the enzyme that catalyzes the formation of citrulline from ornithine, is absent from nervous tissue (10). Nonetheless, arginine enters readily from the blood stream (14), and urea is formed in the brain by the arginase reaction 1 (5,15). The specific activity of arginase in

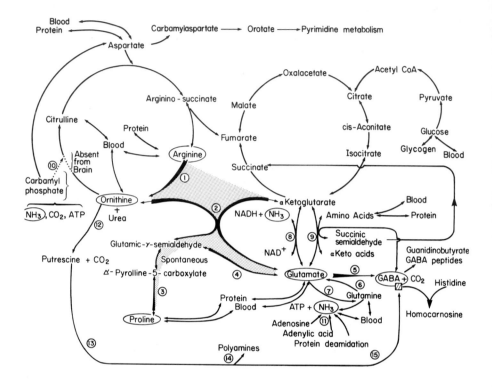

FIG. 1.   Pertinent Metabolic Relationships in Nervous Tissue

brain is higher than that of the ornithine aminotransferase
(reaction 2) (20), suggesting that the latter might be the
rate-limiting reaction in the metabolism of arginine in brain
and, therefore, in the utilization of arginine nitrogen in the
biosynthesis of glutamate via the linked pathway (reactions 2 and
4) or in the formation of proline from arginine (reactions 2 and
3). The rate-limiting enzyme in proline synthesis is the
Δ^1-pyrroline-5-carboxylate reductase, a cytosolic enzyme, using
NADH as cofactor, that converts Δ^1-pyrroline-5-carboxylic acid to
proline. Proline oxidase, a mitochondrial-bound enzyme, converts
proline to Δ^1-pyrroline-5-carboxylic acid (reaction 3) (7). It
is unclear from published data whether or not the latter two
enzymatic activities are attributable to a single protein that

can exist in animal tissues in two forms--cytosolic and mitochon-
drion-associated. Glutamic-γ-semialdehyde is the common intermediate in proline and ornithine metabolism that can be transformed
to glutamate by the action of a specific NAD^+-dependent dehydrogenase (reaction 4) (24). Although for 25 years glutamate also
has been considered to be a source of the carbon and nitrogen for
ornithine and proline biogenesis in animal tissues, only recently
the reduction of glutamate to γ-glutamic semialdehyde has been
demonstrated directly in homogenates of rat intestinal mucosa
(19), an enzymatic reaction not yet shown to exist in brain. It
can be seen from Fig. 1 that γ-glutamic semialdehyde can give
rise to ornithine and proline by reversal of the reactions by
which it is formed from these amino acids. Thus, in the presence
of the appropriate enzymes, glutamate, ornithine, and proline
would all be potentially interconvertible. However, since the
glutamate decarboxylase reaction 5 is irreversible, it would be
expected that if the requisite enzymes exist in endings of GABA-
ergic neurons, the metabolite flow would go largely in the directions arginine→ornithine→glutamate→GABA or proline→glutamate
→GABA.

Let us now consider available data that may be relevant to the
above proposal. Urea is synthesized from arginine in the living
rat brain (5). All of the enzymes for the requisite transformations are present in homogenates of brain tissue. It is particularly interesting that of the several enzyme activities measured
(20), only arginase and the ornithine-α-ketoglutarate ω-amino-
transferase activities were considerably higher in the cerebellum
than in cerebral cortex and brain stem; the Purkinje, basket,
stellate, and Golgi II cells of the cerebellar cortex all are
proven GABAergic neurons (12,13,21). In unpublished experiments,
Richard Hammerschlag (personal communication) found that arginine,
ornithine, and proline all gave rise to glutamate when incubated
with isolated sensory and sympathetic bullfrog ganglia. There
also is convincing evidence that proline can be converted to
glutamate in dorsal root ganglia, spinal cord, and cerebral
cortex in the cat (8).

In some recently completed experiments, I have obtained data
in whole mice consistent with the hypothesis that the arginine,
ornithine, and proline pathways may, indeed, lead in brain to the
formation of glutamate that may be available for GABA synthesis
(Table 1). Groups of mice were injected intraperitoneally with
α-ketoglutarate, L-arginine, L-ornithine, or L-proline alone at
8 mM/kg, or with mixtures of each of the above amino acids with
α-ketoglutarate, also at 8 mM/kg of the individual constituents.*

---

*
Such relatively large amounts were injected in order to increase
the chances of observing changes in concentrations of brain constituents. Although procedures may be employed that greatly
affect turnover rates of substances in brain, there is a remarkable tendency to maintain constant steady state concentrations
of the various detectable ninhydrin-reactive constituents (18).

TABLE 1. BRAIN AMINO ACIDS IN MICE AFTER INJECTION OF ARGININE, ORNITHINE, OR PROLINE WITH OR WITHOUT α-KETOGLUTARATE[a] (E. Roberts, unpublished)

Treatment	Amino Acid (µM/g fresh wt)				
	Arginine	Ornithine	Glutamate	GABA	Proline
Control (5)[b]	0.10	0.04	10.94	2.19	0.12
α-Ketoglutarate (3)	0.11	0.04	12.53†	2.18	0.13
L-Arginine (4)	0.19†	0.11†	11.89	2.16	0.16†
L-Arginine + α-Ketoglutarate (4)	0.17‡	0.09‡	12.85‡	2.53†	0.11
Ornithine (5)	0.04‡	0.22‡	11.02	2.09	0.21‡
Ornithine + α-Ketoglutarate (4)	0.05‡	0.18‡	12.16‡	2.56‡	0.15
Proline (5)	0.08	0.06	10.77	2.23	0.15
Proline + α-Ketoglutarate (4)	0.10	0.05	11.85	2.59‡	0.20‡

[a]Although the analyses performed included approximately 30 constituents, only the data pertinent to the discussion are presented here.

[b]Number of mice employed in parentheses.

†P <0.05
‡P <0.01

The animals were sacrificed at 60 minutes after injection, and brain amino acids were analyzed by standard methods with an amino acid analyzer. The administration of α-ketoglutarate alone resulted only in an elevation of glutamate content, suggesting that this occurred in "pools" not related to GABA synthesis. Injection of arginine alone resulted in elevation of arginine, ornithine, and proline content in a manner consistent with the operation of the pathways designated between arginine and proline in Fig. 1, while the glutamate and GABA levels were not changed. When arginine and α-ketoglutarate were given together, the increase in glutamate level was not greater than that observed with α-ketoglutarate alone; however, a significant increase in GABA levels was noted, and the increase in proline no longer was found. The latter result is consistent with the interpretation from Fig. 1 that, in the presence of a large excess of α-ketoglutarate, a portion of the ornithine formed from arginine (reaction 1) and used for proline synthesis (reactions 2 and 3) was diverted to glutamate (reaction 4) and thence to GABA synthesis (reaction 5). Essentially the same results were obtained with ornithine administration as with arginine, with the exception that the arginine levels were significantly reduced below the control levels, probably attributable to the fact that the arginine and ornithine share the same transport system. Proline administration alone produced no significant changes in the amino acids listed, but when given with α-ketoglutarate caused a significant increase in GABA levels. Since proline is not known to undergo any direct interactions with α-ketoglutarate, such as transamination, this result would be consistent with the sparing of ornithine from going to proline formation and shunting the ornithine to glutamate and GABA synthesis. Another possibility is that an increase in NAD^+ levels resulting from the formation of glutamate from α-ketoglutarate via reaction 8 might direct the flow from proline to glutamic-γ-semialdehyde and thence to glutamate and GABA. It would be expected that the oxidation of glutamic-γ-semialdehyde to glutamate would be favored if the NAD^+/NADH ratio were increased. Interestingly, GABA was found to inhibit the glutamic-γ-semialdehyde dehydrogenase from ox liver (24). If reaction 4 were in the sequence of GABA formation in brain, this could be a site for feedback control by GABA of its own formation. In concentrations present in the CNS, GABA does not inhibit its own synthesis by the L-glutamate decarboxylase reaction 5.

   There are intriguing data in nervous tissue with regard to asymmetries in the distribution of arginine and proline. For example, much higher concentrations of arginine were found in the dorsal roots of cat spinal cords relative to those in ventral roots (ratio of 5.30) than was the case for any of the other amino acids measured (ratios of 1.63 or less) (18). Proline also occurs in significantly higher concentrations in dorsal roots than in ventral roots (9). Currently, it cannot be ascertained whether the higher levels of arginine and proline are specifically found in the terminals of primary afferent fibers in the spinal

cord, since the latter are associated so closely with GABAergic
interneurons that are numerous in the dorsal horn (1); and GABA-
ergic synaptic terminals are presynaptic to dendrites, cell
bodies, and to primary afferent as well as other axon terminals
in this spinal cord region.

Since the conversion of ornithine to citrulline (Fig. 1, reaction 10) probably does not take place in brain (10), there is
no question from the data cited that arginine potentially is a
good source of glutamate and GABA in brain. Some of the above
circumstantial evidence also suggests a similar possibility for
proline. But the question is whether or not the necessary enzymes are all present in terminals of GABAergic neurons. Currently employed biochemical, pharmacologic, or physiologic analyses
do not allow identification of small pools of commonly occurring
substances of small molecular weight in specific morphological
entities or in defined neuronal regions. Although much progress
has been made in the development of all sorts of analytical tools
in recent years, the situation remains much the same as it was in
1968 when I turned my own activities to the development of immunocytochemical techniques for visualization of components of the
GABA system. Our success in the latter venture (16) gives me
courage to propose the use of a similar approach to visualization
of the enzymes of the metabolic pathways that may lead from arginine or proline to GABA in the vertebrate CNS and to other pertinent enzymes, such as glutaminase and glutamic dehydrogenase.

BASIC STRATEGIES IN ATTEMPTING TO TRACE PERTINENT METABOLIC PATHWAYS WITH IMMUNOCYTOCHEMICAL AND ISOTOPIC PROCEDURES

At the outset, arginase, ornithine aminotransferase, proline
oxidase, glutamic-γ-semialdehyde dehydrogenase, glutamic dehydrogenase, and glutaminase will be prepared from rat tissues. Specific antisera to the above antigens will be made and applied to
suitably prepared material from rat CNS for immunocytochemical
visualization of the above enzymes at the light and electron
microscopic levels by techniques previously established in our
laboratories for GAD, dopamine-β-hydrolase, and substance P, with
modifications as required. Preparations from rat cerebellum,
spinal cord, and substantia nigra, all regions rich in GABAergic
endings with which we have considerable experience, will be examined. Subsequently, studies could be made of other neural
sectors in which localization of GAD has been studied, such as
the olfactory bulb, hippocampus, and retina. The combination of
results that might be obtained in known GABAergic neurons with
the four of the above enzymes that are related to arginine and
proline metabolism is indicated in Table 2. Of the 14 possible
combinations, two options (a and b) would be compatible with the
possibility that GABA could be formed from arginine via ornithine
in such a manner that both the ω-nitrogen and the carbon chain
could be used in its synthesis. In the series of reactions involved, two molecules of glutamate, and therefore of GABA, could

TABLE 2.   Possible Combinations of Immunocytochemical Findings
in Known GABAergic Neurons and Nerve Endings

Arginase	Ornithine-α-Ketoglutarate Aminotransferase	Glutamic-γ-Semialdehyde Dehydrogenase	Proline Oxidase	Possible Glutamate and GABA Precursor Pathways (from Fig. 1)
1	2	4	3	
a) + a/	+	+	+	1. Arginine via 1, 2 + 4 and 5 2. Proline via 3, 4 and 5
b) +	+	+	-	Arginine via 1, 2 + 4 and 5
c) - a/				1. Ornithine via 2 + 4 and 5 2. Proline via 3, 4 and 5
d) +	-	+	+	Proline via 3, 4 and 5
e) -	-	+	+	Proline via 3, 4 and 5
f) -	+	+	+	Ornithine via 3, 4 and 5
g) +	+	-	+	Arginine via 1, 2 and 5
h) +	+	-	-	Arginine via 1, 2 and 5
i) -	+	-	+	Ornithine via 2 and 5
j) -	+	-	-	Ornithine via 2 and 5
k) +	-	-	+	
l) +	-	+	-	
m) -	-	-	-	
n) -	-	+	-	
o) -	-	+	-	
p) +	-	-	-	

a/ Neurons and/or nerve endings containing enzymes 2, 3, and 4
should be capable of interconverting ornithine and proline.

be formed from one molecule of α-ketoglutarate and one of arginine. The same would hold for ornithine alone, if arginase were
absent and ornithine could be available from sources other than
arginine (options c and f). In the absence of glutamic-γ-
semialdehyde dehydrogenase, arginine and ornithine still could
give rise to glutamate, via transamination of ornithine with
α-ketoglutarate, and then to GABA (options g and h). However,
in the latter instance, only the nitrogen from these amino acids
would find its way directly into GABA, and all of the carbon would
have come from α-ketoglutarate. A similar result would be seen
with ornithine alone if arginase were absent (options i and j).
Proline could give rise to GABA in those GABAergic neurons that
contain both proline oxidase and glutamic-γ-semialdehyde dehydrogenase (options a, c, d, and e). In all of the latter instances,
all of the carbon and nitrogen would come from proline, itself,
since it would not interact with α-ketoglutarate in the reaction
sequence postulated.

If unequivocal results were obtained with the above procedures,
e.g., all GABAergic neurons in the cerebellum were found to contain the enzymes in option b, then intracarotid and/or intracis-
ternal administration of U-^{14}C-labeled or U-^{13}C-labeled arginine
or ornithine should lead to the formation of isotope-labeled
glutamate and GABA in cerebellum with the labeling time-course
showing close to typical precursor-product relations at early
times, before mixing with extracerebral pools would have occurred.
Similar results should be obtained with L-arginine [guanidine-^{15}N]
but not with L-arginine-α^{15}N. On the other hand, if option g
were found to be fulfilled, there should be an entry of ^{15}N into
glutamate and GABA from administered guanidine-^{15}N arginine, but
little or no ^{14}C or ^{13}C label should appear in the early time
intervals. Let us suppose that GAD-negative nerve endings of the
hippocampal pyramidal and granule cells are found immunocytochem-
ically to have the combination of enzymes illustrated in option e
and that none of the known GABAergic endings shows the presence of
proline oxidase. It would then be presumed that proline could be
a source of glutamate in the pyramidal and granule cells, but not
in GABAergic neurons, and possibly that either glutamate, itself,
or a substance formed from it might be the transmitter of the
latter excitatory nerves. If this is so, experiments performed
both with ^{14}C- or ^{13}C- and ^{15}N-labeled proline should show a
ready entry of the label into glutamate, but little or none of
the label should be detected in GABA at early times after administration of the labeled amino acid. It has been suggested
recently that glutaminase might be involved in the formation of a
pool of releasable glutamate in hippocampal slices (6). The
latter enzyme is believed to be synaptosomally contained (2,22).
If the latter were related to actual liberation of glutamate as
excitatory transmitter, then positive results for glutaminase
localization might be expected in primary afferent terminals in
the spinal cord and in terminals of cortical neurons responsible
for the entorhinal input to the molecular layer of the dentate

gyrus; and the positive immunocytochemical reaction should disappear or diminish greatly upon dorsal rhizotomy and destruction of the entorhinal cortex, respectively.

The above examples will serve to illustrate how immunocytochemical results and biochemical approaches might be interdigitated in new approaches to detailed localization of reaction sequences at possible transmitter-forming sites.

CONCLUSION

In our laboratory, we have estimated that approximately 30 to 40 percent of all synaptic connections in the rat CNS are GABAergic. One of the barriers to further progress is that there still is little definitive information on the source (or sources) of the glutamate that is the immediate precursor for GABA synthesis in terminals of GABAergic neurons. In spite of much biochemical work on "compartmentation" in the brain, the interpretations from currently available data lack definition because the neural regions studied contain millions of cells of various types--neuronal, glial, and endothelial. The strategy outlined above, combining immunocytochemical and isotopic procedures, is a difficult one, and the road appears arduous. However, it holds out hope for achieving definitive information at the level of communicating nerve processes. If glutamate is truly a major excitatory transmitter in the vertebrate CNS, the approach outlined has the possibility of furnishing us the means with which to visualize and characterize another large population of neurons and nerve endings in the CNS. It is mind-boggling to consider the possibility that in a few years it may be possible to establish the chemomorphology of 80 percent or more of all the neurons in the vertebrate nervous system. There is room for all who wish to join the quest.

ACKNOWLEDGEMENTS

This work was supported in part by USPHS grants NS01615 and NS12116 from the NINCDS.

REFERENCES

1. Barber, R., Vaughn, J.E., Saito, K., McLaughlin, B.J., and Roberts, E. (1978): Brain Res., 141:35-55.
2. Bradford, H.F. and Ward, H.K. (1976): Brain Res., 110:115-125.
3. Costa, E., Guidotti, A., Moroni, F., and Peralta, E. (1979): In: Glutamic Acid:Advances in Biochemistry and Physiology, edited by L.A. Filer, Jr., S. Garattini, M.R. Kare, W.A. Reynolds, and R.J. Wurtman, pp. 151-166. Raven Press, New York.
4. Cremer, J.E., Sarna, G.S., Teal, H.M., and Cunningham, V.J. (1977): In: Amino Acids as Chemical Transmitters, edited by F. Fonnum, pp. 669-689. Plenum Press, New York.

5. Davies, R.K., Defalco, A.J., Shander, D., Kopelman, A., and Kiyasu, J. (1961): Nature, 191:288.
6. Hamberger, A., Chiang, G.H., Sandoval, E., and Cotman, C.W. (1979): Brain Res., 168:531-541.
7. Johnson, A.B. and Strecker, H.J. (1962): J. Biol. Chem., 237:1876-1882.
8. Johnson, J.L. (1975): Brain Res., 96:192-196.
9. Johnson, J.L. and Aprison, M.H. (1970): Brain Res., 24:285-292.
10. Jones, M.E., Anderson, A.D., Anderson, C., and Hodes, S. (1961): Arch. Biochem. Biophys., 95:499-507.
11. Krogsgaard-Larsen, P., Scheel-Krüger, J., and Kofod, H. (1979): GABA-Neurotransmitters. Munksgaard, Copenhagen.
12. McLaughlin, B.J., Wood, J.G., Saito, K., Barber, R., Vaughn, J.E., Roberts, E., and Wu, J.-Y. (1974): Brain Res., 76:377-391.
13. McLaughlin, B.J., Wood, J.G., Saito, K., Roberts, E., and Wu, J.-Y. (1975): Brain Res., 85:355-371.
14. Pardridge, W.M. and Oldendorf, W.H. (1975): Biochim. Biophys. Acta, 401:128-136.
15. Ratner, S., Morell, H., and Carvalho, E. (1960): Arch. Biochem. Biophys., 91:280-289.
16. Roberts, E. (1980): In: Antiepileptic Drugs: Mechanisms of Action, edited by G.H. Glaser, J.K. Penry, and D.M. Woodbury, pp. 667-713. Raven Press, New York.
17. Roberts, E., Chase, T.N., and Tower, D.B., editors (1976): GABA in Nervous System Function. Raven Press, New York.
18. Roberts, E. and Simonsen, D.G. (1962): In: Amino Acid Pools, edited by J.T. Holden, pp. 284-349. Elsevier, Amsterdam.
19. Ross, G., Dunn, D., and Jones, M.E. (1978): Biochem. Biophys. Res. Commun., 85:140-147.
20. Sadasivudu, B. and Rao, T.I. (1976): J. Neurochem., 27:785-794.
21. Saito, K., Barber, R., Wu, J.-Y., Matsuda, T., Roberts, E., and Vaughn, J.E. (1974): Proc. Natl. Acad. Sci. (USA) 71:269-273.
22. Salganicoff, L. and DeRobertis, E. (1965): J. Neurochem., 12:287-309.
23. Simonsen, D.G. and Roberts, E. (1974): Biochem. Med., 10:36-49.
24. Strecker, J.H. (1960): J. Biol. Chem., 235:3218-3223.
25. Van den Berg, J., Matheson, D.F., and Nijenmanting, W.C. (1977): In: Amino Acids as Chemical Transmitters, edited by F. Fonnum, pp. 709-723. Plenum Press, New York.

Glutamate as a Neurotransmitter,
edited by G. Di Chiara and G. L. Gessa
Raven Press, New York © 1981.

Role of Astroglial Cells in Glutamate Homeostasis

A. Schousboe and *L. Hertz

*Department of Biochemistry A, The Panum Institute, University of Copenhagen, DK-2200 Copenhagen, Denmark; and *Department of Pharmacology, University of Saskatchewan, Saskatoon, Saskatchewan, S7N 0W0 Canada*

INTRODUCTION

Glutamate has excitatory activity (cf. 11, 31), occurs in uni-
quely high concentrations in the central nervous system, and it
is a key compound in the connection between amino acid metabolism
and the tricarboxylic acid cycle (for references, see (22, 46)).
Its metabolism is extremely complex as originally demonstrated by
Lajtha et al. (35) in experiments where the specific radioactivity
of glutamine and glutamate in rat brain was followed after feeding
with ^{14}C-labelled acetate. Under certain conditions the specific
radioactivity of glutamine exceeded the peak specific radioactivity of glutamate indicating that the presence of different compartments with different pool sizes and turn-over rates of glutamate and glutamine. It has since then been firmly established that
the metabolism of these amino acids takes place in at least two
different compartments (e.g. 58), and attempts have been made to
correlate these compartments with cellular structures (e.g. 1).
One of the compartments is often presumed to comprise neuronal
perikarya and nerve endings and is referred to as the 'large'
glutamate pool, whereas another compartment, the so-called 'small'
glutamate pool may consist of glial cells. It has been suggested
(4) that there is a flow of glutamate from neurons to glial cells
and a compensatory flow of glutamine, formed in glia, in the
opposite direction.

These hypotheses of the neuronal-glial interactions in the
metabolism of glutamate and glutamine will be discussed in the
light of recent results obtained with primary cultures of astroglial cells and of cortical neurons and cerebellar granule cells
on activities of enzymes involved in glutamate/glutamine metabolism and of the characteristics of the transport mechanisms for
these amino acids.

TISSUE CULTURE

Astrocytes

Primary cultures of astrocytes were prepared essentially as described by Booher and Sensenbrenner (7). Cerebral hemispheres or other specified areas from newborn mice or rats were dissected and dissociated through sterile nylon sieves into a modified Eagle's minimum essential medium with foetal calf serum (25, 48, 49). This cell suspension was inoculated into Falcon or NUNC T-flasks or Petri dishes and the medium was changed 2-3 times a week during the entire culture period. During the third week of cultivation the cultures received medium supplemented with 0.1-0.25 mM dibutyryl cyclic AMP (dBcAMP) and totally or partly deleted for serum. This treatment induces a morphological differentiation leading to cells resembling mature astrocytes with abundant, relatively short, radial processes (e.g. 25, 40, 45, 48). On the basis of immunohistochemical staining for the astrocytic markers, glial fibrillary acidic protein (GFA) and glutamine synthetase (18, 42) 80-95% of the cells in such cultures and analogous cultures from cerebellum have been identified as astrocytes (e.g. 2, 29, 56). A more detailed discussion of the reliability of primary cultures of astrocytes as models for such cells in vivo may be found in reviews by Hertz (20, 21), Schousboe (43, 45), and Schousboe et al. (52).

Neurons

Two types of primary cultures of neurons have been employed. Cerebellar granule cells were obtained from 7 days old mice as described by Messer (39) and cortical neurons from 15 days old mouse embryos as described by Sensenbrenner (54) and Dichter (13). In both cases the tissue was dissected and exposed to 0.5% trypsin in Puck's solution at 37^0C for 10-15 min and subsequently centrifuged for 10 min at 900 × g. The pelleted cells were resuspended in a modified Eagle's minimum essential medium supplemented with 20% horse serum and seeded in polylysine coated Petri dishes or multitest dishes (NUNC or Falcon). After 15 min of incubation at 37^0C unattached cells were removed together with the medium which was then replaced with an analogous medium containing 24.5 mM KCl, 30 mM glucose, 7 μM paraaminobenzoic acid and 100 mU/l insulin. After 4-5 days in culture the cells were exposed for 24 h to 5×10^{-6} M cytosine-arabinoside which led to a virtual disappearance of astroblasts (13). Thereafter the medium was changed to a medium without the mitotic inhibitor and the cells were in most cases used for experiments after 7 days in culture (26). The synaptic marker D2 (28) shows a developmental pattern in cerebellar cultures similar to that in the cerebellum in vivo (2) and both cortical and cerebellar neuronal cultures have been shown to contain synaptin, another synaptic marker (6), although the amount is relatively low compared to whole forebrain (61). Thus, these cultures show some of the characteristics of mature

Table I

Kinetic constants for uptake of glutamate and glutamine in different preparations of astroglial cells and neurons.

Preparation	Glutamate			Glutamine		
	K_m (µM)	V_{max} (nmol × min⁻¹ × mg⁻¹)	Ref.	K_m (mM)	V_{max} (nmol × min⁻¹ × mg⁻¹)	Ref.
Astrocytes (primary cult.)	10 – 200	5 – 75	(22, 46)	0.2 – 3.3	2 – 50	(22, 26)
Astrocytes (bulk-prepared)	10 – 15	0.6 – 2	(22, 46)	0.6	1.6	(22)
Glial cell lines	14 – 66	0.7 – 4	(22, 46)	0.5	29	(22)
Cortical neurons (primary cult.)	27 – 50	6 – 9	(16, 22, 23 46, 61)	3.0	28	(22, 26, 61)
Cerebellar granule cells (primary cult.)	26 – 66	8 – 25	(16, 22, 46, 61)	0.7	10	(22, 26, 61)
Cerebellar granule cells (bulk-prepared)	15	0.6	(22)	–	–	
Neuronal peri-karya	–	–		1.4	11	(22, 26)
Neuroblastoma cells	30 – 50	0.6 – 6	(22, 46)	0.7	50	(22)
Synaptosomes	1.9 – 30	0.3 – 6	(22, 46)	0.3	3 – 9	(22)

Modified from Hertz (22), Schousboe (46), Hertz & Schousboe (23) and Yu (61) where references to additional original papers can be found.

neurons; they nevertheless may to a considerable extent consist of partly immature cells; in addition some glial cells are present, as indicated by at least trace amounts of GFA (61); therefore, results obtained with these cultures should at the present time be interpreted with some caution.

GLUTAMATE AND GLUTAMINE TRANSPORT

Glutamate

Glial cells.
There is little doubt that glutamate is released as a transmitter from specific types of neurons (e.g. 11, 22, 27, 31, 55, 57); it is more disputed whether, or to what extent, glutamate release may, in addition, serve other purposes and maybe also occurs from other cell types (e.g. 22). Since glutamate present in the extracellular space, regardless of its origin, will have an excitatory effect on neurons (cf. above) it is of crucial importance for the termination of the transmitter activity that efficient, high affinity uptake mechanisms exsist in glial cells and/or neurons (cf. 12). As can be seen from Table I such mechanisms are found in different preparations of glial cells. Especially astrocytes in primary cultures have remarkably high capacities (V_{max}) for glutamate uptake (3, 24, 25, 49) suggesting that astrocytes may be of major functional importance for the inactivation of glutamate (cf. 22, 46). This is further supported by a more intense uptake into bulk-prepared astrocytes than into corresponding preparations of neurons (2, 17), by the autoradiographic demonstration that glutamate to a large extent is accumulated into glia (cf. 22, 27, 46), and by the finding (25) that glutamate uptake into astrocytes represents a net uptake and not a homoexchange (cf. below). Moreover, there appears to be a correlation between the extent of glial glutamate uptake in a specific brain region and the presumed quantitative importance of glutamatergic transmission in that particular brain region (47). Thus, cultured astrocytes from prefrontal cortex and neostriatum were found to have the largest high affinity glutamate uptake in agreement with the proposed glutamatergic nature of the major part of the corticostriatal projections (15, 30, 38).

Neurons.
A high affinity uptake of glutamate is also present in synaptosomes and it seems to be confined to unique synaptosomal fractions (6, 37, 60); as can be seen from Table I the V_{max} is, however, distinctly lower than that for glutamate uptake into astrocytes in primary cultures. Uptake of glutamate into neurons has also been demonstrated autoradiographically (3, 27) and different preparations of cultured and bulk-prepared neurons have high affinity uptake of glutamate (Table I). The demonstrations (15, 27) that surgical destruction of glutamatergic pathways in hippocampus and striatum reduces high affinity uptake of glutamate in these areas strongly support a neuronal (nerve ending) uptake of glutamate.

It is also in keeping with the concept of glutamate uptake into glutamatergic neurons that a specially intense uptake has been demonstrated into cerebellar granule cells (Table I) which are presumably glutamatergic (55). East et al. (17) did not observe a corresponding large glutamate uptake into bulk-prepared granule cells but this may possibly be explained by the rather low glutamate uptake in all of the cell fractions in this study (17).

It should be kept in mind that glutamate uptake into synaptosomes to a large extent often represents a 1:1 homoexchange process (36) which can be of no physiological importance for removal of glutamate from the synaptic cleft. A net uptake occurs, however, under certain conditions (10) e.g. when the membrane potential is intact, which obviously is the case in vivo (cf. 53).

Glutamine

From the studies of glutamate uptake (cf. above) it appears that a considerable fraction of the glutamate, which is released from neurons, is likely to be taken up into astroglial cells. Since this also holds true for GABA (22, 23, 44, 46) it must be concluded that a compartment comprising neurons looses tricarboxylic acid constituents to a compartment comprising astroglial cells. According to Benjamin and Quastel (4) this should be compensated for by a quantitatively similar flow of glutamine in the opposite direction, i.e. from astrocytes to neurons. A prerequisite for this hypothesis is that neurons possess a transport mechanism for glutamine which is more efficient than an analogous mechanism in astrocytes. From the kinetic constants for glutamine uptake into different preparations of glial cells and neurons shown in Table I it is, however, clear that none of these preparations including the presumably glutamatergic granule cells from cerebellum, exhibits high affinity uptake characteristics and that only small quantitative differences exist between the uptake systems in neurons and astrocytes. It is accordingly rather unlikely that glutamine should be preferentially taken up by the neurons although a rather rapid release of glutamine from astrocytes does occur (41, 51). These findings, therefore, do not support the hypothesis of a quantitative, compensatory flow of glutamine from astrocytes to neurons and the possibility exists that CO_2 fixation in the neuronal compartment may compensate for the apparent loss of tricarboxylic acid constituents (22, 23, 26). Such a carbon dioxide fixation is known to occur in the brain (59).

GLUTAMATE AND GLUTAMINE METABOLISM

The activities of some of the enzymes directly involved in the formation and degradation of glutamate and glutamine in neurons and glial cells are summarized in Table II. The glutamine synthetase and the phosphate activated glutaminase may be the most important of these enzymes since they catalyze the transformations of glutamate to glutamine and glutamine to glutamate, each of

Table II

Activities of glutamate and glutamine metabolizing enzymes in different preparations of astroglial cells and neurons.

Preparation	Enzyme activity $(nmol \times min^{-1} \times mg^{-1})$					
	GOT	GLDH	GAD	GLU-S	PAG	Ref.
Astrocytes (primary cult.)	154 – 249	3.0 – 16.6	< 0.09	22.0 – 28.1	3.8	(22,43,46,51)
Astrocytes (bulk-prepared)	356	124	0.1 – 11	13 – 15	1.4	(22, 43, 46)
Glial cell lines	–	11 – 56	0.008 – 0.2	1	–	(22, 43, 46)
Neurons (bulk-prepared)	846	326	0.2 – 11	12 – 23	0.5	(22, 46)
Neuroblastoma cells	–	2.5 – 17	0.07	–	–	(22, 46)
Synaptosomes	–	–	1.3	19	5-80	(22, 33, 46)

Modified from Schousboe (43, 46) and Hertz (22) where references to additional original papers can be found.
GOT: glutamic-oxaloacetate-transaminase. GLDH: glutamate dehydrogenase. GAD: glutamate decarboxylase. GLU-S: glutamine synthetase. PAG: phosphate activated glutaminase.

which represents an irreversible reaction. Also the glutamate decarboxylase (GAD) catalyzes an irreversible reaction and the further metabolism of the reaction product, GABA, is brought about by the GABA-transaminase, which is present both in neurons and astrocytes (cf. 22, 23, 44, 46, 50). This part of the glutamate metabolism is, however, outside the scope of this paper, especially since the GAD activity is very low in glia (Table II). As can be seen from Table II both the transamination of glutamate with oxaloacetate and the oxidative deamination of glutamate take place in neurons and astrocytes with similar velocities indicating that only minor differences between the cell types exist as far as the capacity for reversible conversions of glutamate are concerned. On the basis of this it may be appropriate to concentrate the discussion on the glutamine synthetase and glutaminase reactions (cf. above). The finding of a high glutamine synthetase activity in cultured astrocytes (24, 29, 49, 52) is in agreement with the recent immunohistochemical localization of glutamine synthetase in astrocytes (42). It is obviously also in agreement with prevalent compartmentation theories that glutamine is predominantly synthetized in the 'small', glial, glutamate compartment (cf. above). According to this concept, the glutaminase should reside primarily in the neurons and the enzyme has been found to be enriched in synaptosomes (8, 9, 12, 14, 19). It is, however, evident from Table II that this enzyme also is quite active in astrocytes. The activity reported by Schousboe et al. (51) for astrocytes in primary cultures is of such a magnitude that it is incompatible with a large flow of glutamine from astrocytes to neurons, unless the glutaminase is regulated. Kvamme and coworkers (32, 33) have recently showed that the synaptosomal glutaminase consists of a NEM-sensitive and a NEM-insensitive fraction and that these have different properties with regard to regulation by ammonia and calcium. The NEM-insensitive enzyme is activated by Ca^{2+} whereas the NEM-sensitive enzyme is inhibited, and ammonia only affects (inhibits) the NEM-sensitive enzyme. Apparently the astrocytic enzyme behaves in an analogous way except that ammonia has no effect on this enzyme (34). The functional implications of this are at present not clear. In addition, it is also possible that the apparently high glutamate concentration in astrocytes (cf. 22, 46) leads to a considerable inhibition of the glutaminase since the glial enzyme is strongly inhibited by glutamate concentrations around 1-2 mM (34).

CONCLUDING REMARKS

From the available evidence it seems quite clear that astrocytes are capable of taking up a very large fraction of the glutamate, which is released from neurons due to e.g. neurotransmission. It is also evident that astrocytes have the enzymatic machinery for the conversion of glutamate to glutamine. Since astrocytes not only have an efficient uptake system for glutamine, but also have the enzyme, that converts glutamine to glutamate, it is, however, questionable to what extent glutamine may again be transported back to the neurons in stoichiometrically equivalent amounts and accordingly whether a glutamate-glutamine cycle is operating. To what extent glutamine actually is converted to glutamate in situ is at present not resolved, but it is very likely that astrocytes play a much more complex role in glutamate/glutamine metabolism than hitherto believed. Moreover, a distinct identification of neurons and glial cells with the different compartments of glutamate metabolism is likely to be an oversimplification. The possibility exists that nerve endings and astrocytes together could comprise one compartment (cf. 22). Studies of the incorporation of radioactively labelled substrates into glutamate and glutamine in cultured neurons and astrocytes and of ammonia uptake and release may throw more light on these aspects of astrocytic-neuronal interactions.

ACKNOWLEDGEMENT

The expert technical assistance by Miss Hanne Fosmark, Jytte Christiansen and Dr. S. Mukerji is gratefully acknowledged. The work has been financially supported by The Novo Foundation, Carl & Ellen Hertz' Foundation for Medical Research, The Medical Research Council of Canada (MT 5957) and a NATO Research Grant (1017).

REFERENCES

1. Balazs, R., Patel, A.J. and Richter, D. (1972): In: Metabolic Compartmentation in the Brain, edited by R. Balazs and E.J. Cremer, pp. 167-184. MacMillan Press, London.
2. Balazs, R., Regan, C., Meier, E., Woodhams, P.L., Wilkin G.P., Patel, N.J. and Gordon, R.D. (1980): In: Tissue Culture in Neurobiology, edited by E. Giacobini, A. Vernadakis and A. Shahar, pp. 155-168. Raven Press, New York.
3. Balcar, V.J. and Hauser, K.L. (1978): Proc. Eur. Soc. Neurochem., 1:498.
4. Benjamin, A.M. and Quastel, J.H. (1975): J. Neurochem., 25:197-206.
5. Bennett, J.P. Jr., Logan, W.J. and Snyder, S.H. (1972): Science N.Y., 178:997-999.
6. Bock, E., Jørgensen, O.S., Dittmann, L. and Eng, L.F. (1975): J. Neurochem., 25:867-870.
7. Booher, J. and Sensenbrenner, M. (1972): Neurobiology, 2:97-105.
8. Bradford, H.F. and Ward, H.K. (1976): Brain Res., 110:115-125.
9. Bradford, H.F., Ward, H.K. and Thomas, A.J. (1978): J. Neurochem., 30:1453-1459.
10. Bradford, H.F., Jones, D.G., Ward, H.K. and Booher, J. (1975): Brain Res., 90:245-259.

11. Curtis, D.R. and Johnston, G.A.R. (1974): Ergbn. Physiol., 69:97-188.
12. Dennis, S.C., Lai, J.C.K. and Clark, J.B. (1977): Biochem. J., 164:727-736.
13. Dichter, M.A. (1978): Brain Res., 149:279-293.
14. Dienel, G., Ryder, E. and Greengard, O. (1977): Biochim. Biophys. Acta, 496:484-494.
15. Divac, I., Fonnum, F. and Storm-Mathisen, J. (1977): Nature, Lond., 266:377-378.
16. Drejer, J., Divac, I., Schousboe, A. and Larsson, O.M. (1980): Neurosci. Lett., Suppl. in press.
17. East, J.M., Dutton, G.R. and Currie, D.N. (1980): J. Neurochem., 34:523-530.
18. Eng, L.F., Van der Haegen, J.J., Bignami, A. and Gerstl, B. (1971): Brain Res., 28:351-354.
19. Hamberger, A., Cotman, C.W., Sellström, Å. and Weiler, C.T. (1978): In: Dynamic Properties of Glia Cells, edited by E. Schoffeniels, G. Franck, L. Hertz and D.B. Tower, pp. 163-172. Pergamon Press, Oxford.
20. Hertz, L. (1977): In: Cell Tissue and Organ Cultures in Neurobiology, edited by S. Fedoroff and L. Hertz, pp. 39-71. Academic Press, New York.
21. Hertz, L. (1978): In: Dynamic Properties of Glia Cells, edited by E. Schoffeniels, G. Franck, L. Hertz and D.B. Tower, pp. 121-132. Pergamon Press, Oxford.
22. Hertz, L. (1979): Progr. Neurobiol., 13:277-323.
23. Hertz, L. and Schousboe, A. (1980): In: GABA and Other Inhibitory Neurotransmitters, edited by H. Lal, J.B. Malick and E. Usdin. Brain Res. Bull., 5, suppl. 2: in press. Ankho International, New York.
24. Hertz, L., Bock, E. and Schousboe, A. (1978): Dev. Neurosci., 1:226-238.
25. Hertz, L., Schousboe, A., Boechler, N., Mukerji, S. and Fedoroff, S. (1978): Neurochem. Res., 3:1-14.
26. Hertz, L., Yu, A., Svenneby, G., Kvamme, E., Fosmark, H. and Schousboe, A. (1979): Neurosci. Lett., 16:103-109.
27. Hösli, L. and Hösli, E. (1978): Rev. Physiol. Biochem. Pharmac., 81:136-188.
28. Jørgensen, O.S. and Bock, E. (1974): J. Neurochem., 23:879-880.
29. Juurlink, B.H.J., Schousboe, A., Jørgensen, O.S. and Hertz, L. (1980): J. Neurochem., 35:in press.
30. Kim, J.S., Hassler, R., Haug, P. and Paik, K.S. (1977): Brain Res., 132:370-374.
31. Krnjevic, K. (1974): Physiol. Rev., 54:418-540.
32. Kvamme, E. (1979): In: GABA - Biochemistry and CNS Functions, edited by P. Mandel and F.V. De Feudis. Adv. Exp. Med. Biol., 123:111-138. Plenum Press, New York,
33. Kvamme, E. and Olsen, B. (1979): FEBS Lett., 107:33-36.
34. Kvamme, E., Svenneby, G., Hertz, L. and Schousboe, A. (1979): Proc. Int. Soc. Neurochem., 7:436.

35. Lajtha, A., Berl, S. and Waelsch, H. (1959): J. Neurochem., 3:322-332.
36. Levi, G. and Raiteri, M. (1974): Nature, Lond., 250:735-737.
37. Logan, W.J. and Snyder, S.H. (1972): Brain Res., 42:413-431.
38. McGeer, P.L., McGeer, E.G., Scherer, U. and Singh, K. (1977): Brain Res., 128:369-373.
39. Messer, A. (1977): Brain Res., 130:1-12.
40. Moonen, G., Cam, Y., Sensenbrenner, M. and Mandel, P. (1975): Cell. Tiss. Res., 163:365-372.
41. Nicklas, W.J. and Browning, E.T. (1978): J. Neurochem., 30: 955-963.
42. Norenberg, M.D. and Martinez-Hernandez, A. (1979): Brain Res., 161:303-310.
43. Schousboe, A. (1977): In: Cell, Tissue and Organ Cultures in Neurobiology, edited by E. Fedoroff and L. Hertz, pp. 441-446. Academic Press, New York.
44. Schousboe, A. (1979): In: GABA-Neurotransmitters. Pharmaco-chemical, Biochemical and Pharmacological Aspects, edited by P. Krogsgaard-Larsen, J. Scheel-Krüger and H. Kofod. pp. 263-280. Munksgaard, Copenhagen.
45. Schousboe, A. (1980): Cell. Mol. Biol., in press.
46. Schousboe, A. (1980): Int. Rev. Neurobiol., 22:in press.
47. Schousboe, A. and Divac, I. (1979): Brain Res., 177:407-409.
48. Schousboe, A., Fosmark, H. and Svenneby, G. (1976): Brain Res., 116:158-164.
49. Schousboe, A., Svenneby, G. and Hertz, L. (1977): J. Neuro-chem., 29:999-1005.
50. Schousboe, A., Saito, K. and Wu, J.-Y. (1980): In: GABA and Other Inhibitory Neurotransmitters, edited by H. Lal, J.B. Malick and E. Usdin. Brain Res. Bull. 5, Suppl. 2: in press. Ankho International, New York.
51. Schousboe, A., Hertz, L., Svenneby, G. and Kvamme, E. (1979): J. Neurochem., 32:943-950.
52. Schousboe, A., Nissen, C., Bock, E., Sapirstein, V.S., Juur-link, B.H.J. and Hertz, L. (1980): In: Tissue Culture in Neurobiology, edited by E. Giacobini, A. Vernadakis and A. Shahar, pp. 397-409. Raven Press, New York.
53. Sellström, A., Venema, R. and Henn, F. (1976): Nature, Lond., 264:652-653.
54. Sensenbrenner, M. (1977): In: Cell, Tissue and Organ Cultures in Neurobiology, edited by S. Fedoroff and L. Hertz, pp. 191-213. Academic Press, New York.
55. Snyder, S.H., Young, A.B., Oster-Granite, M.L. and Herndon, R.M. (1975): In: Metabolic Compartmentation and Neurotrans-mission. Relation to Brain Structure and Function, edited by S.Berl, D.D. Clarke and D. Schneider, pp. 1-10. Plenum Press, New York.
56. Stieg, P.E., Kimelberg, H.K., Mazurkiewicz, J.E. and Banker, G.A. (1979): Abstr. Soc. Neurosci., 5:759.
57. Storm-Mathisen, J. (1977): Brain Res., 120:379-386.

58. Van den Berg, C.J. Matheson, D.F., Ronda, G., Reijnierse, G.L.A., Blokhuis, G.G.D., Kroon, M.C., Clarke, D.D. and Garfinkel, D. (1975): In: Metabolic Compartmentation and Neurotransmission. Relation to Brain Structure and Function, edited by S. Berl, D.D. Clarke and D. Schneider, pp. 515-543, Plenum Press, New York.

59. Waelsch, H., Berl, S., Rossi, C.A. Clarke, D.D. and Purpura, D.P. (1964): J. Neurochem., 11:717-728.

60. Wofsey, A.R., Kuhar, M.J. and Snyder, S.H. (1971): Proc. natl. Acad. Sci. U.S.A., 68:1102-1106.

61. Yu, A. (1980): M. Sc. Thesis. University of Saskatchewan, Canada.

Glutamate as a Neurotransmitter,
edited by G. Di Chiara and G. L. Gessa
Raven Press, New York © 1981.

Regulation of Glutamate Biosynthesis and Release by Pathophysiological Levels of Ammonium Ions

A. Hamberger, I. Jacobsson, S.-O. Molin, B. Nyström, and M. Sandberg

Institute of Neurobiology, University of Göteborg, S-400 33 Göteborg, Sweden

Ammonia, including the ammonium ion, is principally produced in the gastrointestinal tract during protein breakdown. The maintenance of normal blood levels of ammonia is essentially taken care of by the liver, and its end product, urea, is secreted with the urine. Ammonia is a prominent link in the liver-brain axis and has been known for a long time for its neurotoxicity, but how its action is exerted is only vaguely understood. A defective liver function raises plasma and brain ammonia concentrations and leads frequently to hepatic encephalopathy and the clinical symptoms of confusion, convulsion, coma and eventually death. The brain contains enzyme systems to detoxify ammonia, the end product being glutamine. It appears hardly ideal, however, to involve the glutamate system of amino acids in the brain as a reserve to dispose of gut-derived ammonia, since the ammonium ion is one of the regulators of the formation of quantitatively important putative neurotransmitters.

A striking feature of hepatic coma is the several-fold elevation of glutamine in the CNS and CSF (15). Various short chain fatty acids are elevated in plasma of patients with hepatic coma and may contribute to the syndrome (35). Plasma tryptophane is often increased and brain serotonin levels seem determined by plasma tryptophan (14, 20). Tryptophan appears particularly toxic when given to patients with liver disease (32). The involvement of so called false neurotransmitters appearing during liver damage, and the depletion of brain norepinephrine (15) have also been discussed as etiological agents.

Infusions of ammonia readily reproduce the clinical syndrome of hepatic coma (8, 22), hepatic encephalopathy, dominated by the proliferation of protoplasmic astrocytes (10) and a number of the changes in laboratory data, including the rise in glutamine. Certain conclusions emerge from the study of the current literature on hepatic coma: the ammonium ion is central as a causative agent,

and the most likely site of the ammonia effect is on CNS neurotransmission (19, 45). Neurotransmission would traditionally be
disturbed by interference with the pre- or postsynaptic neuron,
but the astrocytic glia may also be involved, since glia partici-
pates in the inactivation of transmitter glutamate and GABA (18,
36). In addition, glutamine is exclusively synthesized by astrocytes (31), and appears to be an important precursor for glutamate and GABA synthesis (6, 11).

Ammonia exerts a postsynaptic inhibitory effect, which appears
unconnected with transmitter concentrations, but involves increased intracellular Cl^- concentrations (1, 21, 25). The lag period
before suppression of the electrical activity occurs in cerebellar
slices exposed to pathophysiological concentrations of ammonia
(3), and the observation that administration of methionine sulf-
oximine - an inhibitor of glutamine synthesis - doubles the LD 50
for intraperitoneally infused ammonia (41) indicate that the critical factor is not the ammonium ion itself, but the metabolic
changes induced by ammonia.

Schenker et al. (35) suggested that "proof of the neurotransmitter hypothesis will require demonstration of depletion of physiological neurotransmitters in the synaptosomes of patients and
experimental animals in hepatic coma and ideally a response of
the neurological deficit to repletion of these substances". These
criteria appear related to a presynaptic site of action of the ammonium ion and a presumed metabolic effect. The therapeutic mea-
sures other than those directed towards removal of ammonia, are
actually oriented around the theory of transmitter depletion. Patients with hepatic encephalopathy which were treated with levo-
dopa showed significant improvement (24) and glutamate and aspartate infusions have arousal properties when given to such patients
(45).

In this report, the presynaptic effect of ammonia on the biosynthesis and release of glutamate will be evaluated in vitro,
since the electrical and biochemical phenomena of hepatic coma
are produced in a slice with ammonium ions at pathophysiological
concentrations (3).

AMMONIA AND GLUTAMATE METABOLISM IN THE HIPPOCAMPUS

The hypothesis that ammonia might induce neurological disturbances via depletion of the transmitter pool of glutamate, was
originally proposed by Bradford and Ward (6) and Matheson and van
den Berg (27), and the basis was the inhibition by ammonia of
glutamine utilization for glutamate synthesis. The elevated glutamine concentration seen during hyperammonemia is then as much a
consequence of decreased glutamine breakdown as of an increased
glutamine synthesis. Since the latter occurs in glia (31) and the
former in nerve terminals (33), hepatic coma may be a clinical
example of how the glutamate compartmentation (5) works, or rather
doesn't work.

Hippocampal slices were used for the experimental work, since

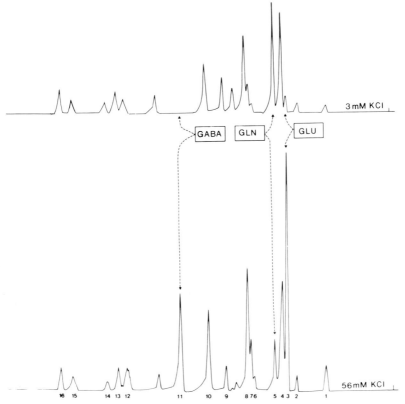

Fig. 1 HPLC analysis of the amino acid pattern in the effluent during perfusion of hippocampal slices with Krebs Ringer bicarbonate medium containing 3 (top) or 56 (bottom) mM KCl, 1 Asp, 2 Asn, 3 Glu, 4 Ser, 5 Gln, 6 Citrulline, 7 Thr, 8 Gly + Arg, 9 Tau, 10 Ala, 11 GABA, 12 Met + NH_3, 13 Val, 14 Phe, 15 Ile, 16 Leu.

even a critical reviewer accepts the tests for transmitter criteria as positive with respect to glutamate for this region (30). A perfusion system was chosen to reflect the time course of changes in various tissue pools as total tissue concentrations are less informative in the compartmented glutamate system. Fig. 1 shows the pattern of endogenous amino acids in the effluent when hippocampal slices are perfused with a Krebs-Ringer bicarbonate medium containing 10 mM glucose. The upper profile represents the results when the medium contains 3 mM K^+ and below is the elution pattern after K^+ was increased to 56 mM in order to depolarise the tissue. It is apparent that the efflux of two amino acids, glutamate and GABA, is increased 30-50-fold with depolarisation, the efflux of the other remains constant or increases only slightly. Glutamine in the effluent was, however, reduced by at least 50 per cent during K^+ depolarisation. The time course of the efflux of a few

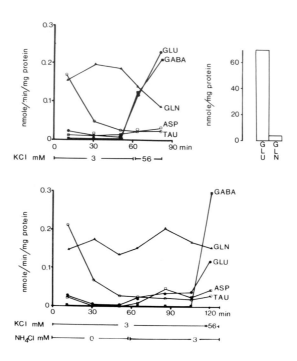

<u>Fig. 2</u> Efflux of endogenous amino acids measured with the HPLC
technique. <u>Top:</u> Effect of 56 mM KCl. <u>Bottom:</u> Effect of 3 mM
NH₄Cl perfusion prior to the 56 mM KCl pulse. <u>Top right:</u> Slice
content of glutamate and glutamine after the perfusion experiment.

amino acids is shown in Fig. 2. The specific and essentially Ca-
dependent efflux of glutamate and GABA (42) is in agreement with
the previous localisation of these amino acids as transmitters in
the hippocampus (12, 37). Glutamine was secreted at high concentrations from the beginning of the experiment and the eventual decrease in glutamine efflux might have occurred even without tissue
depolarisation, as the slice content of glutamine was remarkably
low (Fig. 2). Fig. 2 also shows the effect of introducing 3 mM
NH₄Cl into the perfusion medium for 40 min prior to a pulse with
56 mM K⁺. The ammonium effect <u>per se</u> was a slowly appearing increase in the efflux of glutamine, aspartate and glutamate which may
suggest that they are secreted from the same compartment. This is
most likely glial, since glutamine synthetase seems confined to
astrocytes (31). The increase in glutamine is similarly accompanied by elevated glutamate and aspartate in the CSF of patients
with hepatic coma (26, own unpublished observations). The depolarisation-evoked GABA release was unaffected by the previous ammonia

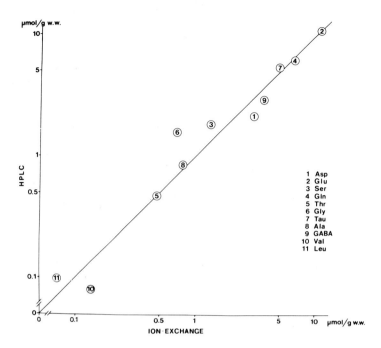

Fig. 3 Correlative analysis of free amino acids in extracts from cerebral cortex measured with ion-exchange and HPLC techniques.

perfusion, but the evoked glutamate release was only 30 per cent of the control (Fig. 2). The principal effect of ammonium ions appears consequently to be a specific inhibition of the depolarisation-evoked glutamate release.

The analysis of endogenous amino acids in the effluent from a few 0.4 mm hippocampal slices requires a sensitivity of the technique in the picomole range. The present data were obtained with precolumn fluorigenic labelling (0-phtaldialdehyde) and reversed phase high performance liquid chromatography (HPLC). The separation and analysis are made in less than 30 min, and the detection limit is in the range of 100 fmol (23). Fig. 3 shows that a comparison with a conventional ion exchange amino acid analyser, employing ninhydrin, gives satisfactory results.

THE INFLUENCE OF EXOGENOUS GLUTAMINE

In a perfusion system the hippocampal slice relatively soon becomes largely depleted of glutamine. Therefore, experiments were performed in which the medium was fortified with 0.5 mM glutamine in addition to 10 mM glucose (16). In analogy with the previous findings, ammonium ions caused a slowly appearing increase in glutamate secretion, and the high K^+-evoked efflux of glutamate

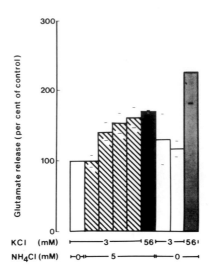

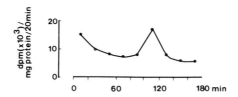

Fig.4 Time course of efflux of endogenous glutamate from hippocampal slices. The KRB medium contained 10 mM glucose and .5 mM
glutamine. ☐ control medium, ◨ + 3 mM NH_4Cl, ▧   + 56 mM
KCl, ■ + 56 mM KCl; 3 mM NH_4Cl. (Top). Time course of efflux
of ^{14}C glutamate radioactivity. The radioactivity was accumulated during incubation of the tissue slice in trace amounts of
label just prior to the start of the time scale.(Bottom).

glutamate was now virtually 100% inhibited (Fig. 4). This inhibition is not immediate but requires 30 - 40 min perfusion with
NH_4Cl. It is also apparent that the ammonia effect is reversible
since an almost normal response of glutamate release was seen when
the high K^+ pulse was given after perfusion for 40 min with ammo-
nia-free media. Fig. 4 (lower graph) shows the efflux of ^{14}C-glut-
amate radioactivity from the same tissue. The radioactivity was
incorporated by preincubation for 10 min with trace amounts of
the isotope. The efflux curve for exogenous glutamate does not
indicate any effect by ammonia either on the "spontaneous" efflux
or on the K^+-induced release. Exogenous glutamate is accumulated
by glia and nerve terminals. The results with exogenous glutamate
are interpreted as indicating that the release mechanisms of the
tissue are unaffected by ammonia, and that the inhibition of the

K$^+$-induced efflux of endogenous glutamate reflects a depletion of the glutamate pool in the nerve terminals. In an attempt to link these observations to the pathogenesis of hepatic coma, rats were subjected to porta-caval anastomosis and the hippocampal tissue tested for ammonia sensitivity 3-4 weeks after the operation. The results showed that ammonia perfusion of the tissue was without effect on either basal or KCl-evoked release of endogenous glutamate, suggestive of an adaptive process in these animals (17).

The glutamate content in the effluent increased severalfold when glutamine was included in the perfusion medium. This increase was, however, mainly seen in the basal efflux. The relative increase in glutamate secretion during K$^+$ depolarisation was considerably smaller than with glutamine-free media. The ammonia inhibition of the depolarisation-induced glutamate efflux was, however, more striking with the glutamine-containing medium, indicating that ammonia efficiently inhibits the utilization of glutamine for glutamate synthesis in the nerve terminals.

GLUCOSE AND ACETATE AS GLUTAMATE
PRECURSORS IN HYPERAMMONEMIA

The ammonia effect was suggestive of an activated glutamate synthesis in the glia as a step in glutamine formation and inhibition of glutamate synthesis in nerve terminals. In order to evaluate this hypothesis, the incorporation of ^{14}C into amino acids from glucose and acetate was studied. The approach was employed since the classical studies on compartmentation indicate that glucose predominantly labels the "large" glutamate pool localised to nerve endings, while the "small" glutamate pool, in which there is an active glutamine synthesis, seems to reside in the glial cells and employs acetate more efficiently as a glutamate precursor (2, 5, 40). The relative incorporation of the two precursors has been employed to demonstrate a biochemical correlate to glial proliferation (29, 39). We have recently used this test system successfully on the outer molecular layer of the dentate gyrus in the rat hippocampus. Twelve days after a lesion in the entorhinal cortex, leading to a degeneration of 70% of the nerve terminals (28) as well as an intense astrocytosis, the glucose incorporation into glutamate was reduced to 50% of the control while the corresponding figure for acetate was over 200%. Fig. 5 shows the effect of ammonium ions on the incorporation of glucose and acetate into amino acids of the hippocampal slice. A significant decrease of acetate-derived ^{14}C radioactivity in amino acids was seen during perfusion with ammonia, while glucose was utilized to an increased extent (Fig. 5). The ammonia effect seemed to be reversible for both precursors. The results appeared, however, definitely to contradict the assumption of an activated glial compartment during hyperammonemia. The increased flow of glucose carbon into amino acids may represent partly an adaptation of the nerve terminals to the restricted availability of the glutamine pool during hyperammonemia, since glutaminase activity is

inhibited by ammonium ions (7, 44). Apparently conflicting data
are reported in the literature on the influence of ammonium into-
xication on the energy metabolism of the brain   (38). The fixation
of CO_2 into glutamine is, however, stimulated <u>in vivo</u> (4). The
increased labelling of glutamate from ^{14}C glucose parallels the
efflux of endogenous glutamate and glutamine during ammonia

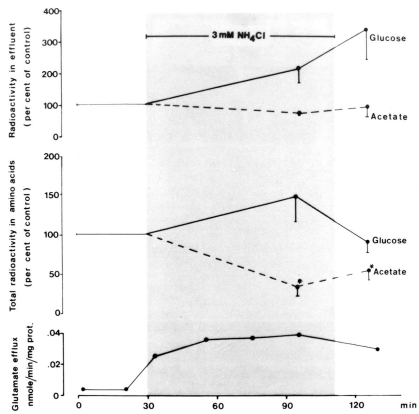

Fig. 5 Utilization of ^{14}C-glucose and ^{14}C-acetate for amino
acid synthesis by hippocampal slices during perfusion with glutamine -free medium. 3 mM NH_4Cl was included as indicated. The
efflux of endogenous glutamate is indicated at the bottom. The
labelled precursors were included in the medium for 20 min during the final period of the NH_4Cl perfusion and in other experiments upon the return to normal medium. The amino acid fraction
was eluted from an AG 50 column with 1 mM NH_4OH. TLC separation
of amino acids showed that 75% of the radioactivity migrated
with glutamic acid. Total radioactivity in amino acids is shown
in per cent of a control which was perfused without NH_4Cl (center). The proportion of the radioactivity which was present in
the medium (medium/medium + slice x 100) is indicated at the
top.

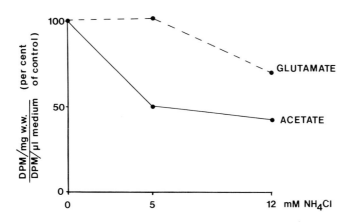

Fig. 6 Effects of NH$_4$Cl on the accumulation of ^{14}C-glutamate (8.5x10^{-7} M) and ^{14}C-acetate (1.8 x 10^{-5}M) by hippocampal sli-ces. The slices were perfused with 0, 5 or 12 mM NH$_4$Cl for 45 min, and then transferred to normal Krebs-Ringer bicarbonate medium containing the isotope for 10 min at 37°. The incubation was terminated by a quick wash in fresh medium after which the wet weight was determined. Tissue and media radioactivity was determined.

perfusion, so the newly formed glutamate may be secreted from a glutamine-synthesizing pool. The results would then indicate that either the "large" pool of glutamate produces glutamine in the presence of elevated ammonia, or that the "small" (glial) pool is the site of the increased glucose utilization. The increasing pro-portion of the newly synthetized glucose-derived glutamate which appears in the medium (Fig. 5, top) during ammonia perfusion, would point towards the glia as the place of glutamate synthesis, since the Vmax's for glutamate uptake are lower in glia than in synaptosomes (43). These considerations are essentially in agree-ment with the work of Cavanagh (9) and of Cremer (13) who studied glucose and acetate metabolism in rats subjected to porta-cava-anastomosis.

The results with ^{14}C-acetate as a glutamate precursor seems largely due to the effects of ammonium ions on the transport of acetate. While glucose transport into the brain is unaffected in rats with a porta-cava anastomosis, that of acetate is reduced by 40-50% (9, 34). This was reproduced in hippocampal slices when ammonia was included in the medium (Fig. 6), while no similar ef-fect was seen on glucose transport. The effect of ammonium ions was also tested on glutamate uptake (Fig. 6), since increasing concentrations of ammonium ions influence its uptake in a similar fashion as increasing concentrations of K$^+$ ions (16).

CONCLUSIONS

The perfused hippocampal slice is a useful in vitro model in which a number of features characteristic of hepatic coma can be reproduced when the slice is subjected to pathophysiological concentrations of ammonium chloride. The spontaneous action potentials are suppressed in a reversible fashion, glutamine and glutamate production is increased, and acetate transport is inhibited. The present results indicate that a depletion of the releasable pool of transmitter glutamate may be an important factor for the etiology of hepatic coma, since the decreased possibility to utilize glutamine for glutamate biosynthesis is not adequately compensated for by the increased rate of glucose metabolism.

Acknowledgements

This work was supported by grants from the Swedish Medical Research Council (B80-12X-00164-16A) and from Axel & Margaret Ax:son Johnsons Stiftelse. The skilful secretarial assistance of Miss G. Grönstedt is acknowledged.

REFERENCES

1. Aickin, C.C., Deisz, R.A., and Lux, H.D. (1980): J.Physiol. (Lond.), 300: 40.
2. Balasz, R. and Cremer, J.E. (eds.)(1973): Metabolic Compartmentation in the Brain. MacMillan, London
3. Benjamin, A.M., Okamoto, K., and Quastel, J.H. (1978): J. Neurochem., 30, 131-143.
4. Berl, S. (1971): Exp.Biol. Med., 4: 71-84.
5. Berl, S., Takagaki, G., Clarke, D.D., and Waelsch, H. (1962): J. Biol. Chem., 237: 2562-2569.
6. Bradford, H.F.,and Ward, H.K. (1975): Biochem.Soc.Trans., 3: 1223-1226.
7. Bradford, H.F.,and Ward, K.K. (1976): Brain Research,110: 115-125.
8. Breen, K.J.,and Schenker, S. (1972): Progr. in Liver Disease, 4: 301-331.
9. Cavanagh, J.B. (1974): In: Brain Dysfunction in Metabolic Disorders, edited by F. Plum, Vol. 53, pp. 13-38, Raven Press, New York.
10. Cole, M., Rutherford, R.B., and Smith, F.O.: Arch.Neurol.,26: 130-136.
11. Cotman, C.W.,and Hamberger, A. (1978): In: Amino Acids as Chemical Transmitters, edited by F. Fonnum, pp. 379-413. Plenum Press, New York.
12. Crawford, I.L., and Connor, J.D. (1973): Nature, 244: 442-443.
13. Cremer, J.E. (1976): In: Advances in Experimental Medicine and Biology, Vol. 69, Transport Phenomena in the Nervous System, edited by G.Levi, L.Battistin, and A. Lajtha, pp.95-102. Plenum Press, New York and London.

14. Fernström, J.D., and Wurtman, R.J. (1972): Science, 178: 414-416.
15. Fischer, J.E. (1974): In: Res.Publ.Assoc.Nerv.Ment.Dis., Vol. 53, Brain Dysfunction in Metabolic Disorders, edited by F. Plum, pp. 53-73. Raven Press, New York.
16. Hamberger, A., Hedquist, B., and Nyström, B.: J. Neurochem., 33, 1295-1302.
17. Hamberger, A., Hedquist, B., Lundborg, H., and Nyström, B. (1980): J. Neurosci. Res. (in press).
18. Henn, F.A., Goldstein, M.N., and Hamberger, A. (1974): Nature, 249: 663-664.
19. Hindfelt, B.: (1975): Ann.N.Y.Acad.Sci., 252: 116-123.
20. Hirayama, C. (1971): Clin.Chim. Acta, 32: 191-197.
21. Iles, J.F., and Jack, J.J.B. (1978): J. Physiol. (Lond.), 280, 20.
22. Ishida, Y. (1967): Jap.J.Pharmac.,17: 6-18.
23. Lindroth, P., and Mopper, K. (1979): Analyt.Chem.,51: 1667-1674
24. Lunzer, M.James, I.M., Weinman, I., and Sherlock, S. (1974): Gut., 15: 555-561.
25. Lux, H.D., Loracher, C., and Neher, E. (1970): Exp.Brain Res., 11, 431-447.
26. Maiolo, A.T., Bianchi Porro, G., Galli, C., Sessa, M., and Polli, E.E. (1971): Exp Biol. Med. 4: 52-70.
27. Matheson, D.F., and Van den Berg, C.I. (1975): Biochem. Soc. Trans. 3: 525-528.
28. Matthews, D.E., Cotman, C., and Lynch, G. (1976): Brain Research, 115: 1-21.
29. Nicklas, W.J., Nunez, R., Berl, S., and Duvoisin, R.(1979): 33: 839-344.
30. Nicoll, R.A., and Iwamoto, E.T. (1978): In: Neuronal Information Transfer, edited by A.Karlin, V.M.Tennyson and H.J.Vogel, pp. 241-267. Academic Press, New York.
31. Norenberg, M.D., and Martinez-Hernandez, A. (1979): Brain Research, 161: 303-310.
32. Ogihara, K., Mozai, T., and Hirai, S. (1966): N.Engl.J.Med., 275: 1255-1256.
33. Salganicoff, L., and De Robertis, E. (1965): J.Neurochem., 12: 287-309.
34. Sarna, G.S., Bradbury, N.W.B., Cremer, J.E., Lai, J.C.K., and Teal, H.M. (1979): Brain Research, 160: 69-83.
35. Schenker, S., Breen, K.J., and Hoyumpa, A.M.(1974): Gastroenterology, 66: 121-151.
36. Sellström, Å., and A. Hamberger (1975): J. Neurochem. 24: 847-852.
37. Storm-Mathisen, J. (1972): Brain Research 40, 215-235.
38. Tsukada, Y. (1971): In: Handbook of Neurochemistry, Vol. 5, Metabolic Turnover in the Nervous System, edited by A. Lajtha, pp. 215-233. Plenum Press, New York.
39. Tursky, T., Ruscak, M., Lassanova, M., and Ruscakova, D. (1979): J. Neurochem., 33: 1209-1215.

40. Van den Berg, C.J., and Garfinkel, D.A. (1971): Biochem.J., 123: 211-218.
41. Warren, K.S., and Schenker, S. (1964): J.Lab.Clin.Med., 64: 442-449.
42. White, W.F., Nadler, J.V., Hamberger, A., and Cotman, C.W. (1977): Nature, 270: 356-357.
43. Weiler, C.T., Nyström, B., and Hamberger, A. (1979): J.Neurochem., 32: 559-565.
44. Weiler, C.T., Nyström, B., and Hamberger, A. (1979): Brain Research, 160: 539-543.
45. Zieve, L., and Nicoloff, D.M. (1975): Ann.Rev.Med., 26: 143-157.

Glutamate as a Neurotransmitter,
edited by G. Di Chiara and G. L. Gessa
Raven Press, New York © 1981.

GABA Potentiates the Depolarization-induced Release of Glutamate from Cerebellar Nerve Endings

Giulio Levi, Vittorio Gallo, and *Maurizio Raiteri

*Laboratorio di Biologia Cellulare, 00196 Rome, Italy; and *Istituto di Farmacologia e Farmacognosia, Facoltà di Farmacia, University of Genova, Italy*

The nature of the excitatory neurotransmitters in the cerebellum has not yet been determined with certainty. There are good indications that glutamate or aspartate may be the transmitters of the parallel fiber and of the climbing fiber terminals (10, 13, 18, 19, 20, 26), but not all the data of the literature are fully consistent with this hypothesis (15, 20). Much more agreement exists on the idea that GABA is the major inhibitory transmitter in the cerebellar cortex (5, 7, 14, 23, 25). The putative "glutamergic" excitatory cells and nerve terminals are thus embedded in a milieu which is largely GABAergic. In this particular anatomical situation, the possibility that GABA might interfere with the neurotransmission mediated by the excitatory fibers seemed to us likely and worth being analyzed.

In the present paper we shall first provide additional biochemical evidence in favor of the hypothesis that glutamate has a neurotransmitter role in the cerebellum, and then we shall show data suggesting that cerebellar "glutamergic" neurotransmission is potentiated by GABA through a mechanism involving GABA receptors localized in glutamate-releasing nerve terminals.

BIOCHEMICAL EVIDENCE IN FAVOR OF A NEUROTRANSMITTER ROLE OF GLUTAMATE

It is generally accepted that a neurotransmitter candidate must satisfy, among others, the following biochemical criteria: i) It must be synthesized and stored in nerve endings. ii) It must be released by depolarizing stimuli in a Ca^{2+}-dependent way. iii) After being released, it must interact with postsynaptic receptors. In the following paragraphs we shall try to verify whether gluta-

mate satisfies these criteria in the cerebellum. Some aspects of
these problems have been previously analyzed by others (8, 12, 20).

Ca^{2+}-dependent release and synthesis of glutamate in cerebellar nerve endings

Glutamate may be present in nerve endings in at least three
pools, which may have different functional significance: a "storage" pool, a "reuptake" pool (deriving from accumulation of exogenous glutamate), and a "new synthesis" pool (consisting of the
most recently synthesized amino acid). In our experiments, we labelled the last two pools with different isotopes, and monitored
simultaneously the depolarization-induced release from the three
pools. In most cases, the "reuptake" pool was labelled by allowing
cerebellar synaptosomes to take up ^{3}H-D-aspartate, rather than radioactive L-glutamate. D-aspartate offers the advantage of not
being metabolized, utilizes the same transport system as L-glutamate (1) and, in our release experiments, always showed the same
behavior as ^{14}C-L-glutamate. The "new synthesis" pool was labelled
by exposing the synaptosomes to ^{14}C-glutamine, a glutamate precursor which is particularly useful to measure the synthesis of glutamate occurring in nerve endings, since the enzyme responsible
for the conversion, g l u t a m i n a s e , seems to be localized
specifically in these structures (3) and has been proposed as a
marker of "glutamergic" nerve terminals. The superfusion conditions utilized in these experiments were such to assure that any
^{14}C-glutamate present in synaptosomes at any time derived only
from new synthesis, and not from reuptake of the newly formed
^{14}C-glutamate which is progressively released from synaptosomes
(11, 16, 17).

Figure 1 shows that depolarization of synaptosomes with 30 mM
KCl caused a release of ^{3}H-D-aspartate which was apparently not
potentiated by the presence of Ca^{2+} in the superfusion medium.
Sandoval and Cotman (20) had previously shown that exogenous radioactive glutamate is not released from cerebellar synaptosomal
preparations in a Ca^{2+}-dependent way. Fig. 1 demonstrates also
that a substantial release of ^{3}H-D-aspartate was evoked by Ca^{2+}
removal, independently of depolarization. As ^{3}H-D-aspartate is
actively taken up by cerebellar glial cells and is promptly released from glial cultures into Ca^{2+}-free media (Gordon, Wilkin,
Gallo, Levi and Balàzs, in preparation), and since our synaptosomal preparations might contain functional "gliosomes", the results
of Fig. 1 do not tell us clearly whether the ^{3}H-D-aspartate present in nerve endings is released in a Ca^{2+}-dependent way. Table 1,

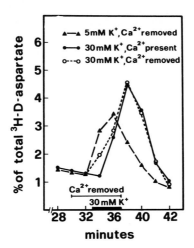

FIG. 1. Effect of Ca^{2+} on the depolarization-induced release of ^{3}H-D-aspartate from cerebellar synaptosomes. Crude
synaptosomal fractions (P_2) preincubated for 10 min in the
presence of 90 nM ^{3}H-D-aspartate were superfused on Milli-
pore filters in parallel chambers thermostated at 37°C (17),
first for 5 min with standard medium, and then for 15 min
with a medium containing 24 µM ^{14}C-glutamine (0.5 µCi/ml).
After washing for 6 min, the superfusion was continued, and
2 min fractions were collected into cooled vials. The superfusion medium was changed as and when indicated in the figure. Aliquots of perchloric acid extracts of the filters and
of the various fractions were counted for radioactivity, the
rest was used for the glutamate determinations reported in
Table 1. The ^{3}H-D-aspartate released in each fraction is given as a percentage of the total ^{3}H-D-aspartate recovered
(total fractions from the time of collection (min 28) plus
filter at the end of superfusion). Each curve is the average
of 4 experiments (dark circles) or of 2 experiments (triangles), all run in duplicate.

however, demonstrates that the release of endogenous glutamate was
Ca^{2+}-dependent, in agreement with the findings of others (20).
Table 1 also shows that the newly synthesized ^{14}C-glutamate, which
should be the most representative of the glutamate present in
nerve endings (3), had a release pattern which was practically su-
perimposable to that of endogenous, unlabelled glutamate. Moreover,
the third column of Table 1 presents data supporting the existence
of an active synthesis of ^{14}C-glutamate from ^{14}C-glutamine in the

TABLE 1. Ca^{2+}-dependent, depolarization-induced release of endogenous and newly synthesized glutamate from cerebellar synaptosomes

	endogenous (pmol/mg prot.)	neo-synthesized (cpm/0.25 mg prot.)	^{14}C-glu as % of total ^{14}C	N
Synaptosomes (start of release)	12,400 ± 600	10,000 ± 800	59 ± 2	7
Ca^{2+} present				
Spontaneous release	201 ± 17	275 ± 24	29 ± 3	14
Stimulated "	1,550 ± 70	1,400 ± 144	61 ± 1	10
Ca^{2+} removed				
Spontaneous release	385 ± 30	372 ± 70	27 ± 3	4
Stimulated "	734 ± 46	699 ± 53	50 ± 2	8

Experimental details are described in the legend for Fig. 1. Total glutamate (column 1) and newly synthesized ^{14}C-glutamate (column 2) were measured in synaptosomes at the 30th min of superfusion and in the fractions collected at the 38th min (that is at the time at which the release induced by 30 mM KCl was highest, see Fig. 1). The third column shows the counts of ^{14}C-glutamate as a percentage of the total ^{14}C-radioactivity present in the various samples analyzed. Means ± S.E.M. are presented.

synaptosomal preparation used. At the start of the release phase of the experiment (that is after 15 min of superfusion with 24 μM ^{14}C-glutamine), over half of the radioactivity present in synaptosomes was represented by ^{14}C-glutamate. In the absence of stimulation, ^{14}C-glutamate accounted for less than 30% of the radioactivity released, but during depolarization the relative amount of ^{14}C-glutamate released became similar to that present in synaptosomes at the beginning of the release period.

In conclusion, these results indicate that glutamate is actively synthesized in cerebellar nerve endings and is released from them by depolarization in a Ca^{2+}-dependent way.

Interaction of endogenously released glutamate with glutamate receptors

It has been suggested that the interaction of glutamate with cerebellar postsynaptic receptors results into an increase of the concentration of cGMP. The evidence supporting this suggestion

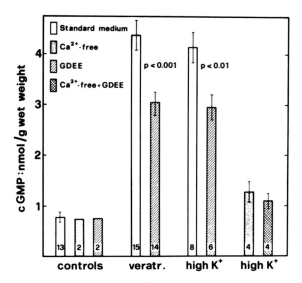

FIG. 2. Inhibition by GDEE (glutamate diethylester) of the depolarization-induced increase of cGMP level in cerebellar slices. Sagittal slices (0.42 mm thick) were incubated at 37°C in a glucose-containing Krebs–Ringer medium, in O_2 atmosphere. After 100 min, the incubation medium was replaced with new, prewarmed medium or, when indicated, with a Ca^{2+}-free medium containing 0.5 mM EGTA. After another 10 min, 1 mM GDEE was added to the appropriate incubation flasks. At min 120 the slices were depolarized with 75 μM veratridine or 45 mM KCl, and at min 125 the incubation was stopped by filtering the slices and transferring them, within few seconds, in Tris–EDTA buffer (pH 7.5) at 95°C. Cyclic GMP was determined by radioimmunoassay (Amersham Radiochemical Centre). Means ± S.E.M. are presented. The number of experiments is given at the bottom of each bar. The statistical significance of the effect of GDEE on the depolarization-induced increase of cGMP was calculated by the Student's "t" test.

consists essentially of the observation that <u>exogenous</u> glutamate causes a rise in the cGMP level in the cerebellum (4, 8, 12, 21), and that this rise is prevented by the glutamate antagonist GDEE (glutamic acid diethylester) (4, 21). The experiment reported in Fig. 2 was planned to determine whether the release of <u>endogenous</u> glutamate elicited by depolarizing stimuli could elevate the concentration of the cyclic nucleotide in cerebellar slices. It has been previously shown that depolarization of cerebellar slices leads to a severalfold increase in the level of cGMP (21). If this increase were partly due to the glutamate released, it should be counteracted in part by GDEE, which is, by itself, without effect (21, see also Fig. 2). The data of Fig. 2 show that, in the presence of GDEE, the rise of cGMP observed in cerebellar slices depolarized with either veratridine of high K^+ was substantially lowered. Interestingly, when the depolarizing stimulus was applied in the absence of Ca^{2+}, cGMP level increased much less than in the presence of the cation, and this increase was not prevented by GDEE. The data are thus consistent with the idea that the endogenous glutamate released by depolarization in a Ca^{2+}-dependent way from nerve terminals evokes an elevation in the level of cGMP, through an interaction with postsynaptic glutamate receptors.

EFFECT OF GABA ON THE DEPOLARIZATION-INDUCED RELEASE OF GLUTAMATE FROM CEREBELLAR NERVE ENDINGS

The data presented up to now support the idea that glutamate functions as a neurotransmitter in the cerebellum. Since the putative "glutamergic" nerve terminals are localized in an environment which is largely GABAergic, we analyzed whether GABA could have a role in the control of glutamate release.

The results reported in Fig. 3 (panels A, B and C) show that GABA caused a substantial increase of the depolarization-induced release of ^{3}H-D-aspartate and ^{14}C-glutamate from cerebellar synaptosomal preparations. The effect was present at micromolar GABA concentrations and was concentration-dependent. The GABA agonist muscimol behaved similarly to GABA, and the effect of both substances was largely prevented by picrotoxin and bicuculline, two classical antagonists at the level of GABA receptors (6, 22, 24).

GABA and, to a lesser extent, muscimol stimulated somewhat also the spontaneous release of radioactive D-aspartate and glutamate, but this effect was not inhibited by the two antagonists.

The specificity of the antagonistic effect of picrotoxin and bicuculline in the experiments reported above was corroborated by the observation that neither one inhibited the K^+-induced release of D-aspartate or L-glutamate when GABA or muscimol were not present (data not shown).

The potentiating effect of GABA on ^{3}H-D-aspartate release showed a regional specificity, since it was not detectable with synaptosomes prepared from the cerebral cortex (Fig. 3, panel D). Experiments with other brain areas are now in progress.

In view of the possibility outlined above that ^{3}H-D-aspartate

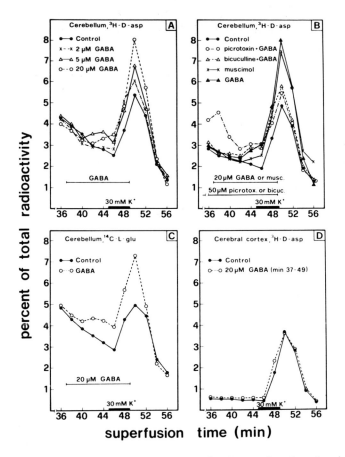

FIG. 3. Effect of GABA and muscimol on the depolarization -induced release of ^{3}H-D-aspartate and ^{14}C-glutamate from cerebellar synaptosomes (panels A, B and C), and lack of effect with cortical synaptosomes (panel D). P_2 fractions were equilibrated in a Krebs-Ringer medium at 37°C for 10 min, and then superfused, first with standard medium for 5 min, then for 15 min with a medium containing 6 nM ^{3}H-D-aspartate (panels A, B and D) or 1-^{14}C-L-glutamate (panel C). In some experiments of panel B, the superfusion medium contained, in addition to ^{3}H-D-aspartate, 24 μM ^{14}C-glutamine (see Table 2 for results). After washing for 6 min, the superfusion was continued, and 2 min fractions were collected. The superfusion medium was changed as indicated in the various panels. The results are expressed as in Fig. 2. Each curve is the average of 2 experiments (panels A and C), 3 experiments (panel D) or 4-6 experiments (panel B), all run in duplicate.

TABLE 2.   Effect of GABA on the depolarization-induced release of glutamate from cerebellar synaptosomes

	endogenous (pmol/mg prot.)	neo-synthesized (cpm/0.25 mg prot.)
Prestimulation		
Control	160 ± 10 (4)	113 ± 19 (6)
20 μM GABA	190 ± 60 (3)	187 ± 24 (4)
20 μM GABA + 50 μM picrotoxin	180 (2)	200 ± 42 (3)
Stimulation (30 mM KCl)		
Control	1,040 ± 50 (9)	897 ± 42 (6)
20 μM GABA	1,110 ± 70 (9)	1,545 ± 34 (7)
20 μM GABA + 50 μM picrotoxin	1,020 ± 90 (7)	1,094 ± 103 (6)

The release of endogenous glutamate and that of ^{14}C-glutamate synthesized from ^{14}C-glutamine was determined in fractions collected at min 46 (prestimulation) and at min 50 (stimulation) of superfusion, in experiments reported in Fig. 3, panel B. Means ± S.E.M. are presented. The number of determinations is given in parentheses.

is taken up also by "gliosomes" contaminating the synaptosomal preparations, it seemed necessary to determine whether GABA potentiated the K^+-induced release of endogenous glutamate and of glutamate recently synthesized from glutamine. The results of these experiments (Table 2) show that GABA caused a picrotoxin sensitive increase in the release of ^{14}C-glutamate previously synthesized from ^{14}C-glutamine, but did not affect the overall release of endo genous glutamate elicited by depolarization with 30 mM KCl. Thus, only the "reuptake" and the "new synthesis" pools of glutamate appear to be released in a way which is susceptible to modulation by GABA. This modulation is likely to occur at the level of GABA receptors located in presynaptic "glutamergic" nerve endings, since this is the structure where most of the synthesis of glutamic acid from glutamine takes place (3).

The lack of effect of GABA on the total release of endogenous glutamate is probably due to the fact that the "new synthesis" plus the "reuptake" pools represent only a small fraction of the total glutamate releasable by depolarization. What, in our opinion, remains to be established is whether all the endogenous glutamate released by depolarization in a Ca^{2+}-dependent way (Table 1)

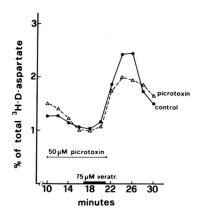

FIG. 4. Effect of picrotoxin on the veratridine-induced release of ³H-D-aspartate from cerebellar slices. Slices (1.5 x 0.3 x 0.3 mm) were incubated at 37°C in glucose-containing medium for 25 min (the last 10 min in the presence of 0.17 μM ³H-D-aspartate), then washed and superfused for 10 min with standard medium. The composition of the medium was then changed as indicated in the figure. Fractions were collected every 2 min. The release of ³H-D-aspartate is expressed as in Fig. 1. Each curve is the average of 5 duplicate or triplicate experiments.

specifically belongs to the glutamate "neurotransmitter" pool.

We have previously mentioned that, in experiments with cerebellar synaptosomes, picrotoxin antagonizes the effect of GABA on the high K⁺-induced glutamate release, but has no influence on the depolarization-induced release of glutamate in the absence of GABA. In order to determine whether the stimulus-coupled release of glutamate could be potentiated by <u>endogenously</u> released GABA, we depolarized cerebellar slices (which may maintain the anatomical connections between GABA-releasing and glutamate-releasing sites) with veratridine (a depolarizing agent which should act mainly on neuronal membranes (2)), and analyzed the effect of picrotoxin on the evoked release of ³H-D-aspartate. Since the GABA antagonist inhibited ³H-D-aspartate release (Fig. 4), this experiment gives additional, although indirect support to the idea that the release of glutamate in the cerebellum is regulated in part by the release of GABA through a mechanism mediated by GABA receptors present in presynaptic "glutamergic" terminals.

The anatomical connections that are at the basis of this regulation can be, so far, only matter of speculation. GABA might be released on parallel fiber or climbing fiber terminals either by cells receiving the "glutamergic" innervation (e.g. Purkinje cells might release GABA from collaterals of their axons or, if release from dendrites (9) is a general phenomenon, from their ramified dendritic tree). Alternatively, GABA might reach the "glutamergic" terminals after being released from GABAergic interneurons (e.g. from the dendrites of Golgi cells or from the stellate cells of the molecular layer). According to the first hypothesis, Purkinje cells would be subject to a sort of positive feed-back mechanism, whereby GABA release would result into a potentiation of the excitation of these cells, and thus into greater GABA release. The circuit could be interrupted only when the activity of the excitatory cells (granule cells or cells of the inferior olive projecting to the cerebellum) comes to a stop. According to the second hypothesis, the GABAergic interneurons would control the GABAergic output of the cerebellum grace to their ability to modulate the release of glutamate from the excitatory terminals innervating the Purkinje cells. Certainly, one can hypothesize other models, but in any case it should be considered that the ultimate result of the potentiating effect of GABA on glutamate release described in the present report would be a potentiation of inhibition, because "glutamergic" terminals inpinge upon GABAergic cells.

ACKNOWLEDGEMENTS

We thank Mrs. M.T. Ciotti and Mr. A. Coletti for excellent assistence. Muscimol was kindly donated by Ciba-Geigy, picrotoxin and bicuculline by Dr. M. Massotti. This investigation was supported in part by NATO Research Grant n. RG 058.80 and by Grant CT79. 01889.04 of the Italian National Research Council.

REFERENCES

1. Balcar, V.J., and Johnston, G.A.R. (1972): J. Neurochem., 19: 2657-2666.
2. Benjamin, A.M. and Quastel, J.H. (1972): Biochem. J., 128: 631-646.
3. Bradford, H.F., Ward, H.K. and Thomas, A.J. (1978): J. Neurochem., 30: 1453-1459.
4. Briley, P.A., Konyoumdjian, J.C., Haidamous, M. and Gonnard, P. (1979): Eur. J. Pharmacol., 54: 181-184.
5. Curtis, D.R. and Johnston, G.A.R. (1974): Ergebn. Physiol., 69: 97-188.
6. Enna, S.J., Collins, J.F. and Snyder, S.H. (1977): Brain Res.,

124: 185-190.

7. Fonnum, F.I., Storm-Mathisen, J. and Walberg, F. (1970): Brain Res., 20: 259-275.

8. Garthwaite, J. and Balàzs, R. (1978): Nature, 275: 328-329.

9. Geffen, L.B., Jessel, T.M., Cuello, A.C. and Iversen, L.L. (1976): Nature, 260: 258-260.

10. Guidotti, A., Biggio, G. and Costa, E. (1976): Brain Res., 109: 632-635.

11. Levi, G. and Raiteri, M. (1978): Proc. Natl. Acad. Sci. (USA), 75: 2981-2985.

12. Mao, C.C., Guidotti, A. and Costa, E. (1974): Brain Res., 79: 510-514.

13. Mc Bride, W.J., Nadi, N.S., Altman, J. and Aprison, M.H. (1976): Neurochem. Res., 1: 141-152.

14. Mc Laughlin, B.J., Wood, J.G., Saite, K., Barber, R., Vaughen, J.E., Roberts, E. and Wu, J.P. (1978): Brain Res., 76: 377-391.

15. Patel, A.J. and Balàzs, R. (1975): Radiat. Res., 62: 456-469.

16. Raiteri, M., Angelini, F. and Levi, G. (1974): Eur. J. Pharmacol., 25: 411-414.

17. Raiteri, M. and Levi, G. (1978): In: Reviews of Neuroscience, Vol. 3, edited by S. Ehrenpreis, and I. Kopin, pp. 77-130. Raven Press, New York.

18. Roffler-Tarlov, S. and Sidman, R.L. (1978): Brain Res., 142: 269-283.

19. Rhode, B.H., Rea, M.A., Simon, J.R. and Mc Bride, W.J. (1979): J. Neurochem., 32: 1431-1435.

20. Sandoval, M.E. and Cotman, C.W. (1978): Neuroscience, 3: 199-206.

21. Schmidt, M.J., Ryan, J.J. and Molloy, B.B. (1976): Brain Res., 112: 113-126.

22. Simmonds, M.A. (1980): Neuropharmacology, 19: 39-45.

23. Storm-Mathisen, J. (1976): In: GABA in Nervous System Function, edited by E. Roberts, T.N. Chase and D.B. Tower, pp. 149-168. Raven Press, New York.

24. Ticku, M.K., Ban, M. and Olsen, R.W. (1978): Molec. Pharmacol., 14: 391-402.

25. Wilkin, G.P., Wilson, J.E., Balàzs, R., Schon, F. and Kelly, J.S. (1974): Nature, 252: 397-399.

26. Young, A.B., Oster-Granite, M.L., Herndon, R.M. and Snyder, S.H. (1974): Brain Res., 73: 1-13.

Glutamate as a Neurotransmitter,
edited by G. Di Chiara and G. L. Gessa
Raven Press, New York © 1981.

Action of Baclofen and Pentobarbital on Amino Acid Release

S. J. Potashner and *N. Lake

*Department of Anatomy, University of Connecticut Health Center,
Farmington, Connecticut 06032; and *Department of Research in Anaesthesia,
McGill University, Montreal, Quebec, H3G 1Y6, Canada*

The action of drugs which depress activity in the CNS commonly includes effects on synaptic function. Although it is often hypothesized that such compounds may exert their effects by potentiating inhibitory transmission mediated by GABA, other actions could be involved. For example, such drugs might conceivably alter tissue stores of transmitters, suppress or enhance the release of transmitters, alter the postsynaptic response to transmitters, or interfere with the removal of transmitters from the region of the synapse.

Both baclofen, an antispastic agent, and pentobarbital, a sedative-hypnotic, depress excitatory transmission in the CNS. At doses useful in antispastic therapy (i.e. $\leq$ 2 mg/kg), baclofen is particularly effective in depressing synaptic transmission in the spinal cord and cuneate nucleus (3,10,15,30-32). This action could be mediated largely by a suppression of excitatory transmitter release from primary afferents, since baclofen does not significantly increase the efficacy of inhibitory transmission, or alter the excitability of primary afferents, spinal motoneurons, and cuneothalamic cells (10,15,29,31). On the other hand, anaesthetic doses of barbiturates apparently depress central excitatory transmission by several mechanisms. They enhance pre- and postsynaptic inhibition mediated by GABA(2,11,22,24-28), depress the electrical and chemical excitability of neurons (2,5, 7,8,21,25,27,28,38,43), inhibit the release of acetylcholine from brain (39), and inhibit transmission at several synapses in a manner suggesting a block of excitatory transmitter release (2,6,16,23,37,41,42,44).

Because the actions of baclofen and barbiturates suggested effects on transmitter release, it was of interest to determine directly if these drugs altered the release of several amino acids considered to be central transmitters.

Amino acid release from slices of cerebral neocortex

Using a Stadie-Riggs microtome, tangential slices (300μ thick) were taken from the neocortex of male, albino guinea pigs (300-400g), and preincubated (37°C, 30-45 min) in Elliott's B medium (12). Tissues were then incubated in fresh, glucose-free medium containing either D-(U-^{14}C)glucose or a labelled amino acid. After 45 min, slices were superfused with fresh isotope-free medium for 30 min, while superfusate was collected as fractions. Following 10 min of superfusion, slices were stimulated electrically for 4 min to evoke amino acid release. Other details have been given elsewhere (33-35) of the preparation, incubation, superfusion, and stimulation of the tissue slices. The levels and the radioactivity of amino acids in tissue slices, and in collected superfusate fractions, were analyzed as described previously (33-35).

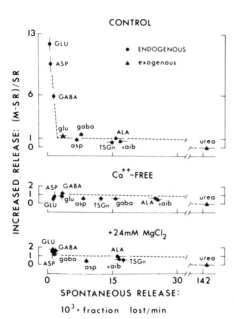

FIG. 1. Amino acid release from cerebral cortex slices. Electrical stimulation of slices resulted in a transient increase in release. The maximum increase in release was plotted on the ordinate as a function of the prestimulation spontaneous release (SR) on the abcissa. The increased release (IR) was calculated using the equation IR = (M-SR)/SR, where M is the maximum release attained on stimulation. In experiments with high Mg^{++}, $MgCl_2$ was added to control media. Data are means ± S.E.M., and are taken from ref. (34). GLU,glutamate; ASP, aspartate; GABA,γ-aminobutyrate; ALA, alanine; TSGn, threonine-serine-glutamine (unseparated);α-AIB, α-aminoisobutyrate.

Electrical stimulation of the slices resulted in a transient increase in the release of endogenous ^{14}C-glutamate, ^{14}C-aspartate, ^{14}C-GABA, ^{14}C-alanine, and ^{14}C-threonine-serine-glutamine (unseparated), which were synthesized via metabolism of the D-(U-^{14}C)glucose (33). Stimulus-evoked transient increases were also observed in the release of exogenous glutamate, aspartate, GABA and α-aminoisobutyrate, which had been taken up by the tissue during the previous incubation period (33). In addition, the increases in the release of endogenously synthesized ^{14}C-glutamate, ^{14}C-aspartate, and ^{14}C-GABA were considerably larger than those of the other compounds (upper plot in Fig.1). All increases in release, except those of ^{14}C-threonine-serine-glutamine, were abolished by tetrodotoxin (34), suggesting that the electrical stimulus produced excitation mainly in axons by opening voltage-sensitive Na^+ channels.

On arrival of the excitation at axon terminals, the entry of Ca^{++} into the nerve endings (1) is an apparent prerequisite to the coupling of the excitation to the release of transmitter(40); Ca^{++}-deprivation, or antagonism of Ca^{++} entry into terminals, blocks the synaptic release of transmitter. Both Ca^{++}-deprivation, and treatment with high Mg^{++} to block Ca^{++} entry into terminals, suppressed selectively the large stimulus-evoked increase in the release of endogenously synthesized ^{14}C-glutamate, ^{14}C-aspartate, and ^{14}C-GABA (Fig. 1). These findings are consistent with the stimulus-evoked release of endogenous ^{14}C-glutamate, ^{14}C-aspartate, and ^{14}C-GABA originating from a synaptic site.

Baclofen.
The action of baclofen was measured by including the drug in the incubation and superfusion media. A concentration of 4 µM was used; this approximated the peak plasma level resulting from the largest subsedative doses administered in the clinical trials of Knutsson et al (19). Stimulus-evoked release of all amino acids could still be observed in the presence of baclofen. However the drug selectively inhibited the evoked release of endogenous ^{14}C-glutamate and ^{14}C-aspartate (Fig. 2), without changing their concentrations in the tissue, their synthesis from ^{14}C-glucose, or their turnover (35).

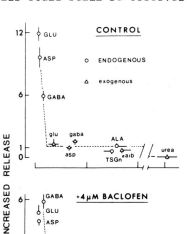
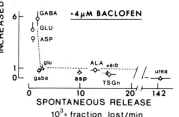

FIG.2. Baclofen and amino acid release from cortex slices. Release is quantitated as in Fig. 1. Data are means ± S.E.M. and are taken from ref. (35).

In view of the possibility that glutamate is the transmitter of some primary afferents projecting to the spinal cord and cuneate nucleus (4,9,18,20), and that aspartate may be the transmitter of some spinal interneurons (9,18,20), the present findings (Fig. 2) are consistent with the inhibition by baclofen of mono- and polysynaptic reflex transmission in the spinal cord, and of transmission through the cuneate nucleus (3,10,15,29,31, 32). Also, the lack of effect on the evoked release of endogenous GABA (Fig. 2) is in accord with the preservation of inhibitory transmission in the spinal cord when EPSPs in motoneurons were inhibited by baclofen (15,31). Therefore should the selective inhibition by baclofen of glutamate and aspartate release obtain in the spinal cord, it may at least partly underlie the antispastic action of the drug.

Pentobarbital.
The action of pentobarbital was also measured by adding the drug to the incubation and superfusion media which, for these experiments, contained 3mM glucose. A concentration of 100μM pentobarbital was used, which is near the level of free pentobarbital found in plasma during surgical anaesthesia (13,14,17), and is without effect on the electrical excitability of neurons (2,37,43,44). Pentobarbital decreased the evoked release of endogenous ^{14}C-glutamate and ^{14}C-aspartate, and increased the release of endogenous ^{14}C-GABA (Fig. 3). There were no significant changes in the evoked release of the other endogenous labelled amino acids (Fig. 3), or in the evoked release of the exogenous amino acids. Similar results were obtained when the experiments were performed in glucose-free media.

The effects above were not due to a primary inhibitory action on GABA uptake which might have resulted in more GABA in the extracellular tissue space and in the collected superfusion fluid. 100μM pentobarbital stimulated, rather than inhibited, the uptake of 10μM GABA (also see 45), and had no effect on the uptake of 1mM GABA or 10μM glutamate. Also, pentobarbital did not change the tissue levels of glutamate, aspartate, and GABA, or the incorporation and turnover of ^{14}C in glutamate and GABA. However, the drug did increase the incorporation and turnover of ^{14}C in tissue aspartate. Since the specific radioactivity of aspartate released by stimulation was unaffected by pentobarbital (Fig. 3), changes in aspartate metabolism in the tissue were probably confined to pools other than those released by the electrical stimulus.

Therefore, pentobarbital probably alters cortical transmission mediated by amino acids in two ways: first, by direct action on inhibitory neurons to facilitate the synaptic release of GABA; second, by inhibiting the synaptic release of the excitatory amino acids, glutamate and aspartate. The latter may involve a direct action of the drug on excitatory neurons, an enhanced synaptic release of GABA, a potentiation of the

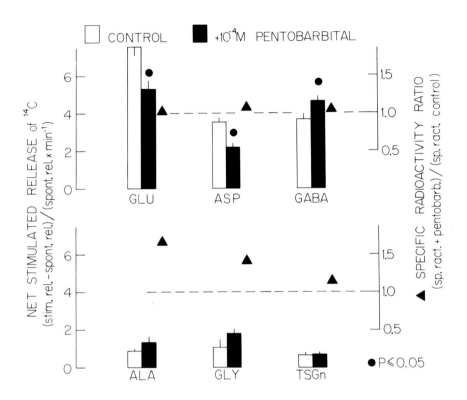

FIG. 3. Pentobarbital and evoked release of endogenous amino acids from cortex slices. The Net Stimulated Release (NSR) and the Specific Radioactivity Ratio (SRR) for each amino acid in the superfusion medium were calculated as indicated above. Pentobarbital changes of the NSR's of five amino acids. However, the increases in the NSR's of ALA and GLY are accompanied by equivalent parallel shifts in their SRR's. Therefore, changes in the NSR's of these compounds reflect only an enrichment of ^{14}C-content rather than an increase in the amount released. Since changes in the NSR's of GLU, ASP, and GABA occur with no shifts in their SRR's, these changes reflect alterations in the amounts released. Data are means ± SEM of 4 experiments; SEM's of SRR's lie within the symbol used.

postsynaptic response to GABA, or a combination of the above. Further investigation is needed to distinguish between these possibilities.

The authors are grateful to the Medical Research Council of Canada and to the University of Connecticut Research Foundation for financial support.

REFERENCES

1. Baker, P.F. (1975): Calcium movement in excitable cells,edited by P.F. Baker and H. Reuter, pp. 7-53, Pergamon Press, Oxford.
2. Barker, J.L., and Ransome, B.R. (1978): J. Physiol. (Lond.), 280:355-372.
3. Bein, H.J. (1972): In: Spasticity - a topical survey, edited by W. Birkmayer, pp. 76-82, Huber, Vienna.
4. Berger, S.J., Carter, J.G., and Lowry, O.H. (1977): J. Neurochem., 28:149-158.
5. Bloom,F.E., Costa, E., and Salomiraghi, G.C. (1965): J. Pharmac. Exp. Therap., 150:244-252.
6. Brooks,C.M., and Eccles, J.C. (1947): J. Neurophysiol., 10:349-360.
7. Catchlove,R.F.H., Krnjeviċ, K., and Maretiċ, H. (1972): Can. J. Physiol. Pharmacol.., 50:1111-1114.
8. Crawford, J.M. (1970): Neuropharmacology, 9:31-46.
9. Davidoff, R.A., Graham, L.T., Shank, R.P., Werman, R., and Aprison,M.H. (1967): J. Neurochem., 14:1025-1031.
10. Davidoff,R.A., and Sears, E.S. (1974): Neurology, 24:957-963.
11. Eccles, J.C., Schmidt, R.F., and Willis, W.D. (1963): J. Physiol. (Lond.), 168:500-530.
12. Elliott,K.A.C. (1969): In: Handbook of Neurochemistry, Vol.2, edited by A. Lajtha, pp. 103-114, Plenum Press, New York.
13. Fisher, R.S., Walker, J.T., and Plummer, C.W. (1948): Am. J. Clin. Pathol., 18:462-469.
14. Forbes, A., Battista, A.F., Chatfield, P.O., and Garcia, J.P. (1949): EEG Clin. Neurophysiol., 1:141-175.
15. Fox, S., Krnjeviċ, K., Morris, M.E., Puil, E., and Werman, R. (1978): Neuroscience, 3:495-515.
16. Galindo, A. (1969): J. Pharmac. Exp. Therap., 169:185-195.
17. Goldbaum, L.R., and Smith, P.K. (1954): J. Pharmac. Exp. Therap., 111:197-209.
18. Johnson, J.L. (1978): Prog. in Neurobiol., 10:155-202.
19. Knutsson, E., Lindblom, U., and Martensson, A. (1974): J. Neurol. Sci., 23:473-484.
20. Krnjeviċ, K. (1974): Physiol. Rev., 54:418-540.
21. Krnjeviċ, K. (1974): In: Molecular mechanisms of general anaesthesia, edited by M. J. Halsey, R.A. Millar, and J.A. Sutton, pp. 65-89, Churchill-Livingston, New York.
22. Larson, M.D. and Major, M.A. (1970): Brain Res., 21:309-311.
23. Lǿyning, Y., Oshima, T., and Yokota, J. (1964): J. Neurophysiol., 27:408-428.

24. Nicoll, R.A. (1972): J. Physiol. (Lond.), 233:803-814.
25. Nicoll, R.A. (1975): Brain Res., 96: 119-123.
26. Nicoll, R.A. (1975): Proc. Nat. Acad. Sci. (Wash.) 72:1460-1463.
27. Nicoll, R.A., Eccles, J.C., Oshima, T., and Rubia, F.(1975): Nature, 258:625-627.
28. Nicoll, R.A., and Wojtowicz, J.M. (1980): Brain Res., 191:225-237.
29. Ono, H., Fukuda, H., and Kudo, Y. (1979): Neuropharmacology, 18:647-653.
30. Pierau, F.K., Matheson, G.K., and Wurster, R.D. (1975): Exp. Neurol., 48:343-351.
31. Pierau, F.K., and Zimmerman, P. (1973): Brain Res., 54:376-380.
32. Polc, P. and Haefely, W. (1976): Naunyn-Schmiedeberg's Arch. Pharmac., 294:121-131.
33. Potashner, S.J. (1978): J. Neurochem., 31:177-186.
34. Potashner, S.J. (1978): J. Neurochem., 31:187-195.
35. Potashner, S.J. (1979): J. Neurochem., 32:103-109.
36. Potashner, S.J., and Knowles, J.D. (1975): Anal. Biochem., 65:435-444.
37. Richards, C.D. (1972): J. Physiol. (Lond.), 227:749-767.
38. Richards, C.D., and Smaje, J.C. (1976): Br. J. Pharmac., 58:347-357.
39. Richter, J.A., and Waller, M.B. (1977): Biochem. Pharmacol., 26:609-615.
40. Rubin, R.P. (1974): In: Calcium in the secretory process, Plenum Press, New York.
41. Somjen, G.G. (1963): J. Pharmac. Exp. Therap., 140:393-402.
42. Somjen, G.G., and Gill, M. (1963): J. Pharmac. Exp. Therap., 140:19-30.
43. Staiman, A., and Seeman, P. (1974): Can. J. Physiol. Pharmacol., 52:535-550.
44. Weakley, J.N. (1969): J. Physiol. (Lond.), 204:63-77.
45. Weinberger, J., Nicklas, W. J., and Berl, S. (1976): Neurology, 26:162-166.

Glutamate as a Neurotransmitter,
edited by G. Di Chiara and G. L. Gessa
Raven Press, New York © 1981.

Effects of Pentobarbitone on the Synaptically Evoked Release of the Amino Acid Neurotransmitter Candidates Aspartate and GABA from Rat Olfactory Cortex

G. G. S. Collins

Department of Pharmacology, University of Sheffield, Sheffield, S10 2TN, United Kingdom

Two consistent actions of the barbiturates on the central nervous system are a potentiation of GABA – mediated inhibition and a depression of excitatory transmission (12). Conceivably, barbiturates may achieve these effects by either a presynaptic (changes in transmitter release) or postsynaptic (effects on receptor/membrane functioning) site of action. Using a synaptically intact preparation, the aim of the present study was to simultaneously assess the effects of pentobarbitone both on evoked electrical activity and neurotransmitter release in order to distinguish between these two possibilities.

For the following reasons, the preparation chosen for these studies was the isolated rat olfactory cortex slice (see Fig. 1). First, the basic neuronal circuitry is known. Second, at least some of the neurotransmitters (aspartate, glutamate and GABA) have been identified. Third, there is a specific afferent input (the lateral olfactory tract (LOT) which, when activated, evokes a series of field potentials which reflect excitatory and inhibitory synaptic activity within the slice. Fourth, because it is possible to measure release of the endogenous neurotransmitter candidates, it is possible to relate directly alterations in transmitter release with changes in evoked electrical activity – the primary aim of the present study. Finally, pentobarbitone dramatically affects synaptic transmission in this brain area (15,16,19).

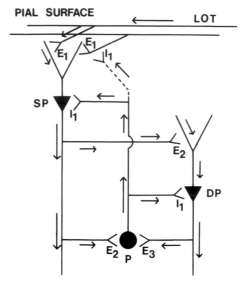

FIG. 1. Basic neuronal circuitry of the olfactory
cortex (not to scale). The lateral olfactory tract
(LOT) lies on the pial surface. The excitatory
transmitter (E_1) of the LOT collaterals depolarizes
the dendrites of the superficial pyramidal (SP) cells
(9,10,17,18) thereby giving rise to a massed
excitatory post synaptic potential recorded as the
surface N-wave (14,16,17,18,21). Chronic denervation
experiments (5,6,7) and release studies (5,6,8)
suggest that in the rat E_1 might be aspartate.
Collaterals from the SP cells release a second
excitatory transmitter (E_2) which excites both the
deep pyramidal (DP) cells and the deeper lying
polymorph (P) inhibitory interneurones (1). The
identities of E_2 and E_3 are unknown but they may be
aspartate and/or glutamate (3,6). Neuropharmacological investigations (15,19), release experiments
(5,6,8) and a depth distribution study (7) all
suggest that the inhibitory transmitter of the P
cells (I_1) is GABA. Once released, the GABA
depolarizes both DP and SP cells, thereby giving rise
to a massed depolarizing recurrent inhibitory postsynaptic potential recorded as the surface I-wave
(15). The GABA also depolarizes the LOT terminals,
thereby reducing release of E_1 (8) and giving rise to
the late N-wave (14).

METHODS

Rat olfactory cortex slices were prepared, preincubated and perfused at room temperature using the procedures described by Pickles & Simmonds (14,15). Evoked field potentials were monitored by a silver ball electrode sited on the pial surface, amplified using a DC preamplifier and the signals fed to a Datalab DL905 transient recorder. Release of endogenous amino acids from the pial surface was monitored using a cortical cup technique (6). The amounts of endogenous glutamate, aspartate, glutamine, GABA and taurine released into the solution within the cup was estimated using a sensitive double-label microdansylation procedure (4). Results have been expressed in terms of the mean total of each amino acid released (in pmole) in excess of or below the mean resting efflux (see refs. 6,8).

RESULTS AND DISCUSSION

Effects of pentobarbitone on evoked field potentials

Simultaneous exposure of both the pial and cut surfaces of olfactory cortex slices to pentobarbitone resulted in characteristic changes in the evoked field potentials (see Fig. 2). First, there was a depression in the amplitude of the N-wave suggesting that excitatory transmission from the LOT fibre terminals to the superficial pyramidal cells (see Fig. 1) was impaired. Second, there was a dramatic potentiation of the duration of the I-wave, suggesting that post-synaptic inhibitory processes were affected. These results are in agreement with previously published work (15,16,19). These effects of pentobarbitone were not accompanied by any depression of the tract action potential amplitude suggesting that a local anaesthetic action was not involved.

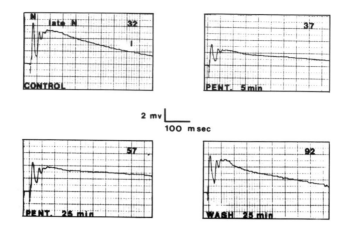

FIG. 2. Effect of pentobarbitone (PENT.,100µM) on the
evoked surface field potentials recorded on LOT
stimulation. Note the depression of the N-wave
(unusually large in this preparation) and the
potentiation of the I-wave. For an explanation of the
neurophysiological basis of the potentials, see legend
to FIG. 1. Readers are referred to Refs. 15 and 19.

Effects of pentobarbitone on the synaptically evoked release of endogenous amino acids

   Supramaximal electrical stimulation of the LOT
(4 stimuli min^{-1} for 20 min) of control preparations
was accompanied by a significant release of aspartate,
GABA and taurine only (Table 1; see Refs. 5,6,8).
Preincubation and perfusion of preparations with
pentobarbitone (10 to 1000µM) resulted in a
concentration dependent inhibition in the evoked
release of aspartate and taurine (Fig. 3). In
contrast, release of GABA was significantly increased
in the presence of up to 250µM pentobarbitone but was
reduced at 1000µM. This potentiation of GABA release
was not the result of inhibition of the re-uptake of
released GABA (not shown; see Refs. 8 and 11).

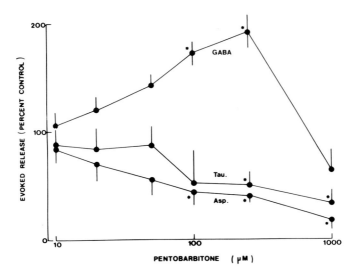

FIG. 3. Effect of pentobarbitone on the release of
endogenous GABA, aspartate (Asp) and taurine (Tau)
accompanying supramaximal LOT stimulation (4 stimuli
min^{-1} for 20 min). An asterisk adjacent to a point
indicates a significant difference (Student $\underline{t}$ test
P <0.05) between that value and the corresponding
control.

Mechanisms of action of pentobarbitone
in affecting amino acid release

Aspartate
In the present experiments, the origin of the
released aspartate is likely to be the LOT fibre
terminals (see legend of Fig. 1 for references). Both
neuropharmacological (13,14) and neurochemical (8)
evidence suggests that release of the excitatory
transmitter is regulated by presynaptic GABA
receptors. For example, structural analogues of GABA
as well as GABA itself depolarize LOT fibre terminals,
an action which is antagonized by picrotoxin (13).
Similarly, the field potential which reflects
presynaptic inhibition is abolished by GABA receptor
antagonists (14). Moreover the release of aspartate
which accompanies LOT stimulation is markedly
inhibited in the presence of muscimol (10µM) and this
effect is antagonised by picrotoxin (15µM) (8).

TABLE 1. Effects of pentobarbitone, picrotoxin and pentobarbitone plus picrotoxin on evoked amino acid release from the rat olfactory cortex slice[a]

| Amino Acid | Control | Lateral olfactory tract stimulation[b] | | |
		Pentobarbitone (100µM)	Picrotoxin (15µM)	Pentobarbitone (100µM)+ Picrotoxin (15µM)
Taurine	651 ± 107	347 ± 106[d]	844 ± 116	767 ± 132
GABA	42 ± 6	99 ± 14[d]	40 ± 8	72 ± 12
Aspartate	208 ± 21	130 ± 22[d]	220 ± 19	145 ± 26
Glutamate	-17 ± 25	31 ± 10	20 ± 15	18 ± 20

Direct stimulation[c]

Amino Acid	Control	Pentobarbitone (100µM)	Picrotoxin (15µM)	Pentobarbitone (100µM)+ Picrotoxin (15µM)
Taurine	609 ± 86	185 ± 103[d]	777 ± 91	467 ± 100
GABA	55 ± 8	55 ± 14	60 ± 7	51 ± 9
Aspartate	433 ± 66	158 ± 27[d]	362 ± 21	105 ± 21[d]
Glutamate	32 ± 55	37 ± 24	9 ± 16	64 ± 50

a Slices were pre-incubated for 2hr either alone (control) or in the presence of the appropriate drugs prior to perfusion. Each value is a mean ± S.E. (n between 9 and 12) total amount of amino acid (p mole) released in excess of or below (negative value) prestimulation resting efflux (not shown). Of the 7 amino acids monitored, only taurine, GABA and aspartate release significantly increased following stimulation; glutamate release is shown for comparison.

b 4 supramaximal stimuli min^{-1} for 20 min.

c Stimulating electrode placed on the surface of the slice within the cortical cup (4 stimuli min^{-1} for 20 min, current of 2mA).

d Significant difference (Student t-test) when compared to control ($P < 0.05$).

Because of this, it is conceivable that the increased GABA released in the presence of pentobarbitone (see Fig. 3) is the cause of the reduced aspartate release.

In order to investigate this possibility, the effects of picrotoxin on the pentobarbitone-induced reduction in aspartate release was assessed (Table 1). That picrotoxin at a concentration known to antagonize the actions of GABA in the olfactory cortex (13) fails to alter the effects of pentobarbitone suggests, first, that the reduced release of aspartate in the presence of pentobarbitone is not a consequence of the increased release of GABA and, second, that pentobarbitone does not interact directly with GABA receptors localised on the LOT fibres and fibre terminals. What is the mechanism of the pentobarbitone-induced reduction in evoked aspartate release? One possibility is suggested by the finding that release of aspartate is calcium-dependent (6) and, moreover, barbiturates are potent inhibitors of excitation-secretion coupling, probably by antagonizing the increased calcium-permeability which accompanies terminal depolarization (2). Whatever the mechanism involved, the reduced release of the presumed excitatory transmitter of the LOT terminals is in full accord with the pentobarbitone-induced depression of the N-wave (Fig. 2 and Refs. 15,16).

GABA

It is likely that the major sites of GABA release in the present experiments are the deeper lying inhibitory interneurones (see legend of Fig. 1). Potentiation of evoked GABA release by pentobarbitone only occurs in preparations which are synaptically activated (Table 1); this might suggest that the site of action of the pentobarbitone is not necessarily the GABA-releasing neurones themselves. Potentiation of GABA-mediated processes by pentobarbitone might be expected to reduce GABA release for there is evidence that GABA release in the rat olfactory cortex is regulated (inhibited) by presynaptic autoreceptors (8). The release of GABA from interneurones reflects a balance between excitatory input from pyramidal cell collaterals and inhibitory inputs from other interneurones (1). By reducing aspartate release and by as yet unknown effects on release of the excitatory transmitter of the pyramidal cell collaterals, pentobarbitone will alter this balance, conceivably leading to increased GABA release.

Taurine
All experimental evidence (5,6) suggests that taurine is unlikely to be a neurotransmitter in the olfactory cortex and that its likely origin is glial cells. It is not clear whether the changes in release reflect direct actions of pentobarbitone and picrotoxin on such cells (unlikely) or whether the changes in taurine release are secondary to some other action of the drugs. As the release patterns of GABA and taurine differ, it is unlikely that the two amino acids are released from the same cells.

SUMMARY

1. In the rat olfactory cortex slice, sub-anaesthetic concentrations of pentobarbitone reduce the amplitude of the N-wave with a concomitant reduction in the release of the excitatory transmitter aspartate. The pentobarbitone induced potentiation of the GABA-mediated I-wave is accompanied by increased GABA release. Although the changes in transmitter release and evoked electrical activity are consistent, there is only circumstantial evidence that the phenomena are related.
2. Pentobarbitone also reduced release of taurine although the significance (if any) of this finding is obscure.
3. The results are discussed in terms of the mechanisms by which pentobarbitone induces the changes in amino acid release.

Acknowledgements. This work was supported by the Medical Research Council (U.K.) and the University of Sheffield Medical Research Fund.

REFERENCES

1. Biedenbach, M.A. and Stevens, C.F. (1969):
   J. Neurophysiol., 32: 193-203.

2. Blaustein, M. (1976): J. Pharmac. exp. Ther.,
   196: 80-86.

3. Bradford, H.F., and Richards, C.D. (1976):
   Brain Res., 105: 168-172.

4. Clark, R.M., and Collins, G.G.S. (1976):
   J. Physiol., 262: 383-400.

5. Collins, G.G.S. (1979a): Br. J. Pharmac., 66:
   109-110P.

6. Collins, G.G.S. (1979b): J. Physiol., 291: 51-60.

7. Collins, G.G.S. (1979c): Brain Res., 171: 552-555.

8. Collins, G.G.S. (1980): Brain Res., 190: 517-528.

9. Haberly, L.B. (1973): J. Neurophysiol., 36:
   762-774.

10. Haberly, L.B. (1973): J. Neurophysiol., 36:
    776-788.

11. Jessel, T.M., and Richards, C.D. (1977):
    J. Physiol., 269: 42-44P.

12. Nicoll, R. (1978): In: Psychopharmacology;
    A Generation of Progress, edited by M.A. Lipton,
    A. DiMascio and K.F. Killam, pp 1337-1348.
    Raven Press, New York.

13. Pickles, H.G. (1979): Br. J. Pharmac., 65:
    223-228.

14. Pickles, H.F., and Simmonds, M.A. (1976):
    J. Physiol., 260: 475-486.

15. Pickles, H.G., and Simmonds, M.A. (1978):
    J. Physiol., 275: 135-148.

16. Richards, C.D. (1972): J. Physiol., 227: 749–767.

17. Richards, C.D., and Sercombe, R. (1968): J. Physiol., 197: 667–683.

18. Richards, C.D., and Sercombe, R. (1970): J. Physiol., 211: 571–584.

19. Scholfield, C.N. (1978): J. Physiol., 275: 547–557.

20. Scholfield, C.N. (1978): J. Physiol., 275: 559–566.

21. Yamamoto, C., and McIlwain, H. (1966): J. Neurochem., 13: 1333–1343.

Glutamate as a Neurotransmitter,
edited by G. Di Chiara and G. L. Gessa
Raven Press, New York © 1981.

The Release of GABA and Glutamate from the Cerebral Cortex Is an Index of the Activity of Underlying Aminoacidergic Neurons

F. Moroni, R. Corradetti, F. Casamenti, G. Moneti, and G. Pepeu

Department of Pharmacology, University of Florence, 50134 Florence, Italy

INTRODUCTION

The release of a putative neurotransmitter from the nerve endings is considered an indication of the activity of the neurons to which the endings belong. This assumption stems from studies performed in the peripheral nervous system (5) and is supported by investigations on acetylcholine (17) and dopamine output (1) from different brain regions. Little information however is available as to whether the release of endogenous amino acid neurotransmitters can also be taken as an indication of neuronal activity. GABA and glutamate (Gl) for instance are also present in the blood (16), and cerebro-spinal fluid (7) from which the tricarboxylic acid cycle and metabolic changes could influence their level.

In this investigation we attempted to ascertain by the use of a very sensitive and specific mass-fragmentographic method (13) whether GABA, GL and glutamine (GLN) output from the cerebral cortex of freely moving and anaesthetized rats originate from the nervous tissue, and, whether it is affected by the activity of the cortical aminoacidergic neurons.

157

MATERIALS AND METHODS

Male Wistar rats 200-250 g body weight fasted 3 hrs before the experiments were used.

Collection of GABA, GL and GLN released from the cerebral cortex

Samples were collected in 1) freely moving rats with intact dura; 2) urethane-anaesthetized rats (1 g/kg i.p.) with intact dura; 3) anaesthetized rats with removed dura.

Freely moving rats

Under ketamine-anaesthesia (100 mg/kg i.p.), a Perspex cylinder containing 0.5 ml of Ringer solution was screwed into the left or right parietal bone so as to exert a slight compression of the dura. The amino-acid output was measured 3 days after surgery. During this time the dura was washed with a terramycin solution (300 ug/ml).

Anaesthetized rats

The rats were placed in a stereotactic apparatus; the skull was opened and the Perspex cylinder was placed either on the dura mater or on the exposed fronto-parietal cortex. The rectal temperature was maintained at 37° C. In several rats the electrocort-icogram (ECoG) was recorded by means of silver ball electrodes applied on the exposed cerebral cortex and connected with a Galileo recorder.

Mass-fragmentographic determination of GABA, GL and GLN output

A Ringer solution with the following composition: NaCl 9.0, KCl 0.42, $CaCl_2$ 0.24, $NaHCO_3$ 0.5, glucose 1 g/l was placed in the collecting cylinder. Every 20 min the solution was removed and stored at -70° C until assayed.

GABA, GL and GLN were measured using the mass-frag-mentographic method described by Costa et al., (4) and Moroni et al., (13). The method can be summar-ized as follows: Deuterated internal standards GABA ($^2H_6$) 0.10, GL ($^2H_5$) and GLN ($^2H_5$) 0.10 nmoles, dis-

solved in perchloric acid (0.4N) were added to the collected samples and loaded into small Dowex columns
(50 x 8, 200-400 mesh in acid form). After washing
with H_2O the aminoacids were eluted from the resin with
0.7 ml of NH_4OH 3N and the eluate transferred into
Kontes vials and evaporated to dryness under a stream of
nitrogen. Fifty ul of 1,1,1,3,3,3, hexafluoroisopro-
panol (Pierce Co.) and 50 ul of pentafluoropropionic
anhidride (Pierce Co.) were added to the dry residue.
The vials were sealed and heated for 30 min at 50° C.
The reaction mixture was then evaporated and the residue dissolved into 10 ul of ethylacetate. Aliquots of
1-2 ul were injected into a gas-chromatograph-mass-
spectrometer LKB 2091 equipped with a multiple ion
detector. The separation was made on a 2.5 m x 1 mm
i.d. silanized glass column packed with 3% OV 1
(Applied Science). The chromatographic conditions were
column temperature 120° C, flask heater 200° C, helium
flow 12 cm^3/min. The following ions were recorded with
the multiple ion detector: m/e 230 for GL and GLN;
m/e 235 for GL ($^2H_5$) and GLN ($^2H_5$) and m/e 232 and 238
for GABA and GABA ($^2H_6$) respectively.

Determination of GABA and GL content in the brain

When the aminoacid content was measured in the cerebral cortex, the rats were killed by microwave radia-
tion, the brain dissected out and the parietal cortex
was omogenized in $HClO_4$ (0.4N) and processed as described above.

RESULTS

The first group of experiments were aimed at clarifying the origin of GABA, GL and GLN. Since these
aminoacids are present in the blood, changes in their
efflux could reflect modifications in blood aminoacid
concentration, cerebral blood flow, or capillary permeability. To rule out these possibilities, attempts
were made to change GABA and GL output from the cerebral
cortex without affecting their level in the blood or
modifying brain circulation.

In order to obtain evidence that GABA, GL and GLN
had a neuronal origin, changes in neuronal activity

were induced by applying on the cortical surface depolarizing KCl solutions, tetrodotoxin, a well known
inhibitor of the inward fast Na^+ channels (15) or
activating cortical neurons by means of amphetamine
administration. Finally the possible functional meaning of aminoacid release was investigated by correlat-
ing its changes with those of the ECoG.

Spontaneous aminoacid output

Table 1 shows the spontaneous GABA and GL output in
freely moving and anaesthetized rats.

TABLE 1. Spontaneous output of GABA and GL

Conditions	aminoacid output nmol/cm^2. 20 min	
	GABA	GL
Freely moving intact dura (5)	0.104±0.08	6.10±0.65[a]
Anaesthetized intact dura (5)	0.072±0.010	4.10±0.40[b]
Anaesthetized removed dura (8)	0.080±0.014	16.4 ±2.1 [c]

Number of animals in parenthesis. The output was
measured in 3 samples for each animal; a versus b
P <0.05; b versus c P<0.01; a versus c P<0.01.

It can be seen that while GABA output was neither
affected by anaesthesia nor by the presence of the dura,
GL output was significantly decreased by urethane anaesthesia and hampered by the presence of the dura.

Effect of aminooxyacetic acid (AOAA) on GABA and GL output

As shown in Table 2 the intracerebroventricular
(i.c.v.) administration of AOAA, an inhibitor of GABA
transaminase (18), was followed by an increase in
cortical GABA level and in its release into the epidural cup. The GABA level in the blood was not affected. A slight sedation was also observed.

TABLE 2.   Effect of intracerebroventricular
administration of AOAA (30 ug)
in freely moving rats

Cortical output	198 ± 5+
Cortical level	148 ± 16+
Blood level	116 ± 12

+ P 0.01; GABA level was measured 60 min after i.c.v
administration of AOAA. Control GABA output
0.10 ± 0.06 nmol/cm^2.20 min; control cortical level:
21.4 ± 0.5 nmol/mg protein; control blood level
0.37 ± 0.042 nmol/ml. From Moroni et al. (14).

Effects of KCl (50 mM) depolarization on aminoacid
release and ECoG in rats with intact dura

As shown in FIG. 1 the substitution of an equimol-
ecular concentration of NaCl with KCl 50 mM in the
Ringer solution filling the epidural collecting

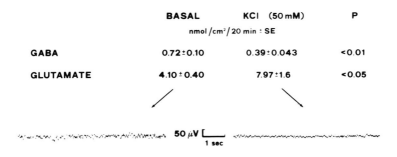

	BASAL	KCl (50 mM)	P
	nmol /cm²/ 20 min ± SE		
GABA	0.72±0.10	0.39±0.043	<0.01
GLUTAMATE	4.10±0.40	7.97±1.6	<0.05

50 µV
1 sec

FIG. 1. Effects of KCl on aminoacid release and on
ECoG in animals with intact dura mater. Each number
is the mean ± S.E. of at least 6 experiments.

cylinder was followed by a short lasting increase in
GL and a decrease in GABA output in both freely moving
and anaesthetized rats. The decrease in GABA output
lasted up to 80 min and was associated with changes in
the ECoG pattern characterized initially by high frequency low voltage waves followed after 5 - 10 min by
a diffuse depression of the electrical activity. The
time-course of ECoG and aminoacid output changes was
similar.

Effect of KCl (50 mM) depolarization on aminoacid release and ECoG in rats with removed dura

When a Ringer solution containing KCl 50 mM was

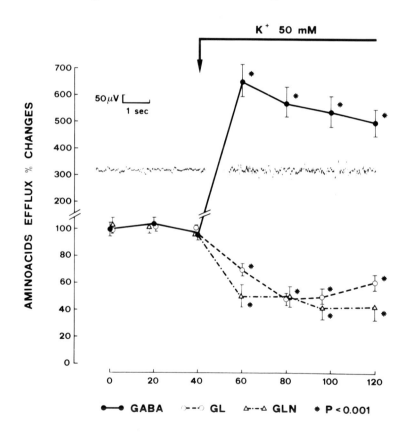

FIG. 2. Effects of KCl on aminoacid release and on
ECoG in animals with removed dura mater. Each point
is the mean ± S.E. of at least 5 experiments.

directly applied on the cortical surface a large increase in GABA associated with a decrease in GL and
GLN output was observed. As shown in FIG. 2 the peak
effect on GABA output occurred in the first 20 min
while the maximum decrease in GL and GLN was observed
40 min after KCl application. The modifications in
aminoacid release rate were associated with the appearance of high voltage low frequency ECoG waves. A relationship between ECoG changes in the pattern of ECoG
and cortical aminoacid output had been previously proposed in the cat and rabbit by Jasper and Koyama (9),
Iversen et al. (8), Blagoeva et al. (2).

Effect of tetrodotoxin (TTX) on KCl (25 mM) induced increase in GABA output

In order to ascertain whether the large increase in
GABA output elicited by the application of KCl Ringer
solution was caused by activation of neuronal firing
an attempt was made to block the rapid Na^+ influx

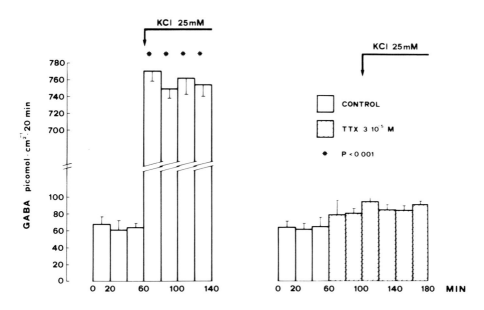

FIG. 3. Effects of tetrodotoxin ($3.10^{-5}M$) on the KCl
(25 mM) induced modifications of GABA release. Each
bar is the mean ± S.E. of at least 5 experiments
*P < 0.01.

associated with depolarization. Na^+ influx may activate the voltage dependent Ca^{2+} channels (11), Ca^{2+} influx triggers in turn the neurotransmitter release (10). TTX ($3.10^{-5}M$) was added to the KCl 25 mM Ringer solution filling the collecting cortical cylinder. As illustrated by FIG. 3, the more than 7 fold increase in GABA output elicited by the KCl was almost completely prevented by the presence of TTX. The decrease in GL and GLN release was also reduced.

The effect of amphetamine on GABA and GL output from the cerebral cortex

Amphetamine administration elicits behavioural and ECoG activation in several animal species (12) associated with an increase in acetylcholine output from the cerebral cortex (16). An attempt was made to ascertain whether amphetamine also modified GABA and GL efflux from the cerebral cortex in urethane anaesthetized rats with removed dura.

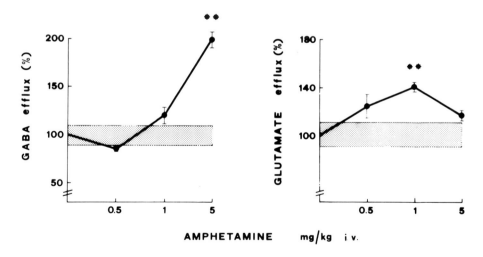

FIG. 4. The effects of amphetamine on GABA and GL release from the cerebral cortex of urethane anaesthetized rats with removed dura mater. The % modifications of aminoacid efflux were calculated in the first 20 min sample after i.v. amphetamine. Shaded areas represent the basal aminoacid efflux $\pm$ S.E. $**P < 0.05$

In FIG. 4 the relationships between increasing doses of amphetamine and the percent changes in GABA and GL efflux are shown. Amphetamine at the dose of 1 mg/Kg i.v. stimulated GL efflux. However, at the dose of 5 mg/Kg i.v. had no effect on GL but doubled GABA efflux. GL increase was short lasting while GABA output increase reached a maximum 20 min after amphetamine administration and was still evident 80 min later.

It should be noted that a marked increase in blood pressure induced in rats by i.v. infusion of noradrenaline (5 ug/Kg.min) was not associated with changes in GABA and GL efflux.

DISCUSSION

Two questions were asked in the introduction. First, where GABA, GL and GLN detected in epidural or cortical collecting cylinder originate from. Second, whether GABA, GL and GLN efflux is related to neuronal activity. Our experiments offer an answer to both questions. GABA, GL and GLN efflux appears to originate from the nervous tissue. This assumption is supported by the observations that 1) AOAA administration increased brain GABA level and GABA efflux without increasing blood GABA level; 2) cortical KCl depolarization modified GABA and GL efflux in opposite directions; 3) the effect of KCl depolarization was antagonized by the presence of TTX which block Na^+ fast inward channels.

The diverging changes in GABA and GL output following KCl application in epidural or cortical cups seem to rule out modifications of cortical blood flow or vascular permeability induced by KCl. It seems unlikely that circulatory or permeability changes could increase the efflux of one aminoacid while decreasing that of the other. Similar considerations and the lack of the effect of noradrenaline would exclude that amphetamine-induced changes in GABA and GL output might depend upon cerebral blood flow changes.

Evidence suggesting a relationship between GABA and GL efflux and neuronal activity comes from two facts: 1) modification in GABA and GL release were associated with ECoG changes; 2) amphetamine and urethane which affect cortical neuronal function brought about changes in GABA and GL release.

Our results on cortical aminoacid release are in line with previous reports (3,8,9). They definitively demonstrate, by means of a very specific and sensitive method, the release of endogenous aminoacids from the cerebral cortex. From the monitoring of the release information can be obtained on the functional activity of underlying GABAergic and glutamatergic neurons and on their possible relationship.

ACKNOWLEDGEMENTS

This work was supported by grant n° 7901950.04 from C.N.R. Mass-spectrometric analysis was carried out at the Mass-spectrometry service of the Medical School, University of Florence.

REFERENCES

1. Besson, M.J., Cheramy, A., Fletz, P. and Glowinski, J. (1971): Brain Res., 32:407-424.
2. Blagoeva, P., Masi, I., Scotti de Carolis, A. and Longo, V.G. (1972): Physiology and Behaviour, 9:307-313.
3. Clark, R.M. and Collins, G.G.S. (1976): J. Physiol. 262:383-400.
4. Costa, E., Guidotti, A., Moroni, R. and Peralta, E (1979): In: Glutamic Acid: advances in biochemistry and physiology, edited by L.J. Filer, S. Garattini, M.R. Kare, W.A. Reynolds and R.J. Wurtman, pp. 151-161, Raven Press, New York.
5. Emmelin, N. and MacIntosh, F.C. (1956): J. Physiol. 131:477-496.
6. Ferkany, J.W., Smith, L.A., Seifert, W.E.Jr., Caprioli, M. and Enna, S.S. (1978): Life Sciences, 22:2121-2128.
7. Huizinga, J.D., Teelken, A.W., Muskiet, F.A.J., Jeuring, H.J. and Wolthers, B.G. (1978): J. Neurochem., 30:911-913.

8. Iversen, L.L., Mitchell, J.F. and Srinivasan, V. (1971): J. Physiol., 212:519-534.
9. Jasper, H.H. and Koyama, I. (1969): Canadian J. Physiol. and Pharmacol., 47:889-905.
10. Kelly, R.B., Deutsch, J.W., Carlos, S.S. and Wagner, J.A. (1980): Ann. Rev. Neurosci., 2:399-446.
11. Kidakora, Y., Ritchie, A.K. and Hagiwara, S. (1978): Nature, 278:63-65.
12. Longo, V.G. and Silvestrini, B. (1957): J. Pharmacol. Exp. Ther., 120:160-170.
13. Moroni, F., Tanganelli, S., Bianchi, C., Moneti, G. and Beani, L. (1980): Pharmacol. Res. Comm., (in press).
14. Moroni, F., Casamenti, F., Moneti, G. and Pepeu, G. (1980): Brain Res. Bull., (in press).
15. Narahashi, T., Moore, J.W. and Scotti, W.R. (1964): J. Gen. Physiol., 47:406-417.
16. Pepeu, G. and Bartolini, A. (1968): European J. Pharmacol., 4:254-263.
17. Pepeu, G. (1973): Prog. Neurobiol., 2:257-286.
18. Wallach, D.P. (1961): Biochem. Pharmacol., 5:323-331.

Glutamate as a Neurotransmitter,
edited by G. Di Chiara and G. L. Gessa
Raven Press, New York © 1981.

Measurement of γ-Aminobutyric Acid Turnover Rates in Brain Nuclei as an Index of Interactions Between γ-Aminobutyric Acid and Other Transmitters

A. V. Revuelta, D. L. Cheney, and E. Costa

Laboratory of Preclinical Pharmacology, National Institute of Mental Health, Saint Elizabeths Hospital, Washington, D.C. 20032

INTRODUCTION

Gamma-aminobutyric acid (GABA) functions as a major inhibitory neurotransmitter in neurons of the mammalian central nervous system (40). Therefore its rate of synthesis in various brain GABAergic neurons is regulated by afferent inputs while GABAergic neurons can in turn regulate the synthesis of other transmitters in the various neurons they innervate. Hence we have decided to use the measurement of GABA turnover rate as a tool to detect how other neuronal systems afferent to various brain nuclei regulate the activity of the GABAergic neurons that are included in these nuclei. In contrast to the dopamine system whose cell bodies are compactly and discretely localized the cell bodies of the GABA neurons are randomly distributed in various brain nuclei. Here they function either as intrinsic interneurons or when provided with long axons they project to other nuclei and function as important links for the transfer of information. Because of inherent technical difficulties electrophysiological studies have been difficult to perform in GABA interneurons intrinsic to the striatum, nucleus (n) accumbens or septum, whereas the long axon GABAergic neurons that link striatum to substantia nigra have been a bit more accessible to detailed electrophysiological investigation. A biochemical method developed for the simultaneous quantitation by mass fragmentography of the glutamate and GABA content in brain tissue (2) has made it possible to measure the turnover rate of GABA in small brain structures (3,24). This has been done by monitoring the changes with time in the enrichment of ^{13}C in glutamate and GABA in various brain nuclei following constant rate infusion of [^{13}C]-glucose (Fig. 1). From the relationship between the precursor and product curves, GABA utilization has been calculated by assuming that immediately after infusion of [^{13}C] glucose the neuronal GABA that is selectively labeled is stored in a

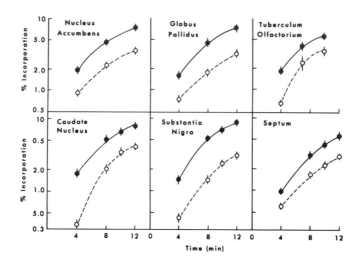

FIG. 1.   Percent incorporation of ^{13}C-glucose (75 μmol/kg/min; 0.1 ml/min) into glutamate (closed circles) and GABA (open circles) of various brain nuclei as a function of time.

single open metabolic compartment.   Thus the equations derived by Racagni et al. (39) have been used to calculate the fractional rate constant for GABA efflux (k_{GABA}).   This value multiplied by the steady-state concentration of GABA will give an estimate of the turnover rate of GABA (TR_{GABA}).   This measurement of GABA turnover is useful for comparative studies of drug or transmitter interactions, but fails to yield absolute values of GABA synthesis rates.   Moreover while this measurement yields a reliable indication of ongoing turnover rates for nuclei that contain terminals of long axon GABA neurons or only a population of GABAergic interneurons that do not synapse with each other, the turnover rate of GABA fails to yield reliable information on rate of activity in the case of brain nuclei that contain GABA interneurons that are interconnected.   The mathematical model used to calculate k_{GABA} implies that the glutamate pool (labelled from glucose at a fast rate) that is present in a brain sample serves as a precursor of GABA.   This assumption is never completely true since glutamate functions not only as a GABA precursor but also as an intermediate metabolite and a primary transmitter.   By collecting the samples very early during the infusion of [^{13}C] glucose and by selecting those tissues where the pool of glutamate which functions predominantly as a GABA precursor prevails over that of the other two glutamate pools, the errors derived from such a generalization can be minimized.   In the studies reported here the turnover rate of GABA has been estimated in n. accumbens, n. caudatus, globus

pallidus, substantia nigra, septum and tuberculum olfactorium
where the rate of change of ^{13}C incorporation into glutamate and
GABA fulfills some minimal criteria for expression as a precursor-
product relationship. Since these criteria were not fulfilled in
cerebellar cortex, deep cerebellar nuclei, colliculus, hippocampus
or in areas of the cortex (frontal parietal, occipital or temporal)
we did not use these areas for turnover measurements. As shown
in Fig. 2 the curves for the incorporation of ^{13}C are superimposed
on the curves for the incorporation of label into glutamate making
it impossible to determine the turnover rate of GABA in these
areas. Table 1 shows the concentration of GABA and glutamate in
various rat brain areas and, where possible, the fractional rate
constant for GABA efflux and the turnover rate of GABA.

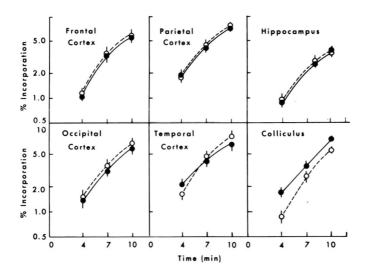

FIG. 2. Percent incorporation of ^{13}C-glucose into glutamate
(closed circles) and GABA (open circles) of various brain
regions as a function of time.

Regulation of GABA Turnover by Impulse Flow

For the reasons mentioned above it is important to establish
whether GABA turnover changes with the activity of the GABAergic
neurons. The strio-nigral pathway was chosen to assess whether
electrical stimulation and surgical deafferentation modify GABA
dynamics using the turnover rate of GABA as an index. The strio-
nigral neurons have been shown to synthesize, store and secrete
GABA (4,9,13,14,35). These GABAergic axons synapse with dendrites
of nigral dopaminergic neurons, thus providing inhibitory feedback
regulation of the nigro-striatal pathway (16). The iontophoretic

TABLE 1. GABA and glutamate concentrations and GABA turnover rate in various regions of rat brain

Region	GABA $\dfrac{nmol}{mg\ prot}$	Glutamate $\dfrac{nmol}{mg\ prot}$	k_{GABA} hr^{-1}	TR_{GABA} $\dfrac{nmol/mg}{prot \cdot hr}$
Accumbens	100±4.8	150±10	17±2.5	1700±240
Caudatus	46±0.30	130±2.9	23±2.0	1100±82
G. Pallidus	62±2.6	80±4.7	13±1.4	790±71
S. Nigra	70±2.1	88±2.2	11±2.1	1000±58
T. Olfactorium	31±2.6	90±4.0	25±2.2	900±48
Septum	87±8.7	160±3.1	16±1.2	1500±140
Colliculus	35±1.8	70±1.4	40±3.2	1400±85
Hippocampus	60±3.0	200±8.8	--	--
CA3	40±1.9	190±6.5	--	--
CA1	30±1.5	160±8.2	--	--
Subiculum	38±1.5	190±9.6	--	--
Dentate Gyrus	44±1.3	210±6.3	--	--
Cortex				
Frontal	40±2.1	132±3.4	--	--
Parietal	37±1.8	120±9.9	--	--
Occipital	32±2.2	121±7.0	--	--
Temporal	26±1.3	110±5.2	--	--

application of GABA to substantia nigra inhibits neuronal activity and this inhibition is nullified by picrotoxin (13). When the head of the nucleus caudatus is stimulated electrically, neuronal firing in substantia nigra is reduced (13) presumably because increased amounts of GABA are being released and this reduction can be blocked by picrotoxin (38). In both rats and baboons a brain hemitransection at the subthalamic level results in a marked decline of the GABA content and the glutamic acid decarboxylase activity in the substantia nigra (14,19) suggesting that GABA is preferentially located in the axon terminals of the descending strionigral pathways. Figure 3 shows that when the head of the n. caudatus is electrically stimulated there is a 3 fold increase in the turnover rate of GABA in the substantia nigra of the stimulated side. Nevertheless the GABA and glutamate concentrations of the substantia nigra remain unchanged (24). The GABA turnover rate values in the substantia nigra of hemitransected rats one week after surgery also are presented in Fig. 3. This surgical procedure separates the n. caudatus and the globus pallidus from the substantia nigra by cutting the strio-nigral pathway. Besides reducing the values for GABA turnover on the lesioned side this surgical procedure reduces also the GABA and glutamate content (24). These observations provide direct evidence that electrical activation or surgical lesion of the strio-nigral GABAergic axons increases and decreases the turnover rate of GABA respectively.

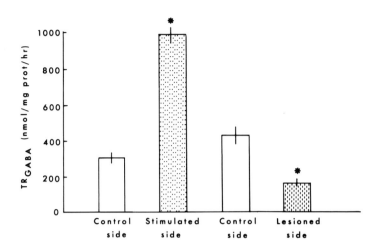

FIG. 3.   Turnover rate of GABA in substantia nigra following unilateral electrical stimulation of the n. caudatus and hemitransection of the strio-nigral pathway.   The following stimulation parameters were used: 8V, 20Hz, 0.5 msec pulse duration, 20 min.   Other
rats were hemitransected by means of a 3 mm wide knife lowered with
an angle of 60° at the level of the coronary suture.   The knife
was inserted next to the midline and subsequently moved outwards
to achieve complete hemitransection.   Uniformly labelled ^{13}C-glu-
cose in saline was infused through the tail vein at a rate of 50
μmol/kg/min (0.1 ml saline/min) for 10, 12 and 14 min.   The rats
were killed by focussed microwave irradiation immediately after
the infusion and the calculations of the turnover rate of GABA and
the k_{GABA} were performed as described by Racagni et al. (39).
Values represent mean±S.E.M. of at least 7 determinations.   Asterisk indicates p<0.05.   Data taken from Mao et al. (24).

Regulation of GABA Turnover by GABAergic Neurons

In order to detect those brain nuclei in which the turnover rate
of GABA fails to parallel the activity of GABAergic neurons because there are synapses between GABAergic neurons, we have decided to determine the presence of GABA receptors on GABAergic
neuronal cell bodies.   To determine the presence of these receptors
it would be necessary to chemically activate the GABA receptors
and then measure the effect of GABA turnover.   Available evidence
indicates that muscimol is a potent and specific GABA receptor
agonist (10,21) and that diazepam and other benzodiazepines can
maximize responses of GABA receptors to the endogenous agonist in
various neuronal systems (4,5; see references 7,8).   The changes
of GABA turnover after treatment with muscimol and diazepam are
shown in Fig. 4 (25).   Since neither diazepam nor muscimol alter

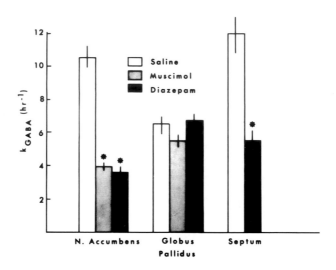

FIG. 4. Effects of muscimol (1 mg/kg; i.v.; 50 min) and diazepam
(1 mg/kg; i.p.; 17 min) on the fractional rate constants of GABA
in n. accumbens, globus pallidus and septum. Uniformly labelled
^{13}C-glucose (50 μmol/kg/min; i.v.) was infused for 10 min. Rats
were sacrificed at 0,2,3.5 and 5 min after the infusion by focussed
microwave irradiation. The change with time of ^{13}C incorporated
into glutamate and GABA was determined by gas chromatography-mass
fragmentography and the fractional rate constants of GABA efflux
in various nuclei were estimated according to the finite difference method (34). Each column represents the mean±S.E.M. of at
least 4 animals. The asterisk indicates p<0.05. Part of the data
taken from Mao et al. (25).

the tissue content of glutamate or GABA, the values of k_{GABA} are
directly related to the turnover rates of GABA in the various
nuclei. Thus the GABA turnover is reduced in n. accumbens and
septum but not in globus pallidus of rats injected with either
muscimol (1 mg/kg; i.v.; 50 min) or diazepam (1 mg/kg; i.p.; 15
min). The results are consistent with the hypothesis that nuclei
in which muscimol and diazepam decrease GABA turnover contain GABA
neurons whose cell bodies or dendrites possess GABA receptors.
Therefore, the reduction of GABA turnover in n. accumbens and
septum of rats treated with muscimol or diazepam suggests the
presence of GABA-GABA synapses in these nuclei. However, this
type of intrinsic neuronal organization is not likely to exist in
globus pallidus because muscimol and diazepam fail to reduce the
GABA turnover in this nucleus. In fact as we will show later
synapses between acetylcholine-GABA appear to occur in globus
pallidus.

Regulation of GABA Turnover by Blockade of Dopaminergic Receptors

Evidence has been accumulating to show that in basal ganglia there is neuronal circuitry involving GABA and acetylcholine secreting neurons that regulates the activity of the nigro-striatal dopaminergic pathway (27). Dopamine turnover in nerve terminals of this pathway is increased when dopaminergic receptors are inhibited presumably via a feedback inhibitory loop (1,5,18,28,33, 36). Thus the GABA neurons forming an integral part of the loop are directly or indirectly under tonic inhibitory dopaminergic control. When rats receive haloperidol (1.5 mg/kg, i.p.) 40 min before the infusion of ^{13}C-glucose, the turnover rate of GABA in n. accumbens and globus pallidus is significantly increased (Fig. 5). Haloperidol slightly decreases the turnover rate in n. caudatus and fails to change that of substantia nigra. It is possi-

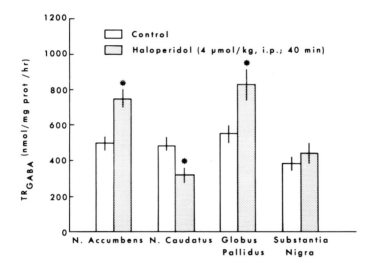

FIG. 5. Effects of haloperidol (4 μmol/kg, i.p.; 40 min) on the turnover rate of GABA in various brain nuclei. Columns represent mean±S.E.M. of at least 7 determinations. See legend under Fig. 3. Asterisk indicates p<0.05. Data taken from Marco et al. (26).

ble to assume that in n. accumbens where GABA turnover is increased by haloperidol, the GABA neurons are directly or indirectly under tonic inhibitory dopaminergic control. However since this structure contains numerous GABA-GABA synapses, it is impossible to draw final conclusions from simple turnover rate measurements. In globus pallidus, the increase of GABA turnover is probably secondary to a drug action on neurons in other structures; perhaps in n. caudatus and n. accumbens. The haloperidol induced de-

crease in GABA turnover rate in caudate suggests that blockade of
dopamine receptors inhibits the firing of a population of GABA
neurons in n. caudatus. However cautionary comments should be
added in the event that this brain structure is found to contain
GABA-GABA synapses.

Antipsychotic drugs with different chemical structures increase
the turnover rate of GABA in n. accumbens and globus pallidus (23).
Those which fail to cause extrapyramidal side effects or tardive
dyskinesis (20,30,37,41,42,43) also increase GABA turnover rate in
n. caudatus and substantia nigra (23). These findings suggest that
drugs which cause antipsychotic activity increase the GABAergic
function in n. accumbens and globus pallidus; those drugs that fail
to affect extrapyramidal function increase GABA turnover in substantia nigra and caudate; the drugs with maximal extrapyramidal
liability fail to change these two parameters.

Regulation of GABA Turnover by Cholinergic Receptors

Intraventricular injection of the cholinergic antagonist,
scopolamine, fails to alter the GABA turnover in any of the brain
regions tested (Fig. 6). Intraventricular administration of the
muscarinic receptor agonist methacholine, increases the GABA
turnover in globus pallidus without altering the GABA turnover in

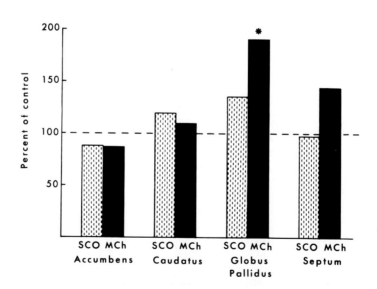

FIG. 6. Effect of intraventricularly injected scopolamine (10 μg;
30 min) and methacholine chloride (10 μg; 30 min) on GABA turnover
in various rat brain nuclei. GABA turnover estimated (39)
following infusion of ^{13}C-glucose (75 μmol/kg/min; 10 min).
Asterisk indicates p<0.05. Significance was determined prior to
expressing data as percent of controls.

any other area. The globus pallidus receives afferents from the
n. accumbens (11) and n. caudatus (probably GABAergic) (14). This
nucleus also contains some cells and tracts which stain for acetyl-
cholinesterase (17) and has high levels of ACh (6) and the acetylcholine turnover rate compares to that of n. accumbens and n.
caudatus (6). However there are no known cholinergic interconnections between n. accumbens, n. caudate, substantia nigra and
globus pallidus. Our results suggest that there is an excitatory
cholinergic input to pallidal GABAergic neurons, but fail to map
this cholinergic pathway. Moreover, our data also indicate that
afferent cholinergic neurons to the spetum do not modulate the
turnover rate of GABA in the medial and lateral septal nuclei.
However the data of Fig. 4 showing the presence of GABA-GABA
synapses in septum should advise one to refrain from any conclusions.

Regulation of GABA Turnover by β-Endorphin

Figure 7 demonstrates that following intraventricular administration of β-endorphin (2.9 nmol; 30 min) the turnover of GABA
decreases in n. caudatus and increases in globus pallidus and substantia nigra. GABA and glutamate concentrations are unaltered
and the changes in GABA turnover can be antagonized by naltrexone

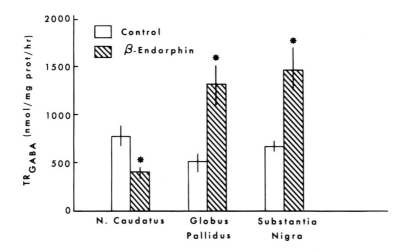

FIG. 7. Turnover rate of GABA following intraventricular adminis-
tration of β-endorphin (2.9 nmol; 30 min). See legend to Fig. 3.
Each column represents mean±S.E.M. of at least 7 determinations.
Asterisk indicates p<0.05. Data taken from Moroni et al. (32).

(32). Similar results are obtained by parenteral injection of
morphine (32). The changes in the turnover rate of GABA in n.

caudatus, globus pallidus and substantia nigra caused by stimulation of opioid receptors suggest that the short axon GABAergic neurons of n. caudatus (29) exert a tonic inhibitory influence on the long axon GABAergic neurons projecting from the n. caudatus to the globus pallidus and to the substantia nigra (14,15). When the opiate receptors in striatum are stimulated, this inhibitory influence on the long axon GABAergic neurons is abolished and the GABAergic activity in the globus pallidus and substantia nigra increases. The increased GABA turnover rate in substantia nigra and globus pallidus elicited by β-endorphin and morphine (32) has been correlated with the catalepsy seen after intraventricular injection of these compounds (31). Lower doses of β-endorphin which cause analgesia but not catalepsy fail to reduce the turnover rate of GABA in n. caudatus (32). Muscimol causes catalepsy when injected into globus pallidus but not when injected into the substantia nigra (32) suggesting that the catalepsy elicited by these opioids is associated with an increased stimulation of GABA receptors located in the globus pallidus.

CONCLUSIONS

The GABAergic neurons located in various brain nuclei are modulated transsynaptically by a number of other transmitter systems. This modulation may be monitored by measuring GABA turnover. We have shown that it is not possible to monitor GABA turnover by our method in areas where glutamate functions as an important primary neurotransmitter. Electrical stimulation and hemitransection experiments have demonstrated that the turnover rate of GABA increases when the activity of the GABAergic strio-nigral pathway is enhanced and decreases when the activity of this pathway is decreased. However such a direct relationship can be substantiated in tissues innervated by long axons GABA neurons but not in tissues with short interneurons. This is particularly true if there are GABA-GABA synapses such as in septum and n. accumbens.

Stimulation of GABAergic receptors with muscimol or facilitation of GABA transmission with diazepam reduces the GABA turnover in septum and n. accumbens indicating the presence of GABA-GABA synapses in these areas which modulate the intrinsic GABAergic activity. Blockade of dopamine receptors with haloperidol appears to increase the turnover and the firing of a population of GABA interneurons in n. accumbens and globus pallidus. The dynamics of this response is not unveiled by the present experiments. Activation of GABAergic receptors in globus pallidus with the cholinergic agonist, methacholine, is consistent with a possible excitatory cholinergic input to the GABAergic neurons of this structure. Opiate receptor agonists increase the GABA utilization in the globus pallidus. This response appears to be associated with the catalepsy caused by opioid receptor agonists. Moreover, stimulation of opiate receptors also exerts an inhibitory influence on the turnover rate of GABA in n. caudatus suggesting that perhaps opiate receptors are located on small GABA neurons which inhibit long axon GABA neurons of n. caudatus. These results, taken as a whole, indicate that the measurement of GABA turnover is a valuable tool in the study of the trans-synaptic modulation of GABA neurons by various neural inputs.

REFERENCES

1. Anden, N.E., Butcher, S.G., Corrodi, H., Fuxe, K., and Ungerstedt, U. (1970): Eur. J. Pharmacol., 11:303-314.
2. Bertilsson, L., and Costa, E. (1976): J. Chromatogr., 118:395-402.
3. Bertilsson, L., Mao, C.C., and Costa, E. (1977): J. Pharmacol. Exp. Ther., 200:277-284.
4. Bunney, B.S., and Aghajanian, G.K. (1976): Brain Res., 117:423-435.
5. Carlsson, A., and Lindqvist, M. (1963): Acta Pharmacol. Toxicol., 20:140-144.
6. Cheney, D.L., Zsilla, G., and Costa, E. (1977): In: Advances in Biochemical Psychopharmacology, Vol. 16, edited by E. Costa and G.L. Gessa, pp. 179-186. Raven Press, New York.
7. Costa, E., Guidotti, A., and Mao, C.C. (1976): In: GABA in Nervous System Function, edited by E. Roberts, T.N. Chase and D.B. Tower, pp. 413-426. Raven Press, New York.
8. Costa, E., Guidotti, A., Mao, C.C., and Suria, A. (1975): Life Sci., 17:167-185.
9. Crossman, A.R., Walker, R.J., and Woodruff, G.N. (1974): Br. J. Pharmacol., 51:137P-138P.
10. Curtis, D.R., Duggan, A.W., Felix, D., and Johnston, G.A.R. (1971): Brain Res., 32:69-96.
11. Domesick, V.B., Smith, G.P., and Nauta, W.J.H. (1976): Anatomy Meeting, Cajal Club.
12. Dray, A., and Straughan, D.W. (1976): J. Pharm. Pharmacol., 28:314-315.
13. Feltz, P. (1971): Can. J. Physiol. Pharmacol., 49:1113-1115.
14. Fonnum, F., Grofova, I., Rinvik, E., Storm-Mathisen, J., and Walberg, F. (1974): Brain Res., 71:77-92.
15. Gale, K., Hong, J.S., and Guidotti, A. (1977): Brain Res., 136:371-375.
16. Goswell, M.J., and Sedgwick, E.M. (1971): J. Physiol. (Lond.), 218:84-85P.
17. Jacobowitz, D.M., and Palkovits, M. (1974): J. Comp. Neurol., 157:13-28.
18. Kebabian, J.W., Petzold, G.L., and Greengard, P. (1972): Proc. Natl. Acad. Sci. USA, 69:2145-2149.
19. Kim, J.S., Bak, I.J., Hassler, R., and Okada, Y. (1971): Exp. Brain Res., 14:95-104.
20. Kline, D.F., and Davis, J.M. (1969): Diagnosis and Drug Treatment of Psychiatric Disorders. Williams and Wilkins, Baltimore.
21. Krogsgaard-Larsen, P., Johnston, G.A.R., Curtis, D.R., Game, C.J.A., and McCullock, R.M. (1975): J. Neurochem., 25:803-809.

22. Mao, C.C., Guidotti, A., and Costa, E. (1975): Naunyn-Schmiedebergs Arch. Pharmacol., 289:369-378.
23. Mao, C.C., Marco, E., Revuelta, A., and Costa, E. (1978): In: Interactions Between Putative Neurotransmitters in Brain, edited by S. Garattini, J.F. Pujol, and R. Samanin, pp. 151-160. Raven Press, New York.
24. Mao, C.C., Peralta, E., Moroni, F., and Costa, E. (1978): Brain Res., 155:147-152.
25. Mao, C.C., Revuelta, A., Marco, E., and Costa, E. (1978): In: Neuro-psychopharmacology, edited by P. Deniker, C. Radouco-Thomas, and A. Villeneuve, pp. 447-452. Pergamon Press, New York.
26. Marco, E., Mao, C.C., Revuelta, A., Peralta, E., and Costa, E. (1978): Neuropharmacology, 17:589-596.
27. McGeer, P.L., Fibiger, H.C., Hattori, T., Singh, V.K., McGeer, E.G., and Maler, L. (1974): In: Advances in Behavioral Biology, Vol. 10, edited by R.O. Myers, and R.R. Druchker-Colin, pp. 27-47. Plenum Press, New York.
28. McGeer, P.L., Fibiger, H.C., Maler, L., Hattori, T., and McGeer, E.G. (1974): In: Advances in Neurology, Vol. 5, edited by F.H. McDowell, and A. Barbeau, pp. 153-163. Raven Press, New York.
29. McGeer, P.L., and McGeer, E.G. (1975): Brain Res., 91:331-335.
30. Miller, R.J., and Hiley, C.R. (1974): Nature (Lond.), 248:596-597.
31. Moroni, F., Cheney, D.L., and Costa, E. (1978): Neuropharmacology, 17:191-196.
32. Moroni, F., Cheney, D.L., Peralta, E., and Costa, E. (1978): J. Pharmacol. Exp. Ther., 207:870-877.
33. Neff, N.H., and Costa, E. (1967): In: Proceedings of the First International Symposium on Antidepressant Drugs, edited by S. Garattini, and M.N.C. Dukes, pp. 28-34. Excerpta Medica Foundation.
34. Neff, N.H., Spano, P.F., Groppetti, A., Wang, C.T., and Costa, E. (1971): J. Pharmacol. Exp. Ther., 176:701-710.
35. Niimi, K., Ikeda, T., Kawamura, S., and Inoshita, H. (1970): Brain Res., 21:327-343.
36. Nyback, H., and Sedvall, G. (1968): J. Pharmacol. Exp. Ther., 162:294-301.
37. Pearl, J., Spilker, B.A., Woodward, W.A., and Bentley, R.J. (1976): J. Pharm. Pharmacol., 28:302-304.
38. Precht, W., and Yoshida, M. (1971): Brain Res., 32:229-233.
39. Racagni, G., Cheney, D.L., Trabucchi, M., Wang, C., and Costa, E. (1974): Life Sci., 15:1961-1975.
40. Roberts, E., Chase, T.N., and Tower, A.B. (1976): GABA in Nervous System Function. Kroc Foundation Series Vol. 5. Raven Press, New York.
41. Shader, R.I., and DiMascio, A. (1970): In; Psychotropic Drug Side Effects, edited by R.I. Shader, and A. DiMascio, pp. 92-106. Williams and Wilkins, Baltimore.
42. Snyder, S.J., Banerjee, S.P., Yamamura, H.I., and Greenberg, D. (1974): Science, 184:1243-1253.

43. Stille, G., and Hippius, H. (1971): Pharmakopsychiatric, 4:182-189.

Glutamate as a Neurotransmitter,
edited by G. Di Chiara and G. L. Gessa
Raven Press, New York © 1981.

Glutamate Synapses and Receptors on Insect Muscle

P. N. R. Usherwood

Department of Zoology, University of Nottingham, Nottingham NG7 2RD, England

My attention during the past two decades has centred on the role of amino acids in transmission at peripheral (nerve-muscle) synapses in insects, in particular the identification of the chemical mediator at excitatory synapses on insect muscle. There are cogent prima facie reasons for gaining an understanding of all facets of nervous function in insects, given the world-wide economic importance of this group of animals. But apart from this, studies of putative amino acid transmitters in any animal may have implications for our understanding of the role of these compounds in the human central nervous system. Comparative neuropharmacology has already made an impact at this level and its catalytic effects on medical research will become increasingly obvious as the search for animal models intensifies.

In an oft-quoted publication on the criteria for identification of synaptic transmitters, Werman (38) warned that criteria "originally mean't to prevent the intrusion of careless work and the neglect of scientific methodology ... now threatens, in some cases to keep out the very information necessary to establish the nature of .... synaptic processes". Perhaps as a result of Werman's strictures, these criteria have been used flexibly as indicators of rather than as dogmatic determinants for transmitter identification at central and peripheral synapses, an approach which has been facilitated by the growing appreciation of the complexities of synapse structure and function. This is not to argue that the criteria have no place in modern neurobiology. Indeed it is important to resurrect them from time to time and to assess their relevance to the contemporary scene.

Despite Werman's timely warnings about the straightjacketing effects of establishing strict criteria for transmitter identification it is comforting to note that identification of the chemical mediator at locust (and other insect) excitatory nerve-muscle junctions as L-glutamate meets most of the criteria as

183

well as some of their more contemporary afterthoughts.

1. Identity of action: Most will agree with Werman that this is the fundamental criterion. It states that a putative transmitter should have an action(s) identical to that (those) of the natural transmitter. The postsynaptic membrane of excitatory synapses on locust muscle is highly sensitive (ca. 100 mV/nC during iontophoresis) to L-glutamate. The postsynaptic receptors gate cation selective ionophores (Na, K, Ca cojointly), the reversal potential of the synaptic current and the L-glutamate current having the same value (Table 1). The mean conductance and life-time of these ionophores are also identical whether they are gated through the action of L-glutamate or the natural transmitter. Inactivation of the receptor/ionophore complex through desensitization blocks the action of L-glutamate and the natural transmitter.

2. Release from nerve-terminals: L-glutamate is released from resting locust nerve-muscle preparations in small quantities (15, 37) and in larger quantities, under certain conditions, from stimulated preparations (37). It has been demonstrated recently that much of the L-glutamate released from stimulated blowfly larval nerve-muscle preparation probably comes from motor nerve terminals (6). Nevertheless the active sequestration of L-glutamate by nerve, muscle and glia continues to complicate efforts to meet the criterion of transmitter collectability in some insect nerve-muscle preparations.

3. Inactivation of transmitter: There is no evidence for an inactivating enzyme(s) at insect nerve-muscle junctions. High-affinity uptake of L-glutamate into nerve terminals has been demonstrated at synapses on some insect muscles, but available physiological data suggests that removal of transmitter from the cleft is diffusional (4, 10). Sequestration of L-glutamate by surrounding cells (muscle, glia and tracheal) may remove extra-cleft transmitter from extracellular space and also protect the synapses from exogenous glutamate. Each nerve terminal on locust muscle makes many synaptic contacts with its end organ. Perhaps the glia cells associated with the terminals serve to protect these synapses from the transmitter which diffuses out of neighbouring synaptic clefts, thereby eliminating cross-talk.

4. Precursors and synthesizing enzymes: Although enzymes and precursors for the synthesis of L-glutamate have not been demonstrated in insect motor nerve terminals, given the ubiquitous distribution of this amino acid their presence at these sites seems highly likely.

5. Presynaptic pharmacology: It could be argued that the presence of presynaptic receptors for L-glutamate at locust excitatory nerve-muscle junctions (29, 35, 36) supports the contention that this compound is the transmitter at these sites. However, receptors for other amino acids are also found here and other putative neurotransmitters (16, 18), such as acetylcholine, also influence the release of transmitters from locust motoneurones. This complex presynaptic pharmacology probably arises

from the presence of synaptic inputs involving different neurotransmitters to the motoneurone rather than its synaptic output to
its target organ (32). In other words the presynaptic receptors represent part of the pharmacologically heterogeneous extrajunctional receptor population of the motoneurone. This does not exclude
the possibility that presynaptic receptors play a modulatory role
in transmission at insect nerve-muscle junctions.

    6. <u>Extrajunctional receptors</u>: Extrajunctional receptors for
specific ligands found on excitable cells may signal the presence
of synapses on those cells at which these ligands or close structural analogues mediate transmission. Extrajunctional receptors
on locust leg muscle comprise topographically heterogeneous populations of two receptor types; D-receptors which are similar
pharmacologically to the junctional receptors found postsynaptically at excitatory junctions and H-receptors which have a dis-
tinctive pharmacology and gate Cl ionophores (14, 22).

    7. <u>Denervation supersensitivity</u>: When locust muscle is de-
nervated there is a significant increase in the sensitivity of
extrajunctional membrane to L-glutamate due to an increase in the
population density of D-receptors (not H-receptors) (11, 30).
The extent of this change depends on the type of muscle; phasic
muscles exhibiting greater denervation sensitivity than their
tonic counterparts. There is a close analogy between the supersensitivity to glutamate which follows denervation of locust
muscle and the supersensitivity to acetylcholine which follows
denervation of some vertebrate skeletal muscles.

    On the basis of the evidence presented in 1-7 above one is
compelled to accept the conclusion that L-glutamate is the transmitter at insect excitatory nerve-muscle junctions.

TABLE 1.   <u>Glutamate-gated ionophores of locust muscle membrane</u>

Site	Ligand	Ions (reversal potential)	Ionophore conduc- tance	Ionophore life-time (Em$\sim$ -60 mV)
Junctional membrane	L-glutamate (5, 35, 36)	Na, K, Ca ($\sim$ 0mV) (3)	120pS (23°C) (1)	$\sim$ 2.5ms (1)
	L-quisqualate (2)	-	$\sim$ 120pS (23°C)(1)	$\sim$ 5.3ms (1)
Extrajunctional membrane	L-glutamate (14)	Na, K, Ca ($\sim$ 0mV) (8)	$\sim$ 120pS (20°C) (12, 20, 26)	$\sim$ 2.5ms (12, 20, 26)
(D-receptors)	L-quisqualate (2)	-	" (12)	$\sim$ 5.2ms (12)
	L-Cysteine sulphinate (12)	-	" (12)	$\sim$ 1.5ms (12)

Em = membrane potential

Junctional and extrajunctional receptors on locust muscle
Junctional glutamate receptors on locust muscle are not homogeneous pharmacologically (19) an observation which has lead to

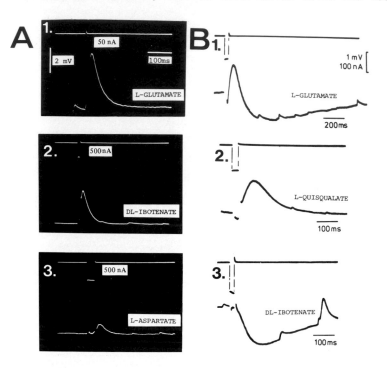

Fig. 1 Pharmacology of glutamate receptors on locust muscle. A;
at some junctional sites depolarizations to L-glutamate, DL-
ibotenate (a rigid isoxazole, similar structurally to fully extended conformation of L-glutamate) and L-aspartate (analogous to
fully folded conformation of L-glutamate) have been recorded (1-
3; recordings from same site). Cross-desensitization studies
showed that receptors for L-ibotenate and L-aspartate are distinct sub-populations of the glutamate receptor population at this
junction, e.g. the L-aspartate sensitive receptors can be desensitized with L-glutamate but not with DL-ibotenate.

    B; when L-glutamate was applied to an extrajunctional site
from one barrel of a multibarrelled iontophoretic pipette, a
biphasic response was evoked; with L-quisqualate the response was
purely depolarising whereas with DL-ibotenate it was hyperpolarizing (1-3 respectively). Miniature excitatory postsynaptic potentials accompany the drug-evoked potentials.

    Voltage and time calibrations same for A (1-3). Voltage and
current calibrations same for B (1-3). A (1-3) from Usherwood
(31); B (1-3) from Usherwood (34), after Clark, Gration & Usherwood (unpublished data).

the suggestion that they may contain a spectrum of receptor types ranging from those which bind L-glutamate in extended conformation to those which accepted the fully-folded conformation of this amino acid (33). The extrajunctional D-receptors are identical to junctional receptors in terms of the ionophores that they gate but it remains to be established whether they are also variable pharmacologically.

The potency of glutamate (agonist) interaction with either junctional or extrajunctional receptor populations will depend on a variety of factors including affinity, and ionophore lifetime. The electrical and ionic properties of the nerve-muscle system will also influence the efficacy of drug action on locust muscle. It is important, therefore, to gain information on the macromolecular events underlying transmitter-receptor interaction at locust nerve-muscle synapses, an approach which will hopefully lead eventually to a molecular view of this system. Since the properties of the extrajunctional D-receptors and their ionophores are, as far as can be estimated, identical to those of junctional glutamate receptors they form a useful starting point to this new approach since they are readily accessible and their population density can be modified by denervation. The patch clamp technique of Neher et al. (24) has been used to study the kinetics of ionophores gated by extrajunctional D-receptors and to gain an understanding of the site and mode of action of compounds such as streptomycin and Philanthus venom which block excitatory nerve-muscle transmission in locusts.

Glutamate-gated ionophores in locust muscle membrane

Whereas noise analysis (21) is ideal for investigating the average properties of membrane receptors in large populations the patch clamp technique enables studies of individual receptor/ionophore complexes. When saline filled patch electrodes containing L-glutamate ($> 10^{-5}$M) are placed against the extrajunctional membrane of a locust muscle fibre transient 'square pulses' of inward current ($\sim$ 6pA at E_m = -60mV and 20°C) are recorded (20, 26). These transients, which are considered to represent the opening and closing of single glutamate-activated membrane channels are not seen when L-glutamate is omitted from the patch electrode. Channel current, but not channel conductance, is voltage dependent. Similar channel currents and conductances to those seen with L-glutamate are seen with its agonists L-quisqualate and L-cysteine sulphinate. However, channel life-time is agonist dependent (11, 12). Although channel life-time is not voltage sensitive it must be remembered that all patch clamp data that have been obtained from locust muscle were recorded in the presence of concanavalin A which may eliminate the voltage dependence of this parameter.

Influence of streptomycin:

Streptomycin and other antibiotics of the aminoglycoside group block transmission at cholinergic and glutamatergic synapses (17, 25) where cationic ionophores are gated. The effects of this compound on glutamate-gated channels in locust extra-junctional muscle membrane (13) support the contention of Onodera & Takeuchi (25) that it blocks transmitter (glutamate) gated ionophores at excitatory synapses on arthropod muscle.

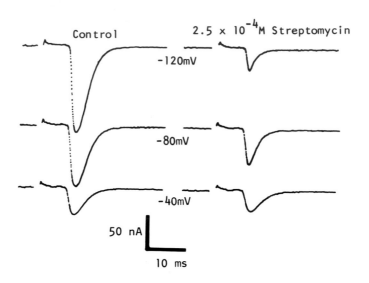

Fig. 2. Effect of streptomycin on e.p.s.c. of locust extensor tibiae muscle. A fibre was **vo**ltage clamped at three different membrane potentials (shown beside traces). Left; control recordings in absence of streptomycin showing increase in amplitude, but no change in decay time of e.p.s.c. with hyperpolarization. Right; records obtained after 5 min. exposure to streptomycin. The amplitude and decay time of e.p.s.c. at -40mV were not greatly different from those of corresponding control e.p.s.c. but with hyperpolarization marked reductions in these parameters were apparent. These was also a voltage dependent reduction in time to peak of the e.p.s.c.

Current and voltage calibrations same for all traces. Resting potential of muscle, ca. -60mV. Temperature ∿ 20°C.

From Clark, Gration, Ramsay & Usherwood (13).

Fig. 2 illustrates the reduction in amplitude of the excitatory postsynaptic current (e.p.s.c.), recorded intracellularly from locust extensor tibiae muscle under voltage clamp (4), by 2.5×10^{-4}M streptomycin. The block is voltage sensitive. In the absence of streptomycin the amplitude of the e.p.s.c. increases linearly with hyperpolarization but the decay of the e.p.s.c. is not voltage sensitive. (N.B. These studies were done with saline containing a high concentration of Mg^{2+} which

may reduce the voltage sensitivity of e.p.s.c. decay.) After 5
min. exposure to 2.5 x 10^{-4}M streptomycin the amplitude of the
e.p.s.c. is unchanged at the resting potential but is significantly reduced with hyperpolarization, which also reduced the
time to peak of the e.p.s.c. and the ½ decay time of this event.
Similar results were obtained with junctional glutamate currents.
The effects of streptomycin were only slowly reversible; 15-20
minutes in drug-free saline being required to reverse the effect
of 2.5 x 10^{-4}M.

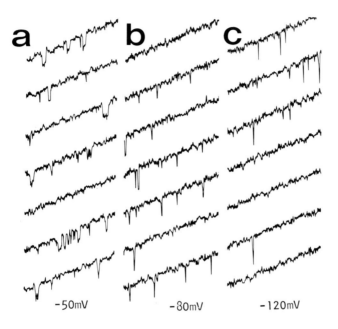

Fig. 3 Patch-clamp recordings of channel in membrane of locust
extensor tibiae muscle gated by L-glutamate in the presence of
10^{-5}M streptomycin (in patch electrode). The membrane of the
muscle fibre (resting potential ca. -60 mV) was clamped at the
levels shown below each sequence of traces (a-c). Note increases in channel current with hyperpolarization (b-c) which
were also seen in the absence of streptomycin. However, the
voltage dependent reduction in channel life-time seen in streptomycin (compare -80mV and -120mV with -40mV) was not characteristic of controls. The muscle was pretreated with 10^{-6}M concanavalin A (23) before recordings were made. Temperature ∿ 20°C.
From Clark, Gration, Ramsay & Usherwood (13).

The conductance of the open glutamate-gated channel was unaffected by the presence of streptomycin in the patch electrode,
but channel life-time became distinctly voltage sensitive (Fig. 3).

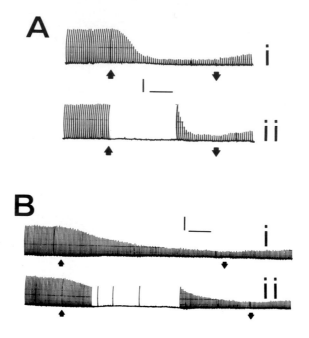

Fig. 4 Effect of δ-PTX on L-glutamate potentials evoked by glutamate iontophoresis at excitatory neuromuscular junctions of locust extensor tibiae muscle. A. (Trace i; saline containing 0.1
U/ml* of δ-PTX was introduced (↑) during repetitive application
of 1.5 nC iontophoretic glutamate doses. Note the rapid reduction
in response amplitude. After 1½ min exposure to δ-PTX,toxin-free
saline was introduced (↓). Trace ii; following 10 min wash with
toxin-free saline, the response was restored to control amplitude.
Saline containing 0.1 U/ml was reintroduced, but iontophoretic
application of glutamate was discontinued for 1 min and then resumed. The amplitude of the first response at the end of the 1
min period was nearly identical to the control amplitude (cf,
trace i). Note the rapid decline in amplitude of response to subsequent glutamate doses. Measurements were made at the resting
potential of the muscle fibre, -60 mV. Calibration bars: potential (vertical), 4 mV; time (horizontal), 20 sec. B. Junctional glutamate potentials from a fibre of a different muscle preparation.
Trace (i); saline containing 0.05 U/ml of δ-PTX was introduced
(↑) during continuous application of 1.4 nC iontophoretic doses
at 0.85 Hz. Following removal of the toxin (↓) the muscle was
washed for 15 min in toxin-free saline to restore the response to
the control amplitude. Trace (ii); saline containing 0.05 U/ml
of δ-PTX was reintroduced, but the iontophoretic pulse was interrupted for various time periods then resumed continuously
after approximately 80 s. From Clark et al. (7).
*Details can be obtained from Piek, et al. (27).

The frequency of channel opening also decreased during hyper-polarization.

It seems likely that streptomycin blocks the open ionophores gated by L-glutamate receptors and that the blocking rate is much higher than the unblocking rate.

Philanthus toxin (δ-PTX):

Crude toxin from the venom glands of the Egyptian wasp (Philanthus triangulum) can be separated into a series of components, some of which block transmission at locust excitatory nerve-muscle junctions (27). The identities of the components are unknown but they have molecular weights of < 700. One component, δ-PTX, depresses the twitch contraction of locust leg nerve-muscle preparations during repetitive stimulation but exerts no measurable effects on these preparations in the absence of neural stimulation (7). It also depresses the amplitude and reduces the $\frac{1}{2}$ decay time of the e.p.s.c. and glutamate potential in a frequency dependent fashion (Fig. 4) which suggests that the toxin exerts its action only on activated junctional receptors or their associated open ionophores. Neuromuscular block with δ-PTX is only slowly reversible and possibly multicomponent (Fig. 4). Similar results were obtained in the presence and absence of concanavalin A so it is unlikely that the effects of δ-PTX are due to enhanced and prolonged desensitization of the postjunctional glutamate receptor/ionophores.

When δ-PTX is included in a patch clamp electrode along with L-glutamate the frequency of glutamate-gated channel openings in extrajunctional muscle membrane under the tip of the electrode was reduced (7). Due to the long blocking time of the venom channel activity appeared as bursts of openings interposed between long (secs) when no channels were seen. The life-time of the channel was reduced in a concentration dependent fashion by the toxin. δ-PTX seems to be a glutamate channel blocker with unusual properties.

Conclusion

At its outset this paper reviews the evidence for assuming that L-glutamate is the transmitter at insect excitatory nerve-muscle junctions. Most of the criteria, established in the 1960s for transmitter identification have been met. Attention has now moved away from establishing a role for glutamate at these sites to the macromolecular aspects of ionophore gating by glutamate receptors and the kinetics of these transient membrane channels. The patch clamp technique affords major opportunities in this new field and already there is a hint of surprises, with receptor/ionophore complexes exhibiting highly individualistic properties which are not appreciated when these structures are viewed as large populations. It had been hoped that studies of δ-PTX would yield a glutamate antagonist of some potency. This has not been realized but the action of the venom on the ionophore gated by glutamate receptors on locust muscle may be a valuable tool in discovering the undoubtedly complex properties of these transient membrane channels.

Acknowledgement

Many of the data reported in this chapter were obtained from studies supported by British Science Research Council Grants to P.N.R.U.

References

1. Anderson, C. R., Cull-Candy, S. G. and Miledi, R. (1978): J. Physiol., 282:219-242.
2. Anis, N., Clark, R. B., Gration, K. A. F. and Usherwood, P. N. R. (1980): (Submitted to J. Physiol.)
3. Anwyl, R. and Usherwood, P. N. R. (1974): J. Physiol., 242: 86-87.
4. Anwyl, R. and Usherwood, P.N.R. (1975): J. Physiol., 254: 46-47.
5. Beranek, R. and Miller, P.L. (1968): J. exp. Biol., 49:83-93.
6. Boden, P., Duce, I., Usherwood, P.N.R. and Wilson, R.G. (1980): (to be published).
7. Clark, R.B., Donaldson, L.A., Gration, K.A.F., Lamb, J., Piek, T., Ramsay, R., Spanjer, W. and Usherwood, P.N.R. (1980): (Submitted to Nature).
8. Clark, R.B., Gration, K.A.F. and Usherwood, P.N.R. (1979): Neuropharmac. 18: 201-208.
9. Clark, R.B., Gration, K.A.F. and Usherwood, P.N.R. (1979). J. Physiol. 290: 551-568.
10. Clark, R.B., Gration, K.A.F. and Usherwood, P.N.R. (1980): Brain Res. (In press).
11. Clark, R.B., Gration, K.A.F. and Usherwood, P.N.R. (1980): J. Physiol., 301: 60-61.
12. Clark, R.B., Gration, K.A.F., Ramsay, R. and Usherwood, P.N.R. (1980): (in preparation).
13. Clark, R.B., Gration, K.A.F., Ramsay, R. and Usherwood, P.N.R. (1980): (in preparation).
14. Cull-Candy, S.G. and Usherwood, P.N.R. (1973): Nature, 246: 62-64.
15. Daoud, A. and Miller, R. (1976): J. Neurochem. 36: 119-127.
16. Dowson, R.J. and Usherwood, P.N.R. (1972): J. Physiol., 229: 13-14.
17. Dretchen, K.L., Sohall, M.D., Gergis, S.D. and Long, J.P. (1973): Eur. J. Pharmac., 22:10-16.
18. Fulton, B.P. and Usherwood, P.N.R. (1977): Neuropharmac. 16:877-880.
19. Gration, K.A.F., Clark, R.B. and Usherwood, P.N.R. (1979): Brain Res., 171:360-364.
20. Gration, K.A.F., Patlak, J.B. and Usherwood, P.N.R. (1979): J. Physiol., 301:60-61P.
21. Katz, B. and Miledi, R. (1972): J. Physiol., 224-665-700.

22. Lea, T.J. and Usherwood, P.N.R. (1973): Comp. gen. Pharmac., 4:333-350.
23. Mathers, D. A. and Usherwood, P. N. R. (1978). Comp. Biochem. Physiol. 59C, 151-155.
24. Neher, E., Sakmann, B. and Steinbach, J.H. (1978): Pflugers Arch. 375:219-228.
25. Onodera, K. and Takeuchi, A. (1976): Neuropharmac. 16: 171-177.
26. Patlak, J.B., Gration, K.A.F. and Usherwood, P.N.R. (1979): Nature, 278:643-645.
27. Piek, T., May, T.E. and Spanjer, W. (1980): In "Insect Neurobiology and Pesticide Action (Neurotox '79)". 219-220. Society of Chemical Industry, London.
28. Rees, D. and Usherwood, P.N.R. (1972): Comp. Biochem. Physiol. 43A, 83-101.
29. Usherwood, P.N.R. (1967): Am. Zool., 7:553-582.
30. Usherwood, P.N.R. (1969): Nature, 223:411-413.
31. Usherwood, P.N.R. (1977): Biochem. Soc. Trans., 5:845-849.
32. Usherwood, P.N.R. (1978): Adv. Comp. Physiol. Biochem., 7: 227-310.
33. Usherwood, P.N.R. (1978). Adv. Pharmacol. Therap 1, 107-116.
34. Usherwood, P.N.R. (1979): Proc. V. Winter School Biophysics of Membrane Transport, Poland. pp78-102.
35. Usherwood, P.N.R. and Machili, P. (1966): Nature, 210: 634-636.
36. Usherwood, P.N.R. and Machili, P. (1968): J. exp. Biol., 49:341-361.
37. Usherwood, P.N.R., Machili, P. and Leaf, G. (1968): Nature, 219:1169-1172.
38. Werman, R. (1966): Comp. Biochem. Physiol., 18:745-766.

Glutamate as a Neurotransmitter,
edited by G. Di Chiara and G. L. Gessa
Raven Press, New York © 1981.

An Analysis of Glutamate-induced Ion Fluxes Across the Membrane of Spinal Motoneurons of the Frog

U. Sonnhof and Ch. Bührle

*I. Physiologisches Institut der Universität, Im Neuenheimer Feld 326,
D-6900 Heidelberg, Federal Republic of Germany*

On the postsynaptic action of GLUT

Intracellular studies of the excitatory action of GLUT
in nerve cells of the vertebrate CNS have so far been
based on the determination of the reversal potential
of the GLUT depolarization and on measurements of
associated changes in neuronal input resistance (Curtis and Johnston, 1974; Krnjević, 1974; Tebecis,1974;
Watkins, 1978).

Comparison of the reversal potential of the GLUT depolarization with that of the EPSP showed considerable
differences, which, however may not necessarily be a
consequence of different ionic mechanisms, but may be
attributed to electronic phenomena resulting from
the complex morphology of nerve cells in the CNS.

Neuronal input resistance in motoneurons (MNs) of both
cat and frog is reported to be increased, decreased
or unchanged during the GLUT action (Altmann, 1976;
Bernardi et al, 1972; Engberg et al, 1979; Shapovalov
et al, 1978).

A decrease of neuronal input resistance was often
found in MNs of the isolated frog spinal cord, when
synaptic transmission was not interfered with. Such
events did not occur consistently, and in many cases
input resistance returned to, or surpassed, control
values when the GLUT depolarization was maximal.

In contrast, no measurable change in input resistance
could be detected during blockade of chemical synaptic
transmission in the presence of Mn^{2+} (2mmol/l), even
when GLUT was applied in very high concentrations
(bath application: 10^{-2} mmol/l; iontophoretic application: 500 nA).

The GLUT depolarization was, however, accompanied by
a considerable accumulation of K^+ in the extracellular

space. The time courses of the GLUT depolarization and of the change in extracellular K^+-activity (aK^+e) measured close to the recorded MN corresponded well (Fig. 1A).

A

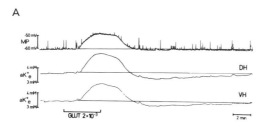

B

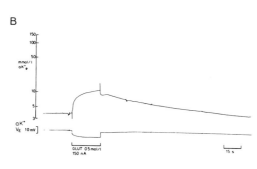

Fig.1

A) GLUT-depolarization of a MN and simultaneous registration of the aK^+e in dorsal (DH) and ventral horn (VH)

B) aK^+e during iontophoretic release of GLUT measured by an ion sensitive electrode incorporated into the iontophoresis pipette

This increase of aK^+e together with the absence of any changes in neuronal input resistance suggested that GLUT might not have any specific action upon the membrane of MNs, and that the observed depolarization may only be a consequence of the decrease of the transmembrane K^+ gradient caused by the liberation of K^+ from surrounding cellular elements susceptible to GLUT.

Furthermore, changes in membrane resistance observed in the state of undisturbed synaptic transmission may be caused by a K^+ mediated depolarization of presynaptic terminals in contact with the recorded MN and a subsequent liberation of transmitter which could lead to marked conductance changes of the postsynaptic membrane.

The conception of such a mode of action is supported by the observation that even iontophoretic application of GLUT with current intensities widely in use (150 nA) induces 4-fold increase of aK^+e at the site of GLUT release in the MN pool (Fig. 1B).

On the basis of these findings, an experimental proof of the postsynaptic action of GLUT in the CNS did not seem to be possible with conventional methods.

According to the work of Lothman and Somjen (1975) the dependence of MP upon changes in aK^+e is unclear in spinal MNs of the cat. The influence of changes in aK^+e upon membrane potential in frog spinal MNs had therefore to be determined to clarify, whether a passive K^+ depolarization was sufficient to explain the phenomena found during the action of GLUT.

An attempt was made to determine, whether the Nernst equation adequately describes the relation between MP and aK^+e or whether other ionic conductances significantly contribute to the generation of the MP and require use of the Goldman equation or related mathematical expressions. If the relation between MP and experimentally elevated aK^+e obeyed the Nernst equation or a similar function in a reproducible manner, any GLUT induced change in membrane permeability should be expressed by a deviation of the measured relation from this function during the action of GLUT, thus demonstrating the postsynaptic action of the amino acid. During blockade of chemical synaptic transmission and superfusion of the preparation with KCl the change of MP per decade elevation of aK^+e ($\Delta MP/dec.\Delta aK^+e$) ranged between 53-56 mV showing only small deviations from the Nernst equation presumably resulting from influences of other ionic conductances upon the generation of the MP (Fig. 2A).

When the same experiment was repeated in a state of intact synaptic transmission, $\Delta MP/dec.\Delta aK^+e$ proved to have an irregular and irreproducible shape with an average slope exceeding by far that predicted by the Nernst equation. Simultaneously prominent fluctuations in neuronal input resistance were found.

These phenomena probably result from discharges of internuncial neurons evoked by the rising level of aK^+e.

The determination of $\Delta MP/dec.\Delta aK^+e$ during synaptic blockade and the action of GLUT, however, yielded values greater than 90 mV, clearly indicating that the depolarization of the MN is not primarily due to a reduction of the transmembrane K^+ gradient nor to liberation of transmitter from depolarized presynaptic structures, but requires an involvement of permeability changes to other ions of the MNs membrane itself (Fig. 2B).

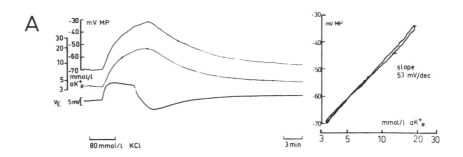

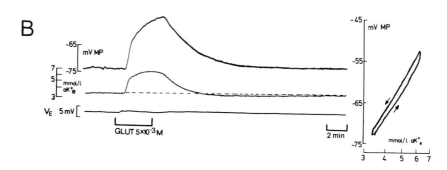

Fig. 2 Dependence of MP upon aK^+_e

    A) Experimental elevation of aK^+_e by super-fusion of KCl (80 mmol/l)

    B) GLUT induced elevation of aK^+_e (slope 9 8mV/dec. $\Delta\ aK^+_e$)

These ion fluxes are obviously too small to be detected by changes of neuronal input resistance, and may therefore be associated with either an increase, a decrease or a combined change of membrane conductances.

An analysis of the ionic processes involved was therefore attempted by simultaneous recording of transient changes of the activity of K^+, Na^+, Ca^{++} and Cl^- in the intra- and extracellular space.

Intracellular ion activity in MNs

Intra- and extracellular measurements of ion activity were performed with conventional double barreled ion sensitive microelectrodes with outer tip diameters of about 1 µm using the following ion exchange resins:

K^+	Corning No. 477 315	
Na^+	Simon, Zürich	
Cl^-	Orion, Corning No.477 317, Simon	
Ca^{++}	Simon, Zürich	

A determination of absolute ion activity with liquid ion exchangers calls for a detailed discussion of cross sensitivities of the respective resins to interfering ions or organic molecules present in the MN. As such a discussion would be beyond the scope of this paper, the uncorrected values of intracellular ion activities and resulting equilibrium potentials are shown in Tab. 1

$a_X i$: mean intracell. ion activity
E_X : mean equilibrium potential

	n	$a\bar{x}i$ SD (mmol/l)	MP SD (mV)	$\bar{E}x$ (mV)
Na^+	37	53.13 ± 13.86	-54.08 ± 8.27	$+ 22.14$
K^+	17	87.82 ± 34.07	-55.87 ± 9.37	$- 80.46$
Ca^{++}	57	$8.25 \times 10^{-2} \pm 6.25 \times 10^{-2}$	-47.21 ± 11.06	$+ 36.51$
Cl^-	42	34.4 ± 9.9	-45.8 ± 10.12	$- 30.4$

Suffice it to say that the true aNa^+_i is presumably 10 mmol/l, the true aK^+_i 5 mmol/l lower than indicated above. Little can be said at present about aCa^{++}_i. The depolarizing deviation of E_{Cl} from the resting potential is due to an inwardly directed Cl^- pump as described by Bührle and Sonnhof (1979)

The ionic mechanism of the GLUT depolarization

As the EMF for Na^+ (76.22 mV) and Ca^{++} (83.72 mV) is quite high, it is conceivable that very subtle increases of membrane permeability to each of these ions result in a considerable membrane depolarization while the associated change of membrane resistance may stay below the threshold of detection. The following findings refer to application of GLUT in the superfusing solution of the preparation (Fig. 3).

Na^+

The GLUT depolarization was accompanied by an increase of aNa^+_i and a decrease of aNa^+_e (Fig. 3A). As with all other ion activities aNa^+_i and aNa^+_e steadily returned to control values after termination of GLUT application. A depolarization equal in amplitude due to experimental elevation of aK^+_e did not lead to measurable changes of Na^+_i.

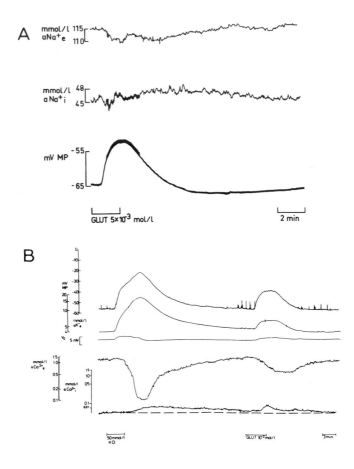

Fig. 3   A) extra- (aNa^+_e) and intracellular (aNa^+_i)
           Na$^+$ activity during GLUT application

         B) voltage dependent and GLUT-induced Ca^{++}-
            changes in a MN and in the extracellular
            space

Ca^{++}

In frog spinal motoneurons as well as in various other nerve cells potential dependent influxes of Ca^{++} are known to exist (Eckert and Lux, 1976). When MNs were passively depolarized by K^+ a marked decrease of aCa^{++}_e was observed. The accompanying rise of aCa^{++}_i shows that at least part of the Ca ions leaving the extracellular space cross the MNs membrane.

This potential dependent Ca^{++} influx was of threshold type and was activated at MP levels between -30 and -25 mV (Fig. 3B).

In opposition to that Ca^{++} influxes during the action of GLUT could already be observed when MP was far below this threshold (Fig. 3B) suggesting that GLUT activates specific Ca^{++} channels in the membranes of MNs.

Cl^-

As E_{Cl} in frog spinal MNs is less negative than MP an increased Cl^- conductance could in theory contribute to the depolarizing effect of GLUT. However, changes in aCl^-_i during K^+ and GLUT depolarizations of comparable amplitude were nearly identical. Therefore, a voltage dependent displacement of Cl^- has to be assumed (Fig. 4B).

K^+

The reduction of aK^+_i during the action of GLUT clearly proves that K^+ leaves the MN and contributes to the increase of aK^+ in the extracellular space (Fig. 4A). An increased K^+ conductance should counteract the depolarization carried by Na^+ and Ca^{++} entering the cell. It is generally assumed that K^+ conductance is the main constituent of membrane conductance in the resting state. Any significant change in K^+ conductance should therefore strongly influence neuronal input resistance. As such influences were not found during the action of GLUT, a passive outward shift of K^+ has to be taken into consideration. Calculations based on values of specific membrane resistance for cat MNs as given by Barrett and Crill (1973) support the idea that such an efflux of K^+ is due to the shift of MP away from E_K during a depolarization essentially carried by an influx of Na^+ and Ca^{++}.

At present, a GLUT induced activation of membrane K^+ conductance at remote dendritic sites cannot be excluded.

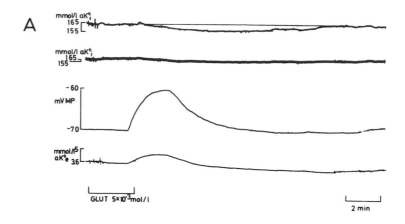

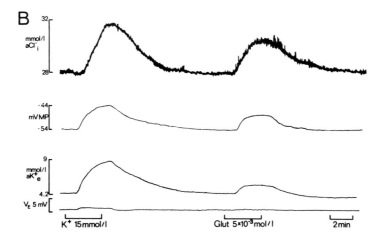

Fig. 4 A) Measurements of intra- and extracellular
aK$^+$ during the action of GLUT

B) Intracellular Cl$^-$ activity during experimental elevation of aK^+_e and during GLUT
depolarization

From these results it is concluded that the depolarizing action of GLUT is a result of a combined influx
of Na$^+$ and Ca^{++}, while GLUT activated conductance
changes are virtually absent for Cl$^-$ and unlikely for
K$^+$.

References

Altmann, H., ten Bruggencate, G., Pickelmann, P. and
   Steinberg, R.: Effects of glutamate, aspartate and
   two presumed antagonists on feline rubrospinal
   neurones.
   Pflügers Arch. 364, 249-255 (1976)

Barrett, J.N. and Crill, W.E.: Specific membrane properties of cat motoneurons.
   J. Physiol. (Lond.) 239, 301-324 (1974)

Bernardi, G., Zieglgänsberger, W., Herz, A. and Puil,
   E.A.: Intracellular studies of the action of L-
   glutamic acid on spinal neurones of the cat.
   Brain Res. 39, 523-525 (1972)

Bührle, Ch.-Ph. and Sonnhof, U.: The ionic mechanism
   of the IPSP in frog spinal motoneurones.
   Pflügers Arch. Suppl. Vol. 382 (1979)

Curtis,D.R. and Johnston, G.A.R.: Amino acid transmitters in the mammalian central nervous system.
   Ergebn. Physiol. 69, 97-188 (1974)

Eckert, R. and Lux, H.D.: A voltage-sensitive per-
   sistent calcium conductance in neuronal somata of
   Helix.
   J. Physiol. 254, 129-157 (1976)

Engberg, I., Flatman, J.A. and Lambert, J.D.C.: The
   actions of excitatory amino acids on motoneurones
   in the feline spinal cord.
   J. Physiol. 288, 227-261 (1979)

Krnjević,K.: Chemical nature of synaptic transmission
   in vertebrates.
   Physiol. Rev. 54, 418-540 (1974)

Lothman, E.W and Somjen, G.G.: Extracellular potassium activity, intracellular and extracellular
   potential responses in the spinal cord.
   J. Physiol. (Lond.) 252 , 115-136 (1975)

Shapovalov, A.I., Shiriaev, B. and Velumian, A.A.:
   Mechanisms of postsynaptic excitation in amphibian
   motoneurons.
   J. Physiol. 279, 437-455 (1978)

Tebecis, A.K.: Transmitters and identified neurons in the mammalian central nervous system. Bristol: Scientechnica

Watkins, J.C.: Excitatory amino acids. Kainic acid as a tool in neurobiology, ed. by EG. McGeer et al, Raven Press, New York (1978)

Glutamate as a Neurotransmitter,
edited by G. Di Chiara and G. L. Gessa
Raven Press, New York © 1981.

Actions of Excitatory Amino Acids on Membrane Conductance and Potential in Motoneurones

J. D. C. Lambert, J. A. Flatman, and I. Engberg

Institute of Physiology, University of Aarhus, DK-8000 Aarhus C, Denmark

Curtis and his colleagues (10,11,12) were the first to demonstrate that central neurones could be excited by iontophoretic application of a range of naturally occurring and synthetic acidic amino acids. The postulate that naturally occurring acidic amino acids might serve as excitatory transmitters was initially discarded (5,10) since virtually all neurones tested were sensitive to the amino acids (whereas selective sensitivity might have been expected for a transmitter candidate). Moreover, the reversal potential for amino acid induced depolarization was found to be lower than that of synaptic excitation (5).

At first it was also assumed that there was only one receptor for acidic amino acids (6,11), and that agonist potency depended upon a) an appropriate interaction of charged groups on the agonist with those of the receptor, b) whether the agonist is taken up into the surrounding tissue (2,7).

More recently, it has been suggested that there are probably at least two distinct receptors for excitatory amino acids. This was first indicated by the differential sensitivity of neurones to L-glutamate and L-aspartate (13) and the subsequent development of antagonists (including Mg^{++} ions) which are able to differentiate between the receptors (30,31,32).

There have hitherto been relatively few direct measurements of membrane conductance (G_M) during the action of excitatory amino acids on mammalian central neurones (but see 1,24,34). Though conductance was not measured directly, an increase in G_M during the action of acidic amino acids was inferred by Curtis et al. (10).

This led to the supposition that all excitatory amino acids cause an increase in membrane permeability, particularly to Na^+ (9).

From detailed studies of the conductance changes underlying motoneuronal responses to a range of acidic amino acid analogues (14,17,25) we have grouped analogues according to the type of response they produce. We will discuss how our grouping compares with the pharmacological classification (30,31).

Detailed description of the methods used in this study has appeared in Engberg et al. (17). Briefly, intracellular recordings were made from lumbar and sacral motoneurones in barbiturate anaesthetized or anaemically decerebrated cats. Amino acids were applied iontophoretically from extracellular barrels surrounding the intracellular recording electrode. G_M was measured by injecting short duration, negative, constant current pulses through the graphite screened (15) recording electrode. The evoked voltage transients were electronically averaged. In some experiments, simultaneous extracellular DC recordings were made from one of the iontophoretic barrels. Hence we simultaneously recorded the intracellular and extracellular potentials (both with respect to a non-polarizable Ag/AgCl electrode buried in the leg muscles). The difference between these potentials gave the "transmembrane" potential.

The presentation will be divided into three sections: I, dealing with the changes in G_M evoked by a range of amino acid analogues; II, dealing with the interaction of barbiturate anaesthetics with excitatory amino acid responses; III, dealing with the extracellular recording of negative going potentials during amino acid release in the grey matter and the significance of these potentials when assessing "membrane potential" changes.

I. MEMBRANE CONDUCTANCE CHANGES

In an earlier project we investigated the action of biogenic amines on motoneurones. These amines caused a hyperpolarization (accompanied by a small decrease in G_M (19,28)) which had a reversal potential of about −20 mV. To see whether a decrease in P_{Na} was involved in the responses, we decided to apply an agent to the motoneurone which would increase P_{Na} and then see if the amines were able to close the channels. As all excitatory amino acids were thought to act, at least in part, by increasing P_{Na} (9), we tried DL-homocysteate (DLH). We were surprised to find that this agent caused a stable <u>decrease</u> in G_M (14). Although precedent existed for agents which could depolarize with a decrease in G_M (e.g. see 33), this was the first time that such a mechanism had been proposed for excitatory amino acids.

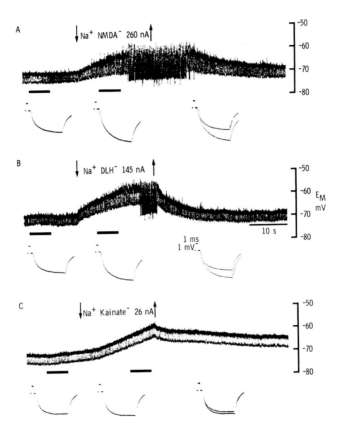

FIG. 1. Membrane potential (E_M) recordings from a motoneurone in a pentobarbitone anaesthetized cat. Current balanced iontophoretic doses of NMDA (A), DLH (B) and kainate (C) were chosen to give similar sized responses. Below each slow speed Mingograph trace are two averaged (50 samples) records of the voltage transients evoked by -3 nA current pulses. These were taken before and during the drug actions, as indicated by bars. The transients are superimposed on the right. The membrane potential records are modulated by the conductance measuring pulses and, in A and B, the afterhyperpolarizations of drug evoked firing.

The depolarization to all agents was accompanied by a decrease in absolute G_M, that during NMDA being the greatest. Note the difference in firing threshold to NMDA and DLH and that kainate did not evoke firing.

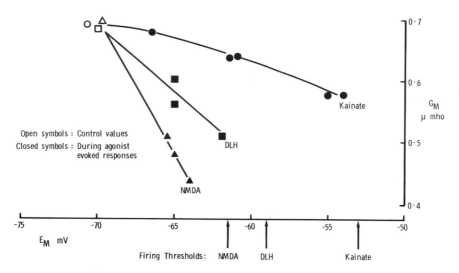

FIG. 2.   Graph from the same experiment as in Fig. 1 showing the membrane conductance (G_M) / potential (E_M) relationship obtained from several applications of each agonist. Arrows on the abscissa indicate the potential at which the neurone just started to fire repetitively in response to each agent.

Since then we have investigated a number of excitatory amino acid analogues. Figs 1 & 2 show results from one motoneurone where the actions of NMDA, DLH and kainate may be quantitatively compared. A range of doses of the three agonists was applied giving depolarizations of increasing size. G_M was recorded at the various levels of membrane potential achieved during the agonist evoked responses. Examples of individual responses are shown in Fig. 1. The depolarization to all three agonists was accompanied by a decrease in G_M – that during NMDA being the greatest, while the G_M during kainate was only slightly less than the control value. The gradients for the three curves in Fig. 2 were: NMDA – 43.3×10^{-9} mho $\cdot$ mV^{-1}; DLH – 21.5×10^{-9} mho $\cdot$ mV^{-1}; kainate – 8.3×10^{-9} mho $\cdot$ mV^{-1} (linear portion of relationship).

Most motoneurones exhibit anomalous rectification – a decrease in G_M when the membrane is depolarized by injected current. In assessing amino acid evoked G_M changes, it is necessary to compare the G_M during amino acid evoked depolarization with that obtained when the neurone has been depolarized to the same level of potential by injected current. Although membrane rectification was not in fact measured in this experiment, it is known from experience that the "membrane curve" would lie between those of DLH and kainate – probably closer to the DLH curve (see Fig. 9 in 17).

On the basis of this type of experiment, we have grouped the amino acids according to the following parameters: a. time course of depolarization; b. effect on G_M; c. ability to maintain stable repetitive firing (Table 1).

TABLE 1. Grouping of amino acids according to response features

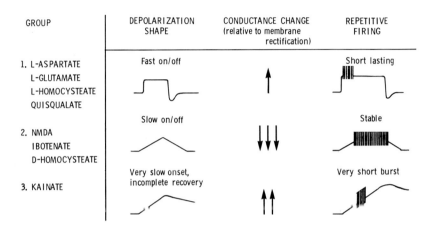

GROUP	DEPOLARIZATION SHAPE	CONDUCTANCE CHANGE (relative to membrane rectification)	REPETITIVE FIRING
1. L-ASPARTATE L-GLUTAMATE L-HOMOCYSTEATE QUISQUALATE	Fast on/off		Short lasting
2. NMDA IBOTENATE D-HOMOCYSTEATE	Slow on/off		Stable
3. KAINATE	Very slow onset, incomplete recovery		Very short burst

Group 1 (L-glutamate, L-aspartate, quisqualate and L-homocysteate)

The responses of this group are typified by those to L-glutamate. Short applications of L-glutamate gave depolarizations with fast onset and recovery with little change in absolute G_M, but usually a small increase in G_M when compared with the current-depolarized membrane. Large, long lasting applications of L-glutamate gave a biphasic change in G_M - an early decrease in G_M followed by a slowly increasing G_M as the depolarization was maintained. We have hypothesized (17) that the high conductance phase may be a manifestation of amino acid uptake - possibly low affinity (see also 4). L-glutamate usually evoked only a short period of repetitive firing. As G_M started to rise the action potential generating mechanism failed. Our studies have revealed that a low background G_M is necessary to support repetitive firing.

Responses to L-aspartate, L-homocysteate and, apart from minor differences in response shape, quisqualate were similar to those of L-glutamate.

Group 2 (NMDA, ibotenate and D-homocysteate)

The agonists belonging to this group are all relatively potent compared with L-glutamate. The evoked depolarizations were slow in onset and recovery and were accompanied by a large, stable decrease in G_M, which was in excess of that accounted for by membrane rectification. When the depolarizations were sufficient to reach the threshold for spike generation, stable repetitive firing resulted,which lasted throughout agonist applications of many minutes. Responses to NMDA (Fig. 1) and ibotenate were virtually identical and, of all the analogues so far tested, evoked the largest decrease in G_M yet seen.

Group 3 (Kainate)

The very potent agonist, kainate, is designated a group of its own since responses to this agent bore no clear resemblance to those featured in the other two groups. Responses to kainate are characterized by a slow onset and very slow recovery, which was usually incomplete unless very small ejecting currents were used (16 and Fig. 3). The rising phase of kainate depolarizations was usually, but not always, accompanied by a short period of repetitive firing, while G_M increased (after allowing for membrane rectification). During continued kainate ejection the membrane potential plateaued. The neurone was then completely inexcitable and G_M immeasurably high.

In Fig. 2 the absolute potential at which each of the agents tested evoked repetitive firing is indicated by arrows. The threshold for firing will be the potential at which inward current exceeds outward current. An agonist which decreases G_K will reduce the outward current, hence firing would occur at a more negative membrane potential. These results illustrate that extracellularly recorded agonist evoked firing is an unreliable indicator of the extent of neuronal depolarization caused by an amino acid.

The two optical isomers of homocysteate appear in different groups in Table 1. The D isomer of homocysteate is about 10 times more potent a neurone excitor than the L isomer, thus, when using the racemic mixture DLH, it is the action of D-homocysteate which dominates.

Current theory (22,32) suggests that there are two distinct excitatory amino acid receptors, the one interacting preferentially with L-glutamate and its analogues and the other with L-aspartate and its analogues.

L-glutamate is likely to interact with both receptors - in its extended form with the glutamate-preferring receptor and in its folded form with the aspartate-preferring receptor (32). Aspartate, being a shorter molecule, should have low affinity for the glutamate preferring receptor. Pharmacological analyses (31) have revealed that kainate is likely to interact exclusively with the glutamate-preferring receptor and NMDA with the aspartate-preferring receptor. These two receptors have recently been named after their most selective agonists - i.e. kainate receptors and NMDA receptors respectively (31). D-α-aminoadipate and Mg^{++} ions have emerged as relatively specific blockers of the NMDA receptors, while L-glutamic acid diethyl ester antagonism (or poor blocking by the aforementioned agents) has been taken to indicate interaction with the kainate receptors (30,31).

According to Watkins'(31) classification, NMDA, ibotenate and L-homocysteate should interact with the NMDA receptor, whereas kainate and quisqualate should interact with the kainate receptor. L-glutamate, L-aspartate and D-homocysteate should overlap to a greater or lesser extent. If two distinct receptors existed, it might be predicted that our grouping in Table 1 might parallel the pharmacological classification. There are, in fact, important discrepancies:

a. We find the responses to L-glutamate, L-aspartate and L-homocysteate to be very similar. While L-homocysteate is thought to be a specific agonist of the NMDA receptor (31, but see 30), the responses to these two agonists bear little resemblance. On the other hand, although not evoking such a large decrease in G_M, D-homocysteate responses are much more similar to NMDA responses than they are to L-glutamate and L-aspartate responses.

b. Since both kainate and ibotenate have a ring structure in which a glutamate moiety held in the extended form can be recognized (22,31), it might therefore be predicted that both these agents would act on the kainate receptor. However, the responses to both these agents were very dissimilar. This might indicate that peripheral parts of the molecule are important in determining the type of response. On the other hand, responses to ibotenate and NMDA were very similar, suggesting that they use the same mechanism of depolarization, and possibly the same receptor.

c. The responses to kainate and L-glutamate are so different as to question whether these two agents in any way share the same receptor (16). Similar doubts have been expressed from pharmacological studies (21,30).

In summary, there is more than one conductance me-

chanism available to the excitatory amino acid analogues. This does not definitively infer the presence
of more than one receptor, though this seems likely.
While correlation of our analogue grouping and the
pharmacological classification is presently poor, it
remains to be seen if active uptake of some of the agonists (3) can explain some of the discrepancies.

II. BARBITURATE ANAESTHETICS

Having demonstrated that a G_M decrease accompanied
the depolarization caused by certain agonists, it was
necessary to investigate whether this decrease was a
function of the presence of barbiturate anaesthetics.
We have investigated the action of pentobarbitone and
thiopentone on the excitatory amino acid depolarizing
responses (25,26). These experiments were performed on
decerebrated cats. Depolarizations to L-glutamate were
usually decreased in size by the barbiturates and the
L-glutamate evoked increase in G_M was markedly reduced.
Depolarizations to DLH and NMDA were always decreased
in size by the barbiturates, but there was no change
in the G_M decrease mechanism underlying the responses.
The pattern of responses to ibotenate depended on
whether barbiturate anaesthetics were present or not.
In barbiturate anaesthetized cats, the first response
to ibotenate was accompanied by a large decrease in G_M.
Subsequent responses to ibotenate (and NMDA) were depressed for many minutes. The depression may be caused
by the conversion of ibotenate to the GABA-agonist,
muscimol (8). In decerebrated cats, regular applications of ibotenate gave similar sized responses with no
tendency to fade. Moreover, NMDA responses were markedly enhanced during or following ibotenate applications.
When pentobarbitone was then applied iontophoretically,
the pattern of responses seen in pentobarbitone anaesthetized cats was obtained. Barbiturates are known to
potentiate responses mediated via GABA receptors. It
therefore seems likely that this is the mechanism underlying the slow, depressive phase of ibotenate's action.

III. EXTRACELLULARLY RECORDED CHANGES IN POTENTIAL DURING IONTOPHORETIC APPLICATION OF EXCITATORY AMINO ACIDS

In a recent study (18) we compared extra- and intracellular recordings during iontophoresis of various
agents. Application of excitatory amino acids regularly
resulted in a slow negative shift of the potential recorded extracellularly (close to the point of agonist

release) with respect to a distant indifferent electrode. Though initially dismissed as artifacts of the iontophoretic technique (see e.g. 23), these focal potentials (FPs) turned out to be manifestations of the responses of nearby neurones to the amino acids. We have previously described in detail (20) why we do not consider the FPs to be artifacts of the iontophoretic technique. FPs, which may be up to -50 mV in size, have been recorded in response to all of the excitatory amino acid analogues tested.

Together with H. Jahnsen (Copenhagen), we have recently recorded FPs in hippocampal slices, as has Lanthorn (27), who reports that sizeable FPs may be evoked by diffusing agonists onto the slice from blunt pipettes. FPs have also been seen previously in the cerebellar cortex (29), though perhaps their relevance for the interpretation of intracellular recordings was not appreciated at the time.

Since the negative going FP will reduce the potential gradient across the neuronal membrane, the question that now arises is: what is the true transmembrane potential (TMP) during the action of excitatory amino acids (and any other agents which produce FPs)? This question is, of course, of crucial importance when trying to relate the reversal potential of a synaptic event to that of the putative transmitter.

Kainate produces the most spectacular FPs which can be up to -50 mV in size and spread for up to 1 mm from the point of release (20). We are thus reasonably confident that the TMP measured at one point is representative for the neurone as a whole. Such an experiment is shown in Fig. 3. During kainate ejection, the "classical" intracellular recording plateaued at -49 mV, where G_M was immeasurably high. The TMP record, however, showed the neurone to be completely depolarized. The experiment also shows that it was necessary to withdraw the electrodes by ca 1 mm before there was no FP.

It remains to investigate the mechanism which generates the FP, though speculations have been made (20). We have detected an increase in tissue resistance during FPs which could be explained by a shrinkage of the extracellular space. During the high conductance state of kainate, there is likely to be little difference between the membrane and extracellular resistances. Kainate could thus be considered to have created an artificial "cell" in the grey matter whose "membrane" would be at the boundary of the FP.

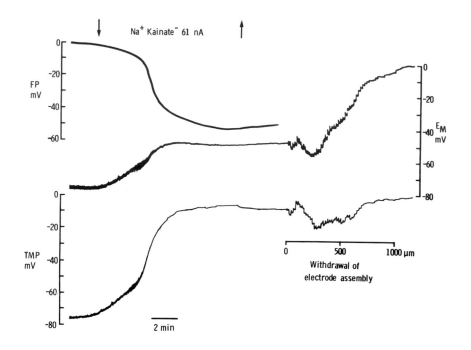

FIG. 3. Simultaneous potential recordings during a current balanced iontophoretic application of kainate onto a motoneurone. Upper trace: the focal potential (FP) recorded just outside the motoneurone from one of the iontophoretic barrels (containing NaCl). Middle trace: the intracellular potential (E_M). Both the FP and E_M were referred to a non-polarizable electrode buried in the leg muscles. Lower trace: the transmembrane potential (TMP), as recorded from a differential amplifier, i.e. the difference of the upper two records. The FP record was replotted from another pen recording. The kainate retaining voltage was turned off shortly before the start of the traces. After a long latent period, kainate ejection produced a depolarization of about 25 mV of the E_M recording, while the transmembrane depolarization was about 75 mV. After the kainate ejection, the electrode assembly was withdrawn in 20 μ steps at 6 steps · min^{-1}. As can be seen from the E_M recording (now extracellular) the volume of grey matter in which the FP could be detected had a radius of about 1 mm.

ACKNOWLEDGEMENTS

We wish to thank the following for gifts of substances: Dr. J. C. Watkins for NMDA, D- and L-homocysteate, Professor C.H. Eugster for ibotenic acid and Professor T. Takemoto for quisqualic acid. Thanks are also due to Finn Marquard for technical assistance and Karen Damgaard Ottesen for typing the manuscript. This work was supported by the Danish Medical Research Council.

REFERENCES

1. Altmann, H., ten Bruggencate, G., Pickelmann, P. and Steinberg, R. (1976): Pflügers Arch., 364:249-255.
2. Balcar, V.J. and Johnston, G.A.R. (1972): J. Neurobiol., 3: 295-301.
3. Cox, D.W.G. and Bradford, H.F. (1978): In: Kainic Acid as a Tool in Neurobiology, edited by E.G. McGeer, J.W. Olney and P.L. McGeer, pp. 71-93. Raven Press, New York.
4. Cox, D.W.G., Headley, P.M. and Watkins, J.C. (1977): J. Neurochem., 29:579-588.
5. Curtis, D.R. (1965): In: Studies in Physiology, Presented to J.C. Eccles, edited by D.R. Curtis and A.J. McIntyre, pp. 34-42. Springer, Heidelberg, New York.
6. Curtis, D.R., Duggan, A.W., Johnston, G.A.R., Tebecis, A.K. and Watkins, J.C. (1972): Brain Res., 41:283-301.
7. Curtis, D.R., Duggan, A.W. and Johnston, G.A.R. (1970): Exp. Brain Res., 10:447-462.
8. Curtis, D.R., Lodge, D. and McLennan, H. (1979): J. Physiol., 291:19-28.
9. Curtis, D.R. and Johnston, G.A.R. (1974): Ergebn. Physiol., 69:97-188.
10. Curtis, D.R., Phillis, J.W. and Watkins, J.C. (1960): J. Physiol., 150:656-682.
11. Curtis, D.R. and Watkins, J.C. (1960): J. Neurochem., 6: 117-141.
12. Curtis, D.R. and Watkins, J.C. (1963): J. Physiol., 166: 1-14.
13. Duggan, A.W. (1974): Exp. Brain Res., 19:522-528.
14. Engberg, I., Flatman, J.A. and Lambert, J.D.C. (1975): Br. J. Pharmac., 55:250-251 P.
15. Engberg, I., Flatman, J.A. and Lambert, J.D.C. (1975): Br. J. Pharmac., 55:312-313 P.
16. Engberg, I., Flatman, J.A. and Lambert, J.D.C. (1978): Br. J. Pharmac., 64:384-385 P.
17. Engberg, I., Flatman, J.A. and Lambert, J.D.C. (1979): J. Physiol., 288:227-261.
18. Engberg, I., Flatman, J.A. and Lambert, J.D.C. (1979): J. Neurosci. Meth., 1:219-233.
19. Engberg, I. and Marshall, K.C. (1971): Acta physiol. scand., 83:142-144.
20. Flatman, J.A. and Lambert, J.D.C. (1979): J. Neurosci. Meth., 1:205-218.
21. Hicks, T.P., Hall, J.G. and McLennan, H. (1978): Can. J. Physiol. Pharmacol., 56:901-907.
22. Johnston, G.A.R., Curtis, D.R., Davies, J. and McCulloch, R.M. (1974): Nature, Lond., 248:804-805.
23. Krnjević, K. (1972): In: Methods of Neurochemistry, edited by R. Fried, pp. 129-172. Marcel Dekker Inc., New York.
24. Krnjević, K. and Schwartz, S. (1967): Exp. Brain Res., 3: 306-319.
25. Lambert, J.D.C., Flatman, J.A. and Engberg, I. (1978): In:

Iontophoresis and Transmitter Mechanisms in the Mammalian Central Nervous System, edited by R.W. Ryall and J.S. Kelly, pp. 375-377. Elsevier/North Holland Biomedical Press, Amsterdam.

26. Lambert, J.D.C., Flatman, J.A. and Engberg, I. (1980): Acta physiol. scand., 108:14A.
27. Lanthorn, T.H., personal communication.
28. Marshall, K.C. and Engberg, I. (1979): Science, N.Y., 205: 422-424.
29. McCance, I. and Phillis, J.W. (1968): Int. J. Neuropharmacol., 7:447-462.
30. McLennan, H. and Lodge, D. (1979): Brain Res., 169:83-90.
31. Watkins, J.C. (1978): In: Kainic Acid as a Tool in Neurobiology, edited by E.G. McGeer, J.W. Olney and P.L. McGeer, pp. 37-69. Raven Press, New York.
32. Watkins, J.C. (1980): Trends in Neurosci., 3:61-64.
33. Weight, F.F. (1974): In: Synaptic Transmission and Neuronal Interaction, pp. 141-151, Raven Press, New York.
34. Zieglgänsberger, W. and Puil, E.A. (1973): Exp. Brain Res., 17:35-49.

Glutamate as a Neurotransmitter,
edited by G. Di Chiara and G. L. Gessa
Raven Press, New York © 1981.

The Actions of Glutamic Acid on Neurons in the Rat Hippocampal Slice

Menahem Segal

Isotope Department, The Weizmann Institute of Science, Rehovot, Israel

Extensive research, in the past two decades has been directed towards the characterization of the excitatory amino acid neurotransmission in mammalian central nervous system (3-5,7,10,16). Compared to the wealth of information accumulated on the glutamate (Glu) receptors in spinal cord (5,6,10) relatively little was known, until recently, about the pharmacology and physiology of these receptors in supraspinal structures (1,9,12,20,25). This was partly due to the lack of a central model system where stable intracellular recording can be achieved for prolonged periods of time and where drug and ionic concentrations can be controlled. The recently developed hippocampal slice preparation offers an ideal test system for the study of central receptor mechanisms (21,24). The hippocampus contains several excitatory input pathways which are presumed to use Glu and/or aspartate (Asp) as excitatory neurotransmitters. Glu is released upon activation of these pathways (14-15,26) and, when applied iontophoretically, excites hippocampal neurons (1,9,20, 22,25). Glu antagonists (e.g. glutamate diethyl ester, GDEE) block responses to Glu or to activation of certain excitatory pathways in the hippocampus (9,20,22). The hippocampal slice preparation preserves the structural organization of the intact hippocampus and thus, allows the study of an excitatory, putative Glu/Asp containing pathway in in-vitro conditions.

The present report summarizes a study of the Glu receptor in the hippocampus. Specifically, the study was addressed to the following questions: 1. Is there one type of response to Glu, or are there several response types, e.g. excitatory vs. inhibitory (17,27). 2. What is the relationship between responses to Glu and Asp. 3. What is the pharmacological profile of the Glu receptor in the hippocampus. 4. What is the physiological basis of action of the neurotoxin kainic acid (KA). Answers to these and related questions were attempted using intracellular recording of neuronal responses to Glu and excitatory afferent stimulation in the hippocampal slice preparation.

METHODS

Adult (250-300 gm) male Wistar rats were decapitated and their brains rapidly removed and placed in cold Ringer solution. The hippocampus was dissected out and sliced into 350μm slices with a McIlwain tissue chopper. The slices were transferred into the recording chamber (21) where they were superfused continuously from the bottom with oxygenated warm (32-34°C) Ringer solution. The warm, humidified gas mixture of 95%O_2, 5%CO_2 was also circulated in the chamber, above the slices. The Ringer solution contained (in mM) NaCl 124, KCl 5, KH_2PO_4 1.25, $NaHCO_3$ 26, $CaCl_2$ 2, $MgSO_4$ 2, glucose 10, and had a pH of 7.4. Intracellular recording was made with glass micropipettes filled with 4M K^+-acetate and having a resistance of 50-100MΩ. Signals were fed through a WPI M707 microprobe system, displayed on an oscilloscope and continuously plotted on a Brush recorder. A monopolar stimulating electrode was placed on stratum radiatum (Fig. 1) to activate the excitatory Schaffer-collateral-commissural system.

Drugs were applied by pressure injection of 5-20nl droplets containing the drug solution from coarse (20-40μm) pipettes on the surface of the slice, near the recording electrode. All electrodes were placed under visual control, using a Nikon dissecting microscope. Further details of the methodology are presented elsewhere (21).

RESULTS AND DISCUSSION

Stable intracellular recording was made from 70 neurons located in stratum pyramidale of region CA1 of the hippocampus. Resting membrane potential, measured upon withdrawal of the electrode from the recorded neurone amounted to -65 to -80 mV. Input resistance, measured by passage of a 0.2-0.5 nA hyperpolarizing current pulse through the recording pipette, was 12-60MΩ. The neurons could discharge action potentials of 80-130mV upon passage of depolarizing current pulses through the recording electrodes. Activating the excitatory afferents to produce sufficiently large (20-30mV) EPSP's could also trigger action potential discharges. Stable recording was maintained for 5-10 minutes before drug application.

Effects of Glu

Three components could be detected in the response of neurons to Glu. The first one was seen in only a few cells, mainly those encountered deep in the slice, and consisted of a fast (1-2 sec) hyperpolarization associated with a marked (20-30%) decrease in input resistance. This response was replaced, when present, by a large depolarization, found in all neurons, which reached a peak within 4-10 sec. This depolarization was accompanied in some neurons by changes in input resistance. There were large differences among neurons in this respect; in some neurons there

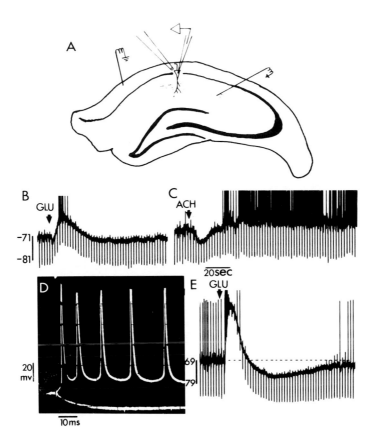

Fig. 1. A. The arrangement of the stimulating, recording and
drug electrodes in the rat hippocampal slice. Monopolar stimulating electrodes are placed in stratum radiatum (right) and in the
alveus (left) while recording is made from CA1 stratum pyramidale.
B & C. Responses of a neuron to application of glutamate (Glu)
and acetylcholine (ACh, c). The drugs were applied at the arrowheads. Downward deflections are voltage changes produced by passage of 100 msec 0.5 nA hyperpolarizing current pulses through
the recording electrode at a rate of 0.5 Hz. Upward deflections
are chopped action potentials. Glu and ACh are applied in droplets which contain 10mM solutions calibration; abscissa time, ordinate potential (mV). D. An oscillographic record of membrane
changes produced by passage of hyperpolarizing and depolarizing
currents. E. An example of another neuron responding to Glu.
Note the difference in conductance changes between B and E. In
E, the depolarization is followed by a marked hyperpolarization.

were no changes in input resistance (Fig. 1B) and in others input resistance was reduced to about 20% of basal levels. Most neurons fell between these two extremes. There was only a partial correlation (r=0.68) between the magnitude of the potential change and the magnitude of the resistance change. Two possible explanations can account for the variability in the resistance changes among the neurons; it is possible that Glu activates two types of receptors, one associated with conductance change and one which is not. Alternatively, the Glu receptors might be located close to or away from the soma, which will result in presence or absence of detected conductance changes.

Following the recovery from the depolarization, there was in many neurones, a marked, up to 15mV, hyperpolarization (Fig. 1E). This hyperpolarization was slow, recovered with 1-2 minutes and was not associated with specific conductance changes. Inhibitory responses to Glu have been noticed before (17,27). Experiments were therefore designed to test whether these are true postsynaptic responses or are they mediated by activation of an inhibitory interneuron.

The application of tetrodotoxin (TTX), a drug known to block fast Na$^+$ currents associated with action potential discharges caused, after a relatively long delay (Fig. 2) the cessassion of spontaneous and depolarization induced action potential dis-

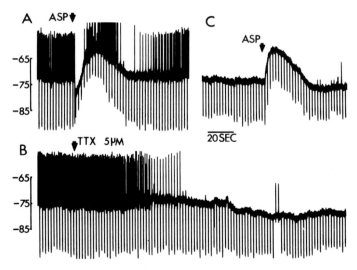

Fig. 2. The effects of TTX on responses to aspartate (Asp). A. Asp produced a fast hyperpolarization accompanied by a reduction in input resistance which was followed by the typical depolarization. B. TTX caused a gradual cessession of spontaneous acctivity and the cell became more polarized. C. In the presence of TTX Asp no longer produced the fast hyperpolarization but the depolarizing response was still marked.

charges. Under these conditions, heterosynaptic effects produced
by activation of an interneuron, are absent. When applied in
presence of TTX, Glu (or, as in Fig. 2, Asp) no longer produced
the initial fast hyperpolarizing response but still caused the
long latency, slow hyperpolarizing response which followed the
depolarization. This indicates that the initial response might
indeed by formed by activation of an inhibitory interneuron which
has a faster reaction time to Glu than the recorded neuron.

The nature of the late hyperpolarization was studied in the
following experiments: Assuming that Glu causes an increase in
Na^+ and K^+ conductances and consequently activates the Na^+-K^+
pump, the possibility that the late hyperpolarization results
from activation of the Na^+-K^+ pump was therefore tested. Ouabain
when applied in relatively low concentrations blocks the Na^+-K^+
pump. The poisoning of the pump is followed by a slow depolarization of the recorded neurons. The recovery from Glu effects
was slower and there was a marked reduction in the late hyperpolarization (Fig. 3). An additional indication that the late
hyperpolarization is caused by activation of an electrogenic Na^+-
K^+ pump is based on the temperature dependency of this energy
requiring pump. Indeed, in slices maintained in low (22°C) temperature, the time to recovery from effects of Glu was longer and
there was a marked attenuation of the late hyperpolarization
(unpublished observations). These observations lend support to
the assumption that Glu causes an increase in Na^+ and K^+ conductance causing Na^+ entry and K^+ exit from the cell and thereby
activating the Na^+-K^+ pump which hyperpolarizes the cell for a

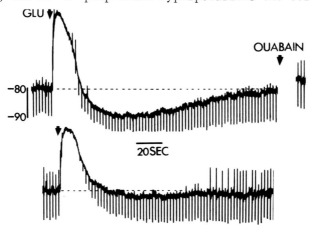

Fig. 3. Effects of ouabain applied in a droplet containing 0.1mM
solution on the hyperpolarization produced by Glu. Initially,
Glu produced an 11mV hyperpolarization yet after ouabain which by
itself depolarized the cell by about 5mV, the hyperpolarization
was markedly attenuated.

long period of time. There is of course the possibility that Glu
activates directly the pump to produce the hyperpolarization independently of its depolarizing action. Further experiments
should clarify this possibility.

The Glu concentration in the droplet required to produce a
maximal effect varied between 1-20mM. This wide range is caused
by the dilution of the agonist while diffusing away from the surface of the slice, where it was placed. An additional factor
might be the efficient active uptake process of Glu into glia and
terminals which might further dilute the agonist concentration at
the receptor sites. It was indeed found that Glu at a concentration of 10mM produced an averaged depolarization of 23.9mV in
neurons located in the top half of the slice whereas it produced
an averaged depolarization of only 9.5mV in cells located in the
bottom half of the slice.

Effects of Glu agonists

The marked variations in potency of Glu prohibited a simple
comparison among different agonists tested in different neurons
and necessitated the comparison of several agonists on the same
neuron. The responses of a neuron to a given agonist were therefore compared with responses of this neuron to Glu.

Marked differences between different agonists were found, both
in the concentrations required to produce similar effects and the
time courses of onset and recovery of these effects. In every
cell tested, Glu and Asp produced almost identical responses.
This was evident for both the time course, response magnitudes
and conductance changes. Furthermore, there were no apparent
potentiating action of Asp on responses to Glu or vice versa as
suggested for other systems (7). In many respects it appeared
that Glu and Asp either share a common receptor or have about
equal number of receptors on most cells. Further experiments are
currently underway to clarify these possibilities. D-glutamate
was about 1.25 times more potent than Glu. Quisqualic acid and
D-L homocisteate (DLH) were about 20 times more potent than Glu.
N-methyl D-aspartate (NMDA) was about 50 times more potent than
Glu. Kainic acid (KA) was the most potent agonist tested; it

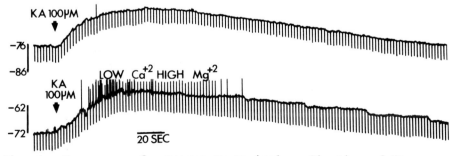

Fig. 4. Responses of a neuron to topical application of KA
before (top) and after (bottom) superfusion of the slice with a
medium containing 0mM Ca$^+$ and 4mM Mg$^+$.

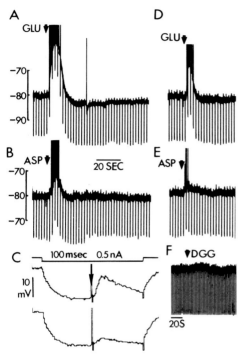

Fig. 5. Effects of DGG on neuronal responses to Glu, Asp and to stimulation of an excitatory input. A & B. Responses to Glu and Asp, respectively, before DGG. Note the uncommon difference between responses to Glu and Asp. C. Computer averages of potential changes produced by passage of 0.5nA 100 msec current pulses through the recording electrode. 50 msec after onset of the current pulse there is a single pulse stimulation of the stratum radiatum to produce an EPSP. Top record, before, bottom after topical application of DGG. D & E. Responses to Glu and Asp after DGG. F. Absence of a direct effect of DGG on potential and input resistance of the recorded neuron. All samples arc from the same neuron. Resting potential is -80mV in all samples.

produced the same depolarization as Glu with 1/100 of the concentrations. The time course of KA was markedly different from that of the other agonists, in that it was much slower to reach the same depolarization produced by Glu. A full recovery from effects of KA was seen, only about 4-10 minutes after KA application. In several cells a recovery was not seen and the cell remained depolarized (by 30-40mV) for the duration of the recording interval. The slow time course of KA indicates that it might exert its neurotoxic action (2,13,18) by releasing excitatory neurotransmitters from preterminal stores. This in fact was already suggested (19). To test this possibility, the effects of KA were measured in cells from slices maintained in 0mM Ca^+ 4mM Mg^+. In these slices synaptic activity was abolished as indicated by the disappearance of EPSP's. The responses to KA were not modified (Fig. 4) suggesting that the physiological effects of KA are exerted postsynaptically.

Glutamate antagonists

It has been suggested recently that certain antagonists act preferentially at a Glu receptor while other block better an Asp receptor (6,9). The following experiments attempted to find such a distinction in the hippocampus. If such a differential action does exist, it will be of interest to find out whether the main excitatory pathways in the slice are of the Glu or the Asp type.

The following antagonists were used: 2-amino 5 phosphonovaleric acid (2APV) GDEE, cis-2,3 piperidine dicarboxylic acid (PDA), and γ-D glutamylglycine (DGG) with the exception of PDA which had a potent agonistic action, all these drugs antagonized both Glu and Asp excitation (Fig. 5). DGG appeared to be the best antagonist, followed by 2APV while GDEE was the least effective antagonist of both Glu and Asp action. The same order of potensy was maintained when the effects of these drugs were tested against the EPSP's produced by stimulation of the excitatory Schaffer collateral-commissural path. These data indicate that if indeed a distinction between Glu and Asp receptor exists in the hippocampus, the receptors for the Schaffer-collateral system is probably of the Glu type.

Summary and conclusions
Effects of Glu and its agonists and antagonists were studied with intracellular recording techniques in the rat hippocampal slice. Topical application of Glu produced a large depolarization accompanied by a marked reduction in input resistance and was followed by a long latency hyperpolarization. This hyperpolarization is probably caused by the activation of an electrogenic Na^+-K^+ pump. Glu and Asp produced similar responses and both were equally antagonized by DGG, 2APV and GDEE in this order of potency. DGG was the best antagonist also of the EPSP's produced by stimulation of the Schaffer collateral-commissural path.

These experiments illustrate that the hippocampal slice is a useful model system for the analysis of the pharmacology and physiology of the glutamate receptor in the brain.

Acknowledgements
I wish to thank Dr. J.C. Watkins for the generous supply of DGG, PDA and 2APV.

REFERENCES

1. Biscoe, T.J., and Straughan, D.W. (1966): J. Physiol., 183: 341-359.
2. Coyle, J.T., and Schwarcz, R. (1976): Nature, 263:244-246.
3. Curtis, D.R., Phillis, J.W., and Watkins, J.C. (1959): Nature, 183:611-612.
4. Curtis, D.R., and Watkins, J.C. (1960): J. Neurochem., 6: 117-141.
5. Davidson, N. (1976): Neurotransmitter Amino Acids. Acad. Press, London.
6. Davies, J., and Watkins, J.C. (1979): J. Physiol. (Lond.), 297:621-635.
7. Freeman, A.R. (1976): Prog. Neurobiol., 6:137-153.
8. Haldeman, S., and McLennan, H. (1972): Brain Res., 45:393-400.
9. Hicks, T.P., and McLennan, H. (1979): J. Physiol. Pharmacol., 57:973-978.

10. Johnson, J.L. (1972): Brain Res., 37:1-19.
11. Johnson, G.A.R., Curtis, D.R., Davies, J., and McCulloch, R.M. (1974): Nature, 248:804-805.
12. Krnjeic, K., and Schwartz, S. (1967): Exp. Brain Res., 3: 320-336.
13. McGeer, E.G., and McGeer, P.L. (1976): Nature, 263:517-519.
14. Nadler, J.V., Vaca, K.W., White, W.F., Lynch, G.S., and Cotman, C.W. (1976): Nature, (London), 260:538-540.
15. Nalder, V.J., White, W.F., Vaca, K.W., Perry, B.W., and Cotman, C.W. (1978): J. Neurochem., 31:147-155.
16. Nistri, A., and Constanti, A. (1979): Prog. Neurobiol., 13: 117-235.
17. Okamoto, K., Quastel, D.M., and Quastel, J.H. (1976): Brain Res., 113:147-158.
18. Olney, J.W., Rhee, V., and Ho, O.L. (1974): Brain Res., 77: 507-512.
19. Ryan, J., and Cotman, C.W. (1978): Soc. Neurosci., Abst., 4: 227.
20. Segal, M. (1976): Br. J. Pharmacol., 58:341-345.
21. Segal, M. (1980): J. Physiol., 303: (in press).
22. Spencer, H., Gribkoff, V.K., and Lynch, G.S. (1978): In: Iontophoresis and transmitter mechanisms in the mammalian central nervous system, edited by R.W. Ryall, and J.S. Kelly, pp. 194-196. Elsevier, Amsterdam.
22. Skrede, K.K., and Westgaard, R.H. (1971): Brain Res., 35: 589-593.
24. Schwartzkroin, P.A. (1975): Brain Res., 85:423-435.
25. Wheal, H.V., and Miller, J.J. (1980): Brain Res., 182:145-155.
26. Wieraszko, A., and Lynch, G. (1979): Brain Res., 160:372-376.
27. Yamamoto, C., Yamashita, H., and Chujo, T. (1976): Nature, (Lond.), 262:786-787.

Glutamate as a Neurotransmitter,
edited by G. Di Chiara and G. L. Gessa
Raven Press, New York © 1981.

A Model for Excitatory Transmission at a Glutamate Synapse

Alan R. Freeman, Richard P. Shank, John Kephart, Michael Dekin, and Michael Wang

Department of Physiology, Temple University School of Medicine, Philadelphia, Pennsylvania 19140

The crustacean has long served as a useful model system for the study of amino acid mediated neurotransmission. In this context the neuromuscular synapse of the lobster, Homarus americanus is well established (24-26). Abundant evidence now exists which supports the candidacy of L-glutamic acid as the excitatory neurotransmitter at the arthropod neuromuscular synapse (1-3,10,11,14, 17,23,27,32,33).

Experiments carried out in this laboratory have suggested the idea that L-glutamate may play a role in a variety of functions. Along these lines, evidence has accumulated favoring not only a role as primary transmitter, but also the ability to act at nonsynaptic and presynaptic sites (8,9,18). The possible functional implications of the existence of these extrasynaptic glutamate receptors has been reviewed elsewhere (19).

We have proposed that the synaptic action of glutamate is modulated by the amino acid L-aspartate (18,19,20,36-39). These experiments demonstrated that when L-glutamate and L-aspartate were applied simultaneously to neuromuscular preparations of the lobster, the glutamate dose-response curve was shifted to the left; no effect on the maximum response elicited by glutamate was seen (36). The ability of aspartate to potentiate the effects of glutamate has been described by a number of investigators (12,29, 30,36,38,39).

The mechanism by which aspartate potentiates the action of glutamate has not been clearly established and a number of explanations have now been proposed. These include: (a) activation of "allosteric" binding sites on the postsynaptic receptors by aspartate which induces an increase in the affinity between glutamate and its binding sites (20,36-38,39), (b) enhancement of the glutamate response due to a capacity of aspartate to act as a glutamate agonist (30), (c) inhibition of glutamate uptake by aspartate, thereby delaying the inactivation process (13,31), (d) displacement of bound extracellular glutamate by aspartate (10,11), and (e) prevention of glutamate induced receptor desensitization by aspartate (15).

227

We have hypothesized that the potentiation of the action of glutamate by aspartate at the lobster neuromuscular junction arises from an increase in the affinity of the receptor for glutamate. We further postulated that this increase in affinity occurs because the receptor possesses an aspartate binding site capable, when aspartate is bound, of allosterically altering the glutamate binding site on the receptor (19,20).

As a consequence of these findings and the fact that aspartate is highly concentrated in excitatory axons, we hypothesized that aspartate might be released from excitatory nerve terminals along with glutamate, and consequently serve as a natural modulator of the excitatory action of glutamate. The observations reported here are the results of experiments undertaken to further investigate the possible role of aspartate as an endogenous neuromodulator.

EXPERIMENTAL PROCEDURES

Tissue Preparation

Our experiments were performed on isolated walking limbs of the lobster, Homarus americanus. The stretcher muscle in the carpopodite was partially exposed by removing some of the overlying carapace. In experiments in which the muscle was neurally stimulated, the nerve innervating the distal musculature was exposed by partially or completely removing the carapace and muscle of the meropodite segment. The limb was then pinned in a chamber and submerged in an artificial sea water (ASW) solution composed of NaCl (450 mM), CaCl (20 mM), $MgCl_2$ (10 mM), KCl (5 mM) and Tris (10 mM). The bathing fluid was adjusted to pH 7.4 $\pm$ 0.1 with 1N HCl. All experiments were performed at 21-23°C.

Electrophysiological Methods

In experiments using electrophysiological techniques, the stretcher muscle in the carpopodite of an isolated walking limb was partially exposed by removing some of the overlying carapace. In some experiments the nerve bundle innervating this muscle was exposed by removing some of the carapace in the meropodite segment. The limb was then anchored in a chamber and immersed in the ASW medium described above.

A superficial muscle fiber was impaled with one or two KCl-filled glass microelectrodes. The electrode resistances ranged from 4 to 15 MΩ. Membrane potentials were recorded from one of the microelectrodes using a standard electronic arrangement. Using the other electrode the membrane could either be voltage or current clamped with the aid of a Dagan 8500 feedback amplifier system. The two intracellular electrodes were placed within a few hundred μm of a neuromuscular junction. A two or three barrel microelectrode was used to iontophoretically apply L-glutamate, L-aspartate and either D-aspartate or D,L-2-amino-4-phosphonobutyrate. Each barrel was filled with a 1 to 2M solution

of the compound in the monosodium or monopotassium salt form.
The iontophoretic electrode was positioned near a junction and
was then manipulated until a sharp and consistent response to a
brief (200 msec or less) pulse of glutamate was obtained. The
iontophoretic electrode resistances ranged between 100 and 300
MΩ and a constant small retaining current (2 nA) was applied to
each barrel to prevent amino acid diffusion from the electrode
tip.

Some experiments determined the effects of substituting Li^+,
Mg^{++}, or methylamine for Na^+ on glutamate and aspartate evoked
responses and on neurally evoked EPSPs. In these experiments
the normal ASW medium was pumped from a reservoir through plastic
tubing and superfused directly onto the muscle fibers. After a
control period the solution was switched to one containing the
substituted ion, and subsequently back to the control solution.
In the ion substituted solutions NaCl was replaced on an equios-
molar basis.

When neurally evoked EPSPs were studied, the exposed nerve in
the meropodite was electrically stimulated with bipolar surface
electrodes.

Glutamate and Aspartate Uptake Experiments

Muscle bundles and their associated nerve fibers and tendons
were removed from the meropodite and carpopodite of the walking
limbs, and placed in cold (0-4°C) normal ASW medium. The strips
of tissue were sectioned at 3 mm intervals, resulting in "slices"
weighing approximately 100 mg. Each tissue slice was blotted,
weighed, placed in a test tube containing 2 ml of cold saline,
and put immediately into a shaking water bath for incubation.
The saline contained 0.025 µCi/ml of $(U-^{14}C)$ glutamate or $(U-^{14}C)$
aspartate (New England Nuclear, Boston MA.). After slices were
incubated for periods of 5 to 40 minutes, the tissue was placed
on filter paper attached to a suction flask. Fluid was drawn off
the tissue by the partial vacuum in the flask. The tissue was
washed rapidly 3 times with 1 ml of cold saline, and placed in a
scintillation vial containing 0.4 ml of hyamine hydroxide. The
tissue was then incubated for 24 hrs at 60°C in order to dissolve
protein. Scintillation fluid (15 ml) was subsequently added to
the vials, and the radioactivity was determined using a Packard
Tri-Carb scintillation counter. The counting efficiency was determined to be 80 to 85% using the external standard.

In some of the uptake experiments LiCl or methylamine Cl was
substituted for NaCl. In other experiments, specified concentrations of glutamate and aspartate analogs were included in the
medium.

In one series of experiments the concentration of glutamate in
the medium was determined using an enzymatic-fluorometric method
(22). In another set of experiments the extent of glutamate and
aspartate metabolism was determined using a thin layer chromatographic procedure (35). For these analyses the tissue was

extracted with 10 volumes of 80% ethanol. The extract was centrifuged, the supernatant dried, and the residue subsequently resuspended in water. For the thin layer chromatographic method
the amino acids in the extract were converted to their dinitro-
phenyl derivatives, and these were subsequently separated on
Analtech (Newwark, Del.) silica gel plates. The separated amino
acid derivatives were scraped off the plates and quantitatively
eluted from the silica gel into a known volume of 0.01 N bicarbonate. Subsequently, the optical density was measured at 360
nanometers to determine the molar amount of each amino acid. The
radioactivity in a portion of the eluate containing each amino
acid derivative was also determined.

RESULTS

Action of Iontophoretically Applied L-Glutamate

In our experience, it is usually possible to find several discrete locations on individual muscle fibers which are highly responsive to iontophoretically applied glutamate. Generally it is
possible to elicit a 2 to 4 mV depolarization response with 20 to
100 nA of iontophoretic current applied for 50 to 100 msec. Frequently the response peaks within 100 to 200 msec of ionotopho-
retic current onset. Occasional preparations have been encountered in which a rapid response to glutamate could not be achieved.
In these preparations there is usually a latency of several hundred msec before any response is observed; this is followed by a
gradual depolarization of only a few mV. It is conceivable that
the slow responses seen in these preparations are due to the
possibility that the junctions are all located at sites relatively
inaccessible to the iontophoretic electrode. However, the actual
meaning of such slow responses remains unexplained at this time.

Dose-response curves obtained with iontophoretically applied
glutamate exhibited remarkably steep slopes. This was observed
when the response was measured as either membrane depolarization
or synaptic current (Figure 1). The data are presented in log-
log format to highlight their relationship to standard chemical
kinetics. The figure demonstrates that, within limits, the log of
the synaptic current varies linearly with the log of applied
glutamate, after which saturation of the current level is observed. The average of 8 experiments obtained in separate animals
shows the slope in the linear region to be 5 with a range of 4 to
6.

Modulation by L-Aspartate Upon Glutamate Responses

In nearly all of our experiments, which include more than 50
individual preparations, aspartate potentiated the responses
elicited by glutamate. This potentiation was evident when changes
in synaptic current were recorded in voltage-clamped muscle fibers,
as well as when membrane depolarization was recorded (Figure 2).

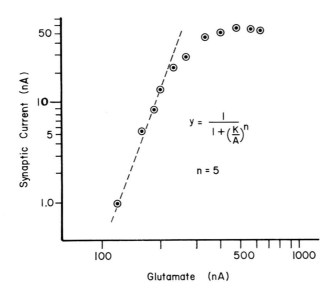

FIG. 1. Log-log display of synaptic currents recorded
under voltage clamp conditions during glutamate application. Ordinate shows synaptic current while abscissa
presents iontophoretic glutamate current. Equation for
n order cooperativity is derived from Werman (42). A
single experiment is shown with n being the average of
8 separate animals. (Graph presents 2 log y for 1 log
x; slope is corrected accordingly).

The potentiative effect of aspartate varied markedly from one experiment to another. This may, at least in part, reflect differences in the relative proximity of the glutamate and aspartate
barrels to the receptors. In some preparations, aspartate alone
could elicit a small response, but this usually required high
iontophoretic currents applied for several hundred msec or longer.
Figure 2 supports the idea that, within certain experimental
ranges, open loop and voltage clamp results are directly comparable. The potentiating effect of aspartate was essentially the
same in the open circuited and voltage clamped modes over the entire experimental range. Thus, transmitter induced alterations
in E_m (i.e., open circuit conditions) could be used in place of
the technically more difficult voltage clamp experiments to obtain meaningful data for the construction of concentration-re-
sponse curves. Another revelation derived from study of wave-
shapes of the synaptic current is the fact that the potentiated
glutamate currents are increased in magnitude but not prolonged
in time.

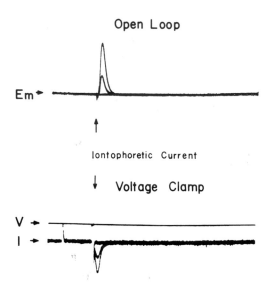

FIG. 2. Membrane responses elicited by glutamate and
aspartate applied by iontophoresis separately and simultaneously from double barrel microelectrodes. The upper
set of traces shows the change in membrane potential in
the open circuited mode, whereas the lower set shows the
change in membrane current of a voltage clamped muscle
fiber. Both sets of data represent three superimposed
traces during which one or both amino acids were iontophoresed for 100 msec. Aspartate alone at 240 nA
elicited no apparent response; glutamate at 80 nA
effected a 4 mV depolarization and an inward directed
current of 15 nA; glutamate (80 nA) plus aspartate
(240 nA) effected a 10 mV depolarization and a 30 nA
inward moving current. The calibration signal in the
upper set of traces is 5 mV and 100 msec.

Figure 3 shows a series of dose-response curves generated by
iontophoretically applied glutamate alone and with varying levels
of iontophoretically applied aspartate. As indicated in the insert, aspartate alone at a current of 10 times the glutamate level
exerts no depolarizing action of its own. This quantitative difference between the activity of glutamate and aspartate cannot be
due to a possible difference in relative amounts applied because
these amino acids have similar transference numbers (21). However, when these two amino acids are iontophoresed simultaneously,
a marked potentiation is observed.
    The dose-response relationship of glutamate alone is depicted
in open circles. When a fixed level of aspartate is ejected from
a second pipette simultaneously with the glutamate current, a

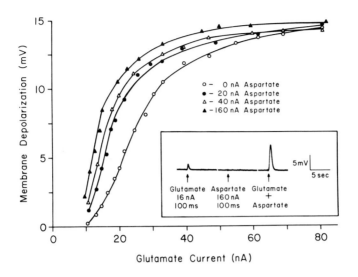

FIG. 3. The effect of L-aspartate on the L-glutamate dose-response curve. The insert shows the oscilloscope trace of responses elicited by single doses of glutamate, aspartate, and glutamate plus aspartate. The amino acids were applied at the current (nA) specified for 100 msec. Note that aspartate by itself did not elicit a response even at a current of 160 nA.

parallel shift to the left of the glutamate response is observed. The degree of this shift is seen to be a function of the magnitude of the aspartate current. Furthermore, neither the contour nor the maximum values of the glutamate curves appear to be significantly altered.

Effect of Ion Substitution on the Actions of Glutamate and Aspartate

In approximately 80% of preparations the responses elicited by glutamate were markedly reduced when Na^+ was replaced by Li^+, Mg^{++}, or methylamine. This reversible effect was observed in the voltage-clamped as well as non-clamped muscle fibers and occurred within a few minutes after Na^+ replacement (Figure 4). In approximately one-fifth of the preparations the glutamate response was not greatly affected when Na^+ was replaced with Li^+, Mg^{++}, or methylamine. These results suggest that at least two types of receptor-channel complexes may exist at lobster excitatory neuromuscular junctions as has been shown previously for crayfish (40). Replacement of Na^+ with Li^+, Mg^{++}, or methylamine did not abolish the potentiating effect of aspartate, although the

potentiation was somewhat less than that observed in the normal
medium.

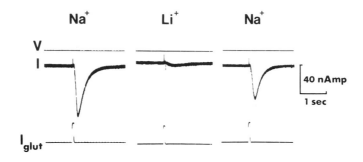

FIG. 4.   Effect of Li⁺ substitution on glutamate
induced membrane current. The muscle fiber was
voltage clamped at the resting potential (-86 mV)
with an intracellular microelectrode located within
a few hundred micrometers of the iontophoretic
electrode. Subsequent to the initial control response, the Li⁺ substituted medium was applied for
approximately 2 minutes during which time the
glutamate induced current declined to that shown.
The post Li⁺ control response was taken approximately 2 minutes after the superfusing fluid was
switched back to the normal saline.

Effects of Glutamate and Aspartate Analogs on the Postsynaptic Responses

We have tested numerous analogs of L-glutamate and L-aspartate
for possible effects on lobster neuromuscular junctions. D-
aspartate exhibited an antagonistic action which was consistently
found to be selective for L-aspartate, in that D-aspartate could
almost totally abolish the potentiating action of L-aspartate at
concentrations which had little effect on glutamate induced responses (Figure 5).

A few compounds were found which appeared to be pure antagonists of L-glutamate; these include D,L-2-amino-4-phosphonobuty-
rate (APB), D,L-β-allo-hydroxyglutamate and γ-methylene L-glutamate. The most potent was APB, which, at concentrations as low
as 0.1 mM, reduced glutamate responses, and similarly reduced
neurally evoked EPSPs. Results obtained with iontophoretically

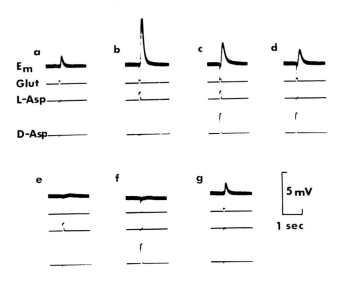

FIG. 5. Depolarization responses elicited by
L-glutamate (80 nA), L-aspartate (240 nA), and
D-aspartate (600 nA) iontophoretically applied
separately and in combination for a period of
100 msec. The responses were elicited sequentially
(a through g) at 30 sec intervals. The preparation
was bathed in the normal saline solution.

applied APB indicate that this analog antagonizes L-glutamate in
a manner similar to that reported previously at insect N-M
junctions, but has little if any ability to antagonize the potentiating action of L-aspartate (Figure 6).

Effect of L-Aspartate on Glutamate Induced Receptor Desensitization

At lobster neuromuscular junctions the glutamate induced membrane response rapidly declines when glutamate is iontophoresed
at high currents for more than a few hundred msec. We have obtained time constants for this desensitization process as short
as a few hundred msec. When L-aspartate was simultaneously iontophoresed the desensitization was not markedly affected (Figure
7).

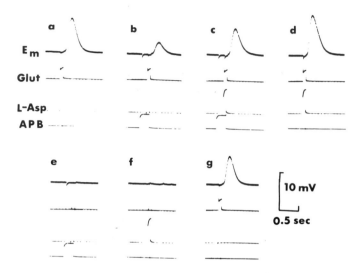

FIG. 6. Effect of D, L-2-amino-4-phosphonobutyrate
(APB) on depolarization responses elicited by L-glutamate
alone and in combination with L-aspartate. These
amino acids were iontophoresed for 100 msec at currents
of 160 and 400 nA respectively, whereas APB was applied
for 300 msec at a current of 500 nA. The response
elicited by glutamate alone (a and g) was approximately 75% of the maximum response. Since aspartate
does not affect the maximum response, the response
to glutamate (a,g) was not greatly potentiated by
L-aspartate (d). However, the APB inhibited glutamate response (b) was markedly potentiated by
aspartate (c).

Effect of L-Aspartate on Neurally Evoked Post-Synaptic Responses

We have previously observed that bath applied aspartate at
relatively high concentrations (≥ 0.5 mM) occasionally increased
the amplitude of evoked EPSPs by as much as 10 per cent. A
similar observation was made by Crawford and McBurney (12,13) in
a crab neuromuscular preparation. In the present experiments we
found that 0.2 mM L-aspartate showed no detectable effect on
neurally evoked post-synaptic responses in either the voltage
clamped or non-clamped muscle fibers. A concentration of 0.2 mM
was chosen for these experiments because aspartate almost completely blocked the Na^+ dependent uptake of glutamate at this
concentration.

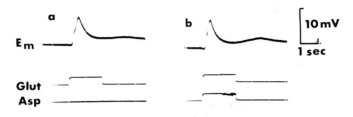

FIG. 7. Effect of L-aspartate on glutamate induced
receptor desensitization. Each amino acid was applied
for 2 sec. at a current of 500 nA.

Uptake of Glutamate and Aspartate by Lobster Nerve and Muscle Tissue

Tissue "slices" obtained from the meropodite and carpopodite
gradually accumulated (U-14C)-L-glutamate and (U-14C)-L-aspartate.
This uptake was not very sensitive to differences in temperature,
and the tissue to medium ratio of ^{14}C (cpm per gm. tissue/cpm per
ml medium) surpassed a value of 1 only when the tissue was incubated for 20 min or longer. The uptake of (U-14C)-L-glutamate by
sections of peripheral nerve and the CNS was similar to that obtained with muscle slices.

When Li$^+$ or methylamine was substituted for Na$^+$ in the incubation medium the uptake of ^{14}C-glutamate was decreased by one-
third to one-half (Table 1). This indicates that less than half
of the uptake observed was Na$^+$ dependent. Both the rate of uptake and the degree of Na$^+$ dependency are similar to values obtained by Baker and Potashner (4), using a crab peripheral nerve
preparation.

TABLE 1.   EFFECT OF Na^+ SUBSTITUTION ON THE UPTAKE OF
$(U-^{14}C)$-L-GLUTAMATE BY LOBSTER
NERVE-MUSCLE TISSUE [a]

Na^+ Substitute	% Uptake in Na^+ Medium ± S.D.
Li^+	65.7 ± 7.2
Methylamine	59.8 ± 25.2

[a] The data represent the mean of 5 experiments in which tissue incubation in each substituted medium was paired to an incubation in the normal Na^+ medium. For the Na^+ substituted media NaCl was replaced with LiCl or methylamine chloride on an equimolar basis. Tissue "slices" ($\sim$ 100 mg. wet wt.) from meropodite and carpopodite muscle bundles were incubated 30 min at 23°C.

TABLE 2.   EFFECT OF FOUR GLUTAMATE ANALOGS ON THE UPTAKE
OF $(U-^{14}C)$-L-GLUTAMATE BY LOBSTER
NERVE-MUSCLE TISSUE [b]

Glutamate Analog	% of Control ^{14}C-Uptake ± S.D.	
	0.2 mM (N=3)	1.0 mM (N=4)
L-Aspartate	61.3 ± 5.8	63.0 ± 11.9
D-Aspartate	61.7 ± 16.8	69.0 ± 14.6
L-Cysteate	54.1 ± 7.2	68.7 ± 13.2
D,L-β-OH-threo-aspartate	56.3 ± 24.1	68.5 ± 7.7

[b] Tissue "slices" ($\sim$ 100 mg) from meropodite and carpopodite muscle bundles were incubated for 30 min at 23°C in the normal Na^+ medium buffered with Tris to pH 7.4. In each experiment a control tissue slice was paired with slices incubated in the presence of each of the specified analogs.

Effect of Glutamate and Aspartate Analogs on the Uptake of Glutamate

A number of compounds were tested for their ability to inhibit the uptake of $(U-^{14}C)$-L-glutamate by the nerve-muscle tissue. Of the compounds tested, the four most potent inhibitors were D,L-threohydroxy-aspartate, L-aspartate, D-aspartate and L-cysteate. These four compounds at a concentration of 0.2 mM caused a 30 to 50% reduction in the uptake of ^{14}C-glutamate (Table 2). At higher concentrations (1.0 and 4.0 mM) there was no further inhibition of ^{14}C-glutamate uptake by these compounds. These results indicate that the Na^+ dependent uptake of glutamate is completely inhibited by these analogs at 0.2 mM. Although all of these four compounds exhibited an ability to potentiate the postsynaptic action of glutamate, the concentration required for a maximum effect, even for L-aspartate, was much greater than 0.2 mM. Several compounds, including kainate, D,L-2-amino-3-phosphonobutyrate, and γ-methyl-L-glutamate, were able to potentiate the action of glutamate but at the same concentrations had little inhibitory effect on the uptake of ^{14}C-L-glutamate.

DISCUSSION

It is now established that transmitter-receptor interaction in many, if not most, instances is cooperative in nature (7,42). Thus, dose-response curves frequently have sigmoid shapes rather than the hyperbolic form characteristic of the Langmuir isotherm model. Although the nature of this cooperativity has not been established for any given receptor, it is assumed that such receptors have multiple transmitter (ligand) binding sites, and/or that receptors are complexes composed of two or more interacting or independent protomers or subunits (7,28,41,42). Werman (42) suggested that ligand-receptor interaction can be considered cooperative if log-log plots of dose-response curves have limiting slopes significantly greater than 1. Werman (42) has further shown that the numerical value of the limiting slope may reflect the number of transmitter binding sites or subunits possessed by individual receptors. In the present study, the limiting slope of such log-log plots for the action of glutamate was approximately 5 (Figure 1). Dudel (14) has reported a similar slope for glutamate at the crayfish synapse. Such a steep slope may prove to play an important role in determining the efficiency of the synaptic process.

The transmitter action of glutamate is modified strikingly by the presence of L-aspartate (Figure 3). Under the conditions reported here, L-aspartate exhibits virtually no activity of its own. However, the presence of this compound in the bathing medium dramatically alters the effect of L-glutamate. This point is evidenced by the shift to the left of the glutamate response with increasing levels of aspartate. It should be pointed out that aspartate causes this shift without appreciably altering the slope of the glutamate curve.

One interpretation of these findings is that L-aspartate may act allosterically as a modulator to increase the affinity of L-glutamate for its post-synaptic receptor sites (19). However, mentioned earlier was the notion that as many as five hypotheses could be invoked to explain these results.

None of the five proposals for the potentiating effect of aspartate is mutually exclusive; therefore, all five possibilities could conceivably contribute to the observed effect. However, it should be possible to experimentally differentiate among these explanations because some differences in the nature of the potentiating effect would be expected. For example, if the potentiation were due to an inhibition of glutamate uptake or the prevention of receptor desensitization then the glutamate induced response should be prolonged appreciably. Such a prolongation would not necessarily be expected if the potentiation were due to a possible agonistic action or to an allosteric modulatory effect. The absence of an apparent prolongation in voltage-clamped muscle fibers (Figure 2) therefore supports the "agonist" and the "allosteric modulatory" mechanisms.

Another theory explaining the potentiative ability of aspartate upon glutamate suggests that this activity is due to an elevation of free glutamate in the synaptic cleft mediated by a displacement of bound extracellular glutamate (10,11). It must be emphasized that aspartate can markedly potentiate the action of glutamate at concentrations where this compound exhibits virtually no effect of its own regardless of the order of amino acid iontophoresis. Therefore, it seems unlikely that the "agonist" or "displacement" explanations can account for the potentiation. Furthermore, these explanations cannot readily explain the ability of D-aspartate to selectively antagonize L-aspartate's potentiating action.

Although our experiments on the uptake of glutamate confirm that aspartate is a strong inhibitor of the Na^+ dependent transport process, our results in general do not support the concept that aspartate's potentiating effect is due to an inhibition of glutamate uptake. The ability of L-cysteate, D-aspartate and D,-L-threo-hydroxy-aspartate to block the Na^+ dependent uptake at a concentration which does not markedly potentiate the postsynaptic glutamate response (0.2 mM) suggests that there is little, if any, correlation between the inhibition of glutamate uptake and the potentiation of its postsynaptic action. This is supported by the observation that some compounds (e.g. kainate and 2-amino-3-phosphonobutyrate) can potentiate glutamate responses at concentrations which do not inhibit the uptake of glutamate. The ability of aspartate to potentiate the glutamate response when Na^+ was replaced with Li^+ in order to prevent uptake is further evidence against the view that the potentiating effect is primarily due to an inhibition of glutamate uptake. Indeed, it is conceivable that reuptake may not contribute appreciably at all to the termination of EPSPs. Along these lines, autoradiographic experiments with other arthropod nerve-muscle preparations indicate that glutamate is taken up primarily by sheath cells surrounding the nerve axons (16,30,34). These results coupled with our finding that L-aspartate has no detectable effect on neurally evoked postsynaptic responses at a concentration which totally blocks the Na^+ dependent glutamate uptake supports the idea that reuptake by the nerve terminal does not contribute appreciably to the termination of EPSPs in these preparations. This conclusion has been reached previously by Anwyl and Usherwood (2) for insect excitatory neuromuscular junctions.

Of the proposed explanations for the potentiative effect of aspartate, only the allosteric modulator mechanism remains consistent with all of our findings.

Although the physiological significance of this transmitter modulation remains to be established, there is mounting evidence that many neurons release more than one active substance from their synaptic terminals (5,6). This supports the possibility that glutamate and aspartate may be released together and may function as a transmitter-modulator pair (19,20).

Strong evidence favoring this idea is seen in the observation that D-aspartate depresses neurally evoked EPSPs at a concentration which shows no blocking action whatsoever upon L-glutamate responses (37). Thus, it is reasonable to suggest that the D-aspartate depression of EPSPs is not directly related to blockade of endogenously released glutamate. Furthermore, while showing no action on glutamate alone, the same D-aspartate level prevented entirely the potentiative effects of L-aspartate (37). Accordingly, these findings support the idea that, with respect to EPSPs, D-aspartate depresses by blocking endogenously released L-aspartate which normally exerts a steady state potentiation on the natural transmitter, glutamate.

ACKNOWLEDGEMENTS

The authors wish to thank Dr. Margaret L. Freeman for her careful editing of this manuscript and Ms. Nancy I. Roman for her excellent typing services.

The research reported in this paper was supported by Research Grant NS13979 from NIH and by Biomedical Research Support Grant N° RR05417 from the Division of Research Sources, NIH.

REFERENCES

1. Anwyl, R. (1977): J. Physiol., Lond., 273: 367-388.
2. Anwyl, R. and Usherwood, P.N.R. (1974): Nature, Lond., 252: 591-593.
3. Anwyl, R., and Usherwood, P.N.R. (1975): J. Physiol., London, 46P-47P.
4. Baker, P.F. and Potashner, S.J. (1971): Biochem. Biophys. Acta, 249: 616-622.

5. Brownstein, M.J., Saavedra, J.M., Axelrod, J., Zeman, G.H., and Carpenter, D.O. (1974): Proc. Natl. Acad. Sci. USA, 71: 4662-4665.
6. Carpenter, D.O., personal communication.
7. Colquhoun, D. (1973): In: Drug receptors, A Symposium, Ed. H.P. Rang, pp. 149-182. University Park Press, Baltimore.
8. Colton, C.K., Freeman, A.R. (1975 a): Comp. Biochem. Physiol. 51C: 275-284.
9. Colton, C.K., Freeman, A.R. (1975 b): Comp. Biochem. Physiol. 51C: 285-289.
10. Constanti, A. and Nistri, A. (1978): Brit. J. Pharmacol., 62: 495-505.
11. Constanti, A. and Nistri, A. (1979): Brit. J. Pharmacol., 65: 287-301.
12. Crawford, A.C. and McBurney, R.N. (1977): J. Physiol., London, 268: 697-709.
13. Crawford, A.C. and McBurney, R.N. (1977): J. Physiol. London, 268: 711-729.
14. Dudel, J. (1977): Pflugers Arch., 368: 49-54.
15. Dudel, J. (1977): Pflugers Arch., 369: 7-16.
16. Faeder, I.R. and Salpeter, M.M. (1970): J. Cell Biol., 46: 300-307.
17. Frank, E. (1974): J. Physiol., London, 242: 371-382.
18. Freeman, A.R. (1976a): In: Electrobiology of Nerve, Synapse, and Muscle, edited by J.P. Reuben, D. Purpura, M.V.L. Bennett, and E.R. Kandel, p. 61-80. Raven Press, New York.
19. Freeman, A.R. (1976 b): Progr. Neurobiol., 6: 137-153.
20. Freeman, A.R., Shank, R.P., Kephart, J., Dekin, M., and Wang, M. (1979): J. Physiol., Paris, 75: 605-610.
21. Gent, J.P., Morgan, R. and Wolstencroft, J.H. (1974): Neuropharmacology, 13: 441-447.
22. Graham, L.T. Jr., and Aprison, M.H. (1966): Analyt. Biochem., 15: 487-497.
23. Gration, K.A.F., Clark, R.B., and Usherwood, P.N.R. (1979): Neuropharmacol., 18: 201-208.
24. Grundfest, H. (1972): In: Neuromuscular blocking and stimulating agents. Ed., Cheymold, J., International Encyclopedia of Pharmacology and Therapeutics, Section 14, Vol. 2 p. 621-654. Pergamon Press, Oxford.
25. Grundfest, H., Reuben, J.P. (1961): In: Nervous Inhibition, Ed. E. Florey, p. 92-104. Pergamon Press, New York.
26. Grundfest, H., Reuben, J.P., Rickles, W.H. Jr. (1959): J. Gen. Physiol., 42: 3101-3123.
27. Jan, L.Y. and Jan, Y.N. (1976): J. Physiol., 262: 215-236.
28. Karlin, A. (1967): J. Theor. Biol., 16: 306-320.
29. Kerkut, G.A., and Wheal, H.V. (1974): Brit. J. Pharmacol., 51: 136P-137P.
30. Kravitz, E.A., Slater, C.R., Takahashi, K., Bownds, M.O., Grossfeld, R.M. In: Excitatory Synaptic Mechanism, edited by P. Anderson and J.K.S. Jansen, p. 85-93. Universitetsforlaget, Oslo.

31. McBurney, R.N. and Crawford, A.C. (1979): Fed. Proc. Am. Soc. Exp. Biol., 38: 2080-2083.
32. Onodera, K., and Takeuchi, A. (1975): J. Physiol., 252: 295-318.
33. Patlak, J.B., Gration, K.A.F., and Usherwood, P.N.R. (1979): Nature, Lond., 278: 643-645.
34. Salpeter, M.M., and Faeder, I.R. (1971): Progress in Brain Research, 34: 103-114.
35. Shank, R.P., and Aprison, M.H. (1970): Analyt. Biochem., 35: 136-145.
36. Shank, R.P., and Freeman, A.R. (1975): J. Neurobiol., 6: 289-303.
37. Shank, R.P., and Freeman, A.R. (1976): J. Neurobiol., 7: 23-36.
38. Shank, R.P., Freeman, A.R., McBride, W.J., and Aprison, M.H. (1975): Comp. Biochem. Physiol., 50: 127-131.
39. Shank, R.P., Wang, M.B., and Freeman, A.R. (1977): Brain Res., 126: 176-180.
40. Taraskevich, P.S. (1975): J. Gen. Physiol., 65: 677-691.
41. Triggle, D.J. (1971): Neurotransmitter-Receptor Interactions, Academic Press, New York.
42. Werman, R. (1969): Comp. Biochem. Physiol., 30: 997-1017.

Glutamate as a Neurotransmitter,
edited by G. Di Chiara and G. L. Gessa
Raven Press, New York © 1981.

Effects of Ibotenic Acid on Amphibian and Mammalian Spinal Neurones *in Vitro*

A. Nistri, *J. F. MacDonald, and **J. L. Barker

*Department of Pharmacology, St. Bartholomew's Hospital Medical College, London EC1M 6BQ, England; *Helen Scott Playfair Neuroscience Unit, Toronto Western Hospital, Toronto M5T 2S8, Canada; and **Laboratory of Neurophysiology, NINCDS, Bethesda, Maryland 20205*

Ibotenic acid (IBO) is a conformationally-restricted analogue of glutamate, an amino acid considered to be a central excitatory transmitter (7). On locust muscle fibres, IBO has excitatory (1) as well as inhibitory (3) effects. On feline spinal neurones IBO has also been found to have mixed effects: an initial excitation followed by a prolonged inhibition (5,6) (cf. Fig. 1): the IBO-induced inhibition has been observed as a sustained depression of neuronal firing and found it insensitive to bicuculline, picrotoxin and strychnine. More recently, Curtis et al. (4) reporting that IBO-induced inhibitions could be antagonized by bicuculline, suggested that IBO was transformed by the nervous tissue into muscimol, a potent analogue of the inhibitory amino acid, GABA. In the present report we examine the effects of IBO on two in vitro preparations, frog spinal motoneurones and mouse cultured spinal neurones. By using in vitro tissues and recording potential changes following IBO applications, it should be possible to gain a more precise understanding of the mode of action of IBO. This has hitherto proved to be difficult in experiments based on iontophoretic applications in vivo and extracellular recordings of spike activity.

METHODS

DC-coupled recordings of lumbar motoneuronal responses of the frog (R. temporaria) to bath-applied drugs were obtained essentially as described earlier (2) from IX or X ventral roots pulled from the cord-containing bath and mounted in paraffin-oil filled side chambers. The main modifications of the method consisted in: 1) the use of 5-6°C bath temperature to block amino acid uptake and to minimize an enzymatic tissue conversion of

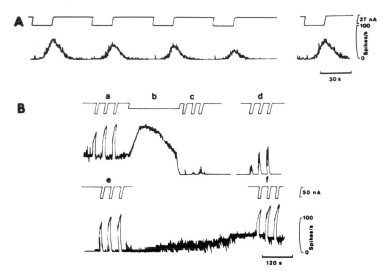

FIG.1. Effects of iontophoretically-applied IBO on the firing rate of a feline spinal interneurone. A: repeated applications of constant IBO currents (monitored on top trace) give progressively smaller responses; recovery 5 min later. B: constant glutamate applications were given before (a), 30 sec (c), 8 min (d), 18 min (e) and 30 min (f) after a sustained application of IBO (b). Note long-lasting depression of glutamate responses and of baseline activity. From (5) with permission of the National Research Council of Canada.

IBO into muscimol; 2) monopolar (rather than differential) recordings from the central end of the ventral root with respect to the bath-ground; 3) the cord was placed in the bath in such a way that practically no length of the ventral root was exposed to the bathing medium. Intracellular recordings from single visually-identifiable neurones grown in dissociated cultures from embryonic mouse spinal cords (8) were obtained with glass microelectrodes (containing 4 M K-acetate); drugs were applied by iontophoresis or by pressure microperfusion.

RESULTS

Excitatory Effects of IBO

On frog motoneurones IBO produced dose-dependent depolarizations with a slow onset and offset. The variation in motoneuronal sensitivity to IBO was fairly large in comparison to the reproducible sensitivity to glutamate. Factors perhaps contributing to such a response variability were the conspicuous

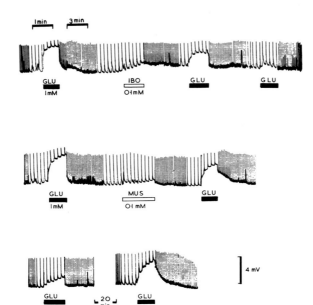

FIG. 2. Responses of frog motoneurones to glutamate (GLU), IBO and muscimol (MUS). Upward deflections are ventral root potentials (VRP) whose amplitude is attenuated by the frequency response of the pen-recorder. Top row: GLU responses are depressed after an IBO application; middle row: recovery of GLU responses (20 min after IBO washout) and subsequent depression following MUS; bottom row: tracing continuous with middle one. Negativity upwards.

fading of depolarizations clearly seen following repeated applications of IBO (cf. similar case in cat neurones - Fig. 1) and/or the concomitant inhibitory effects (v. infra). These complications prevented the construction of complete dose-depolarization curves; nevertheless, the available data suggest that the threshold dose for IBO depolarization is about 20 µM and that IBO is an approximately 7 times more potent depolarizing agent than glutamate (apparent IBO ED_{50} = 45 µM; glutamate (ED_{50} = 300 µM).

On mouse neurones, IBO also evoked membrane depolarizations associated with a small conductance increase. Again depolarization fading was prominent (not shown).

The IBO depolarizations of frog motoneurones were not reduced in the presence of tetrodotoxin (1 µM) but they were strongly depressed by 18 mM Mg^{2+}. In mouse neurone experiments it was also noted that 10 mM Mg^{2+} largely depressed IBO depolarizations.

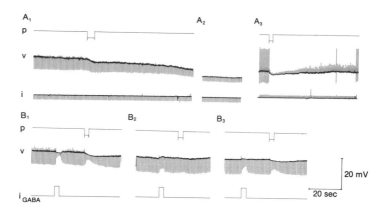

FIG. 3. Two inhibitory responses of cultured spinal neurones
(A and B) to pressure ejections of IBO (5 nM or 50 µM) and to
iontophoretically-applied GABA (13 nA). Letters indicate: p,
pressure ejection of IBO; v, membrane potential; i, applied
intracellular current (0.4 nA in A_1); i_{GABA}, iontophoretic
GABA current. In A_1, IBO (5 nM) causes gradual hyperpolarization from -40 mV to -60 mV (A_2); this response reached a
maximum 2 min after IBO application and was associated with a
decrease in input resistance (compare amplitude of downward
deflections - indicating electrotonic potentials elicited by
constant current pulses - of tracing v in A_1 and A_2). No
recovery of this response during the duration of recording (> 2h).
A second and superimposed inhibitory response to IBO (50 µM) is
illustrated in A_3 where the neurone is depolarized to -45 mV by
steady intracellular current application and it generates action
potentials (upward deflections of v trace; attenuated by the pen
recorder) after short current pulses: this response to IBO is
similar to that evoked by GABA (in B_1). Unlike the long-lasting
response to IBO, the shorter IBO inhibition as well as the GABA
response are blocked by picrotoxin (10 µM; B_2) or bicuculline
(not shown) in a reversible manner (cf. B_3).

Inhibitory Effects

In previous iontophoretic experiments on feline neurones (5,
6) it was found that the inhibitory effects of IBO were more
easily observed as long-lasting neuronal depression following
a few min of IBO application. Attempts were therefore made to
use similarly long bath-applications to frog motoneurones. IBO
(50 µM-1 mM) was applied for periods ranging from 45 sec to 3-4
min. Motoneuronal excitability was tested by repeatedly
administering glutamate (0.5 - 1 mM for 30 sec - 1 min) or K^+
(12 - 17 mM; 30 sec - 1 min) for extended periods (over 60-90
min). Responses to glutamate (but not to K^+) were severely
depressed (never completely abolished) with times for 90%

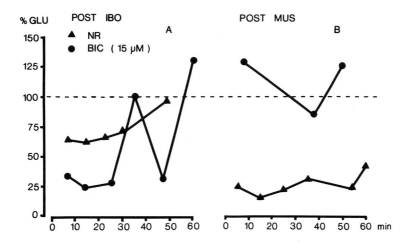

FIG. 4. Frog motoneuronal responses to GLU (0.5 mM) at
different times from washout of a 3 min application of IBO
(50 μM; A) or MUS (50 μM; B). Triangles: responses in Normal
Ringer (NR); circles: responses in the presence of bicuculline
(BIC). Note that bicuculline blocks inhibition of GLU responses
after MUS but not after IBO. The temporary recovery of GLU
responses 35 min after IBO (in A) may be explained by a concomitant large increase in motoneuronal spontaneous activity.

recovery of glutamate response amplitude in the range of 20-45
min as shown in Fig. 2: such a depressant effect was dependent
on the IBO concentration, present when motoneuronal polarization
level returned to the baseline (in some cases a small hyperpolarization was noted during the extended inhibition) and it
was associated with a depression of synaptically-evoked motoneuronal potentials (VRP; produced by orthodromic dorsal root
stimulation). Sustained application of large doses (up to 5 mM)
of glutamate for equivalent periods produced much shorter and
rapidly reversible depressions of motoneuronal glutamate
responses and VRPs. Applications of muscimol (concentration
range as for IBO) for similar periods evoked small depolar-
zations or hyperpolarizations (usually 0.1 - 0.3 mV amplitude) of
motoneurones with concomitant inhibition of their electrical
activity. These muscimol effects were followed by long-lasting
inhibitions of glutamate responses and VRPs which recovered
rather slowly (occasionally after 60 min) (Fig. 2).

On mouse neurones Fig. 3 shows that pressure applications of
IBO (5 nM - 10 μM) induced a sustained hyperpolarization associated with a conductance increase. This hyperpolarization had
a gradual slow onset and could persist for > 1 h. In higher
concentrations (10 - 50 μM) IBO evoked a more rapid hyperpolarization (with conductance increase) whose inversion

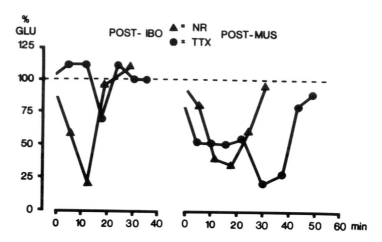

FIG. 5. Frog motoneuronal responses to GLU (1 mM) tested after washout of a 1 min application of IBO (0.1 mM; on the left) or MUS (0.1 mM; on the right) either in Normal Ringer (NR) or in tetrodotoxin (TTX; 1 μM) Ringer. Abscissa: time after IBO or MUS washout; ordinate: GLU response amplitudes as % of control ones. Note that TTX reduces the inhibition of GLU responses after IBO but not after MUS.

potential was similar to that of GABA-induced responses; this short lasting effect was superimposed on the long-lasting hyperpolarization.

On both frog motoneurones and mouse neurones bicuculline (either as a free base or as methiodide salt) evoked a large increase in neuronal excitability (even in the presence of 10 mM Mg^{2+}) characterized by repetitive spontaneous depolarizations (frog motoneurones) or by lowering of the threshold for generation of action potentials (mouse neurones). Bicuculline (and picrotoxin, see Fig. 3) blocked the effects of GABA on mouse neurones and the long-lasting depression of glutamate responses evoked by muscimol in frog motoneurones, (Fig. 4). However, bicuculline did not affect the sustained hyperpolarization evoked by IBO on mouse neurones nor did it significantly alter the long-lasting IBO depression of motoneuronal responses to glutamate (Fig. 4). When propagated interneuronal activity of the frog spinal cord was completely blocked by tetrodotoxin (1 μM) or procaine (1 mM) or when chemical synaptic transmission was fully abolished by 18 mM Mg^{2+}, IBO applications evoked a smaller and shorter motoneuronal inhibition although the inhibition following muscimol was not reduced. Larger IBO concentrations were needed to reproduce in part the degree of inhibition observed in control Ringer. These results thus demonstrate that: 1) a major component of the IBO-evoked inhibition is originated via interneuronal pathways and release of yet unidentified transmitter(s); 2) the use of local anaesthetics allows to separate pharmacologically IBO excitation and inhibition since the former is not significantly altered whereas the latter is reduced (cf. Fig. 5).

DISCUSSION

The present data shows that IBO can excite as well as inhibit (in a sustained manner) amphibian and mammalian neurones in vitro. We therefore confirm our original findings obtained with iontophoretic IBO applications on feline interneurones in vivo (5,6). Our current experiments indicate that the long-lasting inhibitory effect of IBO is very unlikely due to tissue conversion of this substance into muscimol, a GABA agonist, as suggested by Curtis et al. (4). In fact, the long-lasting IBO inhibitions were not blocked by bicuculline (whereas the actions of muscimol and GABA were antagonized) and were sensitive to local anaesthetics and high-Mg^{2+} solutions. It would be difficult to postulate that tetrodotoxin and Mg^{2+} block IBO conversion into muscimol. It is, however, apparent that, at least in the case of mouse neurones, a short-lasting GABA-like inhibition may be evoked by IBO; such a brief inhibition is clearly separated from the most prominent effect of IBO, namely a yet unexplainable long-lasting depression of neuronal excitability.

The present findings do not allow us to establish firmly the precise mode of action of IBO in inducing the sustained neuronal inhibition. It is, however, possible to suggest that such an inhibition might involve an increased membrane permeability to ion(s) whose equilibrium potential is very negative: K^+ is certainly a candidate for this role. Furthermore, from frog cord experiments with tetrodotoxin it is apparent that a significant portion of IBO inhibition is due to activation of inhibitory interneurones releasing a long-acting transmitter (perhaps a peptide?) acting on bicuculline-insensitive receptors of the motoneuronal membrane. Finally, the sensitivity of IBO actions to Mg^{2+} might be taken either as a further confirmation of the presynaptic location of IBO effects or as evidence for an additional Mg^{2+}-dependent mechanism of the postsynaptic membrane involved in the mediation of responses to glutamate-related analogues (9).

ACKNOWLEDGEMENTS

Ibotenic acid and muscimol were generously donated by Prof. C.H. Eugster and Prof. D. Della Bella respectively. Thanks are due to M. Warren, R. Croxton and J.C.R. Gomersall for technical assistance and photography and to Miss Carol Brown for typing.

REFERENCES

1. Clark, R.B., Gration, K.A.F., and Usherwood, P.N.R. (1979): Br. J. Pharmac., 66: 267-273.

2. Constanti, A., and Nistri, A. (1976): Br. J. Pharmac., 57: 347-358.

3. Cull-Candy, S.G. (1976): J. Physiol. (Lond.), 255: 449-464.

4. Curtis, D.R., Lodge, D., and McLennan, H. (1979): J. Physiol. (Lond.), 291: 19-28.

5. MacDonald, J.F., and Nistri, A. (1977): Can. J. Physiol. Pharmac., 55: 965-967.

6. MacDonald, J.F., and Nistri, A. (1978): J. Physiol. (Lond.), 275: 449-465.

7. Nistri, A., and Constanti, A. (1979): Progr. Neurobiol., 13: 117-235.

8. Ransom, B.R., Neale, E., Henkart, M., Bullocks, P.N., and Nelson, P.G. (1977): J. Neurophysiol., 40: 1132-1150.

9. Watkins, J.C. (1978): In: Kainic acid as a Tool in Neurobiology, edited by E.G. McGeer, J.W. Olney, and P.L. McGeer, pp. 37-70. Raven Press, New York.

Glutamate as a Neurotransmitter,
edited by G. Di Chiara and G. L. Gessa
Raven Press, New York © 1981.

On the Nature of the Receptors for Various Excitatory Amino Acids in the Mammalian Central Nervous System

H. McLennan

Department of Physiology, University of British Columbia, Vancouver, British Columbia, V6T 1W5, Canada

Investigation into the actions of the naturally occuring amino acids L-glutamate and L-aspartate upon neurones of the mammalian central nervous system began some twenty years ago when Curtis et al. (9) described the excitation, accompanied by membrane depolarization and a conductance increase, which followed their administration to the extracellular environment of single cells. This initial work was expanded by Curtis and Watkins (10,11) to show that many other compounds possess similar actions insofar as their ability to cause neuronal excitation is concerned. Noting that "The optimum distance between the amino group and one of the acidic groups of the excitatory amino acids is two or three carbon atoms. The other acidic group is optimally situated α with respect to the amino group. The amino group is optimally primary", Curtis and Watkins (10) felt that a three-point attachment site was the most likely config-uration of the receptor activated by these amino acids.

Since these first studies were conducted, more than 75 compounds have been examined, many of considerably greater excitatory potency than L-glutamate itself. Interest has centered particularly on those molecules which possess a degree of conformational restraint, in which the spacing between the presumed three active groups resembles that in glutamate in its extended form (4, 18, 22, 23, 29). Of particular interest in this connection have been kainic acid, ibotenic acid and its derivatives, cis-1-amino-1,3 dicarboxy-cyclopentane (ADCP) and quisqualic acid. Over the

years there developed a tacit assumption that all of
the various compounds examined, including glutamate
and aspartate themselves, probably react with an
homogeneous group of receptors.

One of the first indications that this might not
be the case was the report of McLennan et al. (26) of
a lack of parallelism in the responsiveness of
thalamic neurones to L-glutamate and to two non-
naturally occuring amino acids, DL-homocysteate and
N-methyl-DL-aspartate; and the proposition was
advanced that two populations of receptors, one
specifically activated by glutamate and the second by
the other amino acids as well as by glutamate, might
exist. Recent studies (1,13) which have shown that
the membrane changes induced by glutamate are complicated and are only partially duplicated by homocysteate, may point to a similar conclusion. Thus
the depolarization elicited by homocysteate is
associated with a decreased membrane conductance (13)
rather than with the increase earlier reported to be
caused by glutamate (9). The action of glutamate now
appears as a biphasic one involving both an increase
and a decrease in conductance, which may indeed
indicate reaction with more than one receptor type.

ANTAGONISTS OF THE EXCITATORY AMINO ACIDS

That there exist at least two populations of amino
acid receptors has also been made most evident through
the use of antagonists of the excitatory effects.
Haldeman et al. (16) and Haldeman and McLennan (17)
were the first to report that L-glutamate diethylester
(GDEE) had a selective effect against excitations
induced by glutamate when contrasted with those
produced by aspartate or homocysteate. Although there
have been other reports indicating that the selectivity of action is not always as high as was
originally claimed (1,6,28), it is now generally
accepted that amongst the various amino acids
glutamate is the one most susceptible to blockade by
GDEE.

Another class of antagonist is represented by
certain longer chain mono- and diaminodicarboxylic
acids (2,5,12,14,15,18,20,24,25,27) of which the best
studied has been D-α-aminoadipate (DαAA). Unlike
GDEE, this substance is not very effective against
glutamate-induced excitations but instead has a
preferential action against aspartate and particularly
against the N-methylated derivatives of this compound.
Indeed these two substances, GDEE and DαAA have
largely reciprocal actions as is shown in Table 1;

and the data strongly suggest that there exists one
type of receptor preferentially antagonized by DαAA
and activated by the N-methyl-aspartates, and a second
activated by L-glutamate and blocked by its
diethylester. Compounds appearing towards the centre
of both lists in Table 1, such as the isomers of
homocysteate, presumably can react to an approximately
equal extent with both classes of receptor.

It appears that both types may be of synaptic
importance in the central nervous system. Thus
whereas GDEE may have comparatively weak effects upon
the excitation of spinal neurones evoked by
stimulation of dorsal roots (2,12; but see 17), DαAA
prevents these responses quite effectively. On the
other hand as examples, GDEE but not DαAA blocks the
perforant path input to the hippocampus (21,33), and
the responses evoked by certain corticofugal pathways
are also GDEE-sensitive (31,32). This second group
of synaptic systems may be postulated to use glutamate
as the natural transmitter; while those responses
blocked by DαAA are more likely to be L-aspartate-
mediated on the basis that this compound ranks above
glutamate in the list of DαAA susceptibility shown in
Table 1 and that that list is headed by the N-
methylated derivatives of aspartate. It must be
noted however that the interpretation of these data,
particularly for compounds like aspartate which can
be blocked by suitably large "doses" of either of the
antagonists, must always be somewhat uncertain
inasmuch as the effective concentrations of antagonist
present at a synaptic site cannot be directly
estimated.

Among various other compounds which have been
suggested as selective antagonists of the amino acids,
the longer chain mono- and diaminodicarboxylic acids
are qualitatively similar to DαAA although some are
more potent (2,12,14). L-5,6-dimethoxyaporphine
appears to resemble GDEE in that excitations produced
by L-glutamate and quisqualate are the most easily
affected (8), but McLennan and Wheal (28) could not
distinguish between glutamate, L-aspartate and homocysteate excitations using this material. This last
observation is true too for 1-hydroxy-3-
aminopyrrolidone-2 (7), and N-methyl-D-aspartate
(NMDA) excitations have also been reported to be
strongly depressed by this substance (2) which therefore appears to have rather little selectivity of
action.

TABLE 1.   Antagonism of amino acid-induced
excitations

by GDEE	by DαAA
L-glutamate	⎰N-methyl-D-aspartate
Quisqualate	⎱N-methyl-L-aspartate
D-aspartate	Ibotenate
L-aspartate	⎰ADCP
D-glutamate	⎰L-homocysteate
⎰D-homocysteate	⎱D-homocysteate
⎱L-homocysteate	D-glutamate
Ibotenate	L-aspartate
⎰ADCP	D-aspartate
⎰N-methyl-L-aspartate	Quisqualate
⎱N-methyl-D-aspartate	L-glutamate

Compounds are listed in order of decreasing
susceptibility to blockade, save for those bracketted
together which are indistinguishable one from another.

Data from Hicks et al. (20) and McLennan and
Lodge (27).

Of interest are the actions of the glutamate
analogue 2-amino-4-phosphonobutyrate (2APB) first
reported as an amino acid antagonist in crustacea.
It has been stated that this compound resembles DαAA
although it is considerably weaker, in that NMDA
excitations are preferentially blocked when compared
with those produced by glutamate, and it is said to
have similar effects to DαAA upon the synaptic
responses of spinal cord neurones (12). Davies and
Watkins (12) have also reported that, unlike any of
the other antagonists 2APB attenuates the excitatory
effects produced by kainic acid, while GDEE and DαAA
are both relatively ineffective against this compound
(20,27). The possible significance of this point will
be further considered below.

CONFIGURATION OF AMINO ACID RECEPTORS

The evidence adduced thus far indicates that two
distinct amino acid receptors exist, one antagonized
by GDEE and the other by DαAA. This mode of classification appears more secure than a designation by
agonist for although the GDEE-sensitive receptor
appears preferentially activated by glutamate, the
actions of this substance can also be blocked by
sufficiently large amounts of DαAA (3,20), indicating
that glutamate presumably can react with the second

type of receptor as well. Although it is true that
N-methyl-aspartate excitations are little effected
by GDEE (20,27), the actions of its naturally occuring
analogue L-aspartate are blocked by both antagonists,
as demonstrated by the intermediate position which it
occupies in both lists of Table 1.

Consideration of the dimensions of the various
agonist molecules permits some conclusions to be
drawn regarding the likely configuration of these two
classes of receptor. Table 2 sets forth the maximal
and minimal distances which can exist between the two
acidic groups of a number of excitant molecules of
which three, glutamate, quisqualate (27) and α-amino-
3-hydroxy-5-methyl-4-isoxazolepropionate (AMPA) (23)
are antagonized preferentially by GDEE and little by
DαAA; two, ibotenate and ADCP (20,27) are DαAA-
sensitive and two, L-aspartate (20,27) and 2-
aminomalonate (H. McLennan, unpublished observations)
are affected by both.

TABLE 2. Maximal and minimal distances between the
carboxyl carbon atoms of excitatory amino acids,
in nm.

	Maximum	Minimum
GDEE-sensitive		
Glutamate	0.46	0.18
Quisqualate	0.38	0.20
AMPA	*	0.20
GDEE- and DαAA-sensitive		
Aspartate	0.38	0.25
2-Aminomalonate	0.25	0.25
DαAA-sensitive		
Ibotenate	0.46	0.42
ADCP	0.41	0.41

*Steric interference from the methyl group on the
5-position of the isoxazole ring does not permit a
maximal separation of the acidic groups to occur (23)

The critical difference between the GDEE- and
DαAA-sensitive groups appears to be the minimal
spacing between the two acidic functions, in that
nearly exclusive GDEE sensitivity occurs if that
distance is 0.2 nm or less while preferential
antagonism by DαAA is found only when the distance is
greater than 0.4 nm. The minimal separation in the
aspartate and 2-aminomalonate molecules falls between
these two limits. The implication therefore is that

the GDEE-antagonized receptor accepts amino acid
molecules only when they are fully folded, whereas
that affected by DαAA demands that reaction occurs
with molecules which are in a relatively extended
conformation. Thus the "inflexible" molecules of
ibotenate and ADCP which are unaffected by GDEE,
cannot assume the required minimal separation between
the acidic functions. Flexible molecules such as L-
glutamate can extend to separations greater than
0.4 nm; however it would appear that the affinity of
the "folded" GDEE-sensitive receptor for glutamate is
higher since the excitatory actions of glutamate are
more readily blocked by GDEE. On this basis one could
predict that the excitations produced by the weak
agonist L-α-aminoadipate (18) which possesses a highly
flexible molecule, would be preferentially affected by
GDEE rather than by DαAA and this has been found to be
the case (H. McLennan, unpublished observations).

One further observation indicates the correctness
of the conclusion regarding the conformation of the
receptors. D-glutamate is a neuronal excitant about
one-half as potent as the naturally occuring isomer
(10, 18); however unlike L-glutamate its action is
preferentially blocked by DαAA. When the molecules
are relatively extended D- and L-glutamate could
occupy an identical three-point template, but no such
"fit" is possible in the folded configuration. It is
conceivable therefore that in this latter circumstance
D-glutamate might act as an L-glutamate antagonist.

In a preparation treated with sufficient DαAA to
inactivate the receptors sensitive to this compound
as indicated by the absence of response to NMDA, but
which leaves the reaction to L-glutamate largely
unaffected, the effect of D-glutamate has been to
antagonize the L-glutamate response (H. McLennan,
T.P. Hicks and T.L. Richardson, unpublished observations). In the absence of DαAA D-glutamate is
itself an excitant, as has earlier been shown, and
potentiates other amino acid responses. It seems
likely therefore that D-glutamate reacts preferentially with the extended DαAA-sensitive receptor to
yield excitation, but can act to block the "folded"
type, presumably through steric interference.

KAINIC ACID

The pyrollidine derivative kainate is one of the
more powerful neuronal excitants known, comparable in
potency to quisqualate (4). Its ring structure con-
fers a considerable degree of conformational restraint

upon the molecule, and the distance between the
critical acidic groups can vary only between 0.43 and
0.51 nm. On this basis one would expect kainate-
induced excitations to be insensitive to GDEE as is
the case (12,20,27); however such excitations are also
relatively resistant to the action of DαAA which would
not have been predicted from the above considerations.
A similar insensitivity to blockade by DαAA even when
amounts large enough to affect glutamate are used, is
exhibited also by the much weaker excitant dihydrokainate, but no other substance is presently recognized which shares with kainate this unconventional
pattern of antagonism. The possibility must therefore
be considered that a third type of receptor reacting
preferentially or exclusively with kainate and its
close analogues also exists upon neurones. This
suggestion is strengthened by the claim of Davies and
Watkins (12) to which reference was made earlier, that
2APB alone amongst the recognized antagonists also
depresses kainate excitations while otherwise
resembling DαAA, which would infer that 2APB can
interact both with "kainate" and "N-methyl-aspartate"
activated receptors.

BINDING STUDIES

Further evidence also is forthcoming from binding
studies involving radiolabelled ligands. Membrane
fragments prepared according to Simon et al. (30)
incubated in sodium-free medium specifically bind both
glutamate and kainate. The glutamate binding sites
pharmacologically resemble those receptors here
described as GDEE-sensitive, in that a) bound glutamate can be displaced by quisqualate but not by such
DαAA-antagonized compounds as ibotenate or ADCP, and
b) the binding of glutamate is antagonized by GDEE
but not by DαAA. NMDA does not bind specifically to
this membrane preparation, indicating that DαAA-
sensitive receptors are not present.

Kainate does not interfere with glutamate binding
although it is itself specifically bound, and in this
latter instance again none of the DαAA susceptible
excitants interfere with the process with the
exception of ibotenate to a minor degree. Glutamate
and quisqualate do displace bound kainate but only
with an affinity much less than that exhibited by
kainate itself. These results are set forth in
Table 3, and see also Henke and Cuénod (19).

It thus seems probable that this membrane preparation possesses two distinct types of binding site,

one resembling the GDEE-antagonized, glutamate activated receptor identified in vivo, and the other relatively specific for kainate. The third postulated receptor, that blocked by DαAA and activated most effectively by N-methyl-aspartate, seems not to be present in these isolated membrane preparations, and it therefore must be considered as a distinct third class.

TABLE 3. Potency of various compounds in displacing sodium-independent specific binding of kainate and L-glutamate[a]

Excitants	L-glutamate IC_{50} (µM)	Kainate IC_{50} (µM)
L-glutamate	0.17	1.1
Quisqualate	3.2	3.2
Kainate	>1000	0.073
Ibotenate	>1000	69
NMDA	>1000	>1000
ADCP	>1000	>1000
Antagonists		
GDEE	19	>1000
DαAA	>1000	>300

[a] Unpublished data of H. McLennan

The evidence obtained from an analysis of the antagonism of amino acid-induced excitations in vivo and binding studies in vitro thus point to the existence of (1) a GDEE-sensitive receptor which reacts with molecules in a folded configuration, (2) a DαAA-antagonized receptor accepting relatively extended molecules, and (3) a receptor for kainate which is not readily affected by either GDEE or DαAA but which also must have an "extended" configuration. Certain agonist molecules can react with more than one of the receptor types.

The author is supported by the Medical Research Council of Canada.

REFERENCES

1. Altmann, H., Bruggencate, G. ten, Pickelmann, P., and Steinberg, R. (1976): Pflügers Arch., 364: 249-255.

2. Biscoe, T.J., Davies, J., Dray, A., Evans, R.H., Martin, M.R., and Watkins, J.C. (1978): Brain Res., 148: 543-548.

3. Biscoe, T.J., Evans, R.H., Francis, A.A., Martin, M.R., Watkins, J.C., Davies, J., and Dray, A. (1977): Nature, 270: 743-745.

4. Biscoe, T.J., Evans, R.H., Headley, P.M., Martin, M.R., and Watkins, J.C. (1976): Br. J. Pharmac., 58: 373-382.

5. Collingridge, G.L., and Davies, J. (1979): Neuropharmacology, 18: 193-199.

6. Curtis, D.R., Duggan, A.W., Felix, D., Johnston, G.A.R., Tebecis, A.K., and Watkins, J.C. (1972): Brain Res., 41: 283-301.

7. Curtis, D.R., Johnston, G.A.R., Game, C.J.A., and McCulloch, R.M. (1973): Brain Res., 49: 467-470.

8. Curtis, D.R., Lodge, D., and Bornstein, J.C. (1979): J. Pharm. Pharmacol., 31: 795-797.

9. Curtis, D.R., Phillis, J.W., and Watkins, J.C. (1960): J. Physiol. (Lond.), 150: 656-682.

10. Curtis, D.R., and Watkins, J.C. (1960): J. Neurochem., 6: 117-141.

11. Curtis, D.R., and Watkins, J.C. (1963): J. Physiol. (Lond.), 166: 1-14.

12. Davies, J., and Watkins, J.C. (1979): J. Physiol. (Lond.), 297: 621-635.

13. Engberg, I., Flatman, J.A., and Lambert, J.D.C. (1979): J. Physiol. (Lond.), 288: 227-261.

14. Evans, R.H., Francis, A.A., and Watkins, J.C. (1978): Brain Res., 148: 536-542.

15. Evans, R.H., and Watkins, J.C. (1978): Eur. J. Pharmacol., 50: 123-129.

16. Haldeman, S., Huffman, R.D., Marshall, K.C., and McLennan, H. (1972): Brain Res., 39: 41('25.

17. Hal(an, S., and McLennan, H. (1972): Brain Res.,): 393-400.

18. Hall, J.G., Hicks, T.P., McLennan, H., Richardson, T.L., and Wheal, H.V. (1979): J. Physiol. (Lond.), 286: 29-39.

19. Henke, H., and Cuénod, M. (1979): Neurosci. Letts., 11: 341-345.

20. Hicks, T.P., Hall, J.G., and McLennan, H. (1978): Can. J. Physiol. Pharmacol., 56: 901-907.

21. Hicks, T.P., and McLennan, H. (1979): Can. J. Physiol. Pharmacol., 57: 973-978.
22. Johnston, G.A.R., Curtis, D.R., Davies, J., and McCulloch, R.M. (1974): Nature, 248: 804-805.
23. Krogsgaard-Larsen, P., Honoré, T., Hansen, J.J., Curtis, D.R., and Lodge, D. (1980): Nature, 284: 64-66.
24. Lodge, D., Headley, P.M., and Curtis, D.R. (1978): Brain Res., 152: 603-608.
25. McLennan, H., and Hall, J.G. (1978): Brain Res., 149: 541-545.
26. McLennan, H., Huffman, R.D., and Marshall, K.C. (1968): Nature, 219: 387-388.
27. McLennan, H., and Lodge, D. (1979): Brain Res., 169: 83-90.
28. McLennan, H., and Wheal, H.V. (1976): Neuropharmacology, 15: 709-712.
29. McLennan, H., and Wheal, H.V. (1978): Neurosci. Letts., 8: 51-54.
30. Simon, J.R., Contrera, J.F., and Kuhar, M.J. (1976): J. Neurochem., 26: 141-147.
31. Spencer, H.J. (1976): Brain Res., 102: 91-101.
32. Stone, T.W. (1973): J. Physiol. (Lond.), 233: 211-225.
33. Wheal, H.V., and Miller, J.J. (1980): Brain Res., 182: 145-155.

Glutamate as a Neurotransmitter,
edited by G. Di Chiara and G. L. Gessa
Raven Press, New York © 1981.

Pharmacology of Receptors for Excitatory Amino Acids

*J. C. Watkins, **J. Davies, †R. H. Evans, †A. A. Francis, and †A. W. Jones

*Departments of *Physiology and †Pharmacology, The Medical School, Bristol BS8 1TD, England; and **Department of Pharmacology, The School of Pharmacy, London WC1N 1AX, England*

The recent development of selective antagonists for excitatory amino acids has greatly facilitated investigation of the function of such substances as transmitters in the vertebrate central nervous system (20,39,40). Studies with these antagonists have not only provided strong evidence for amino acid-mediated synaptic excitation, but have also led to the recognition of different types of receptors for excitatory amino acids. Thus, N-methyl-D-aspartate (NMDA), quisqualate and kainate appear to be selective agonists for particular receptor types, while a variety of other amino acids, including L-glutamate and L-aspartate have mixed actions on more than one type of receptor. This paper will summarize the properties of these receptors as observed in experiments in the amphibian spinal cord *in vitro* and the mammalian spinal cord *in vivo*; particular aspects of the mammalian receptors will be illustrated in the companion paper by Davies (14).

SELECTIVE ANTAGONISM BY DIVALENT METAL IONS

The earliest clear differentiation of receptors for excitatory amino acids came from a study of the effect of divalent metal ions on depolarizing responses of frog motoneurones to a range of such excitants (1,17). Low concentrations of Mg^{2+} (threshold, 10 μM) depressed responses to NMDA while having little or no effect on responses to kainate or quisqualate, the latter amino acid being resistant to Mg^{2+} concentrations as high as 20 mM. Responses to L-aspartate were somewhat more sensitive to Mg^{2+} than were responses to L-glutamate, though the major part of the response to each of these putative transmitters were resistant to Mg^{2+} (Fig. 1) Similar results were obtained in experiments in the cat spinal cord *in vivo* (12). Such effects, both *in vitro* and *in vivo* were not reversed by increasing Ca^{2+} concentration, and indeed these latter ions resembled Mg^{2+}, except that they were much less potent (1). The transition metal ions, Co^{2+} and Mn^{2+}, had similar effects to Mg^{2+} in the frog spinal cord, Co^{2+} being stronger and

Mn^{2+} weaker than Mg^{2+} in producing these effects (Table 1)(ref.1). This order of potency is clearly different from that observed for the depression of transmitter release in the peripheral nervous system where Mn^{2+} is considerably stronger than Mg^{2+} (34). The low concentrations of Mg^{2+} required, the resistance of such effects to reversal by Ca^{2+} and the lower potency of Mn^{2+} compared with Mg^{2+} emphasize the difference between these presumably post-synaptic effects and the 'traditional' presynaptic effects (15,34, 41) of the same ions.

NMDA RECEPTORS AND SYNAPTIC EXCITATION

The selective effects of the divalent ions indicates the exist-ence of at least two types of excitatory amino acid receptors, which, for simplicity, we will refer to as NMDA and non-NMDA recep-tors. A range of organic antagonists were soon found to produce

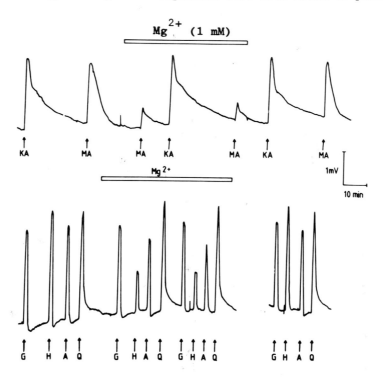

FIG. 1. Selective depression by Mg^{2+} of amino acid-induced depol-arizations of frog motoneurones *in vitro*. The medium contained 0.1 µM tetrodotoxin. The figure shows ventral root recordings, in the presence (bars above records) and absence of 1 mM Mg^{2+}, of depolarizations produced by: top series, 12 µM kainate (KA) and 40 µM N-methyl-D-aspartate (MA): bottom series, 1 mM L-glutamate (G), 100 µM L-homocysteate (H), 1.2 mM L-aspartate (A) and 5 µM quisqualate (Q). From Ault *et al.* (1).

TABLE 1.   Depression of excitatory amino acid-induced depolarization of frog motoneurones by divalent metal ions[a].

	PERCENT CONTROL RESPONSES		
	Mg^{2+} (0.5 mM)	Co^{2+} (0.5 mM)	Mn^{2+} (0.5 mM)
NMDA	22 ± 1	17 ± 3	57 ± 1
L-HOMOCYSTEATE	34 ± 1	40 ± 5	64 ± 3
L-ASPARTATE	82 ± 2	64 ± 11	81 ± 5
L-GLUTAMATE	89 ± 2	93 ± 5	91 ± 3
KAINATE	96 ± 3	96 ± 7	95 ± 1
QUISQUALATE	95 ± 1	105 ± 2	98 ± 1

[a]Method similar to that illustrated in Fig. 1.

similar effects to Mg^{2+}, likewise acting predominantly on NMDA receptors.   These include monoamino and diamino dicarboxylic amino acids, having the D configuration at the amino carboxylate terminals (39,40).   Amongst the most extensively studied of these compounds are D-α-aminoadipate (DαAA)(2-4,13,16,18,21,24,28,30,31), D-α-aminosuberate (DαAS)(13,16) and α,ε-diaminopimelate (α,ε-DAP) (2,3,16,18).   Such antagonists are highly specific, having little or no effect on the depolarizing responses produced by cholinergic, aminergic or peptidergic agonists in the mammalian central nervous system (2-6,18).   They also depress spinal synaptic excitation evoked by dorsal root stimulation, but have no action on the cholinergic excitation of Renshaw cells following ventral root stimulation (2-4), or of sympathetic ganglionic neurones following preganglionic stimulation (18).   Most importantly, the relative potencies of the substances as depressants of spinal synaptic excitation parallel their relative potencies as NMDA antagonists (16).   The simplest explanation of this parallelism is that NMDA receptors are transmitter receptors activated physiologically by an excitatory amino acid transmitter.

MODE OF ACTION OF THE ORGANIC AND INORGANIC NMDA ANTAGONISTS

The relationship between the effects of divalent metal ions and those of organic antagonists at NMDA receptors is unknown, but preliminary experiments suggest that the two types of agent act at different sites in the receptor-ionophore complex (19).   The monoamino and diamino dicarboxylic acids appear to act competitively with NMDA for occupation of the receptors, while the divalent metal ions may act later in the chain of events leading to ionophore activation.   It has been suggested   (18) that changes in extracellular Mg^{2+} concentration may exercise a physiological role in regulating the sensitivity of the receptors to the transmitter during synaptic excitation.

CONFORMATIONAL REQUIREMENTS FOR NMDA RECEPTOR ACTIVATION

Compounds of restricted conformational variability and which resemble either aspartate or glutamate with respect to the separation of charged groups have been used to assess the conformational requirements for NMDA agonist action (7,8,40). The most important finding is that *trans*-2,3- and *trans*-2,4-piperidine dicarboxylates are both NMDA agonists of high potency, whereas the *cis*-2,3- isomer is a partial agonist, and the *cis*-2,4- isomer relatively inactive. The 2,3- compounds are aspartate analogues and the 2,4- compounds are glutamate analogues. However, with respect to the separation of the carboxylate groups, the inactive *cis*-2,4- may be regarded as an 'extended' glutamate analogue and the *trans*-2,4- compound as a 'partially folded' glutamate analogue. Another cyclic compound which can also be regarded as a partially folded glutamate analogue is *cis*-1-amino-1,3-dicarboxycyclopentane and this substance is likewise an NMDA receptor agonist (8,22). It would therefore seem likely that, in conformity with theoretical arguments (26,29) the NMDA receptor is preferentially activated by aspartate analogues or by glutamate analogues that possess, or are able to adopt, a conformation in which the two carboxyl groups are less than maximally separated.

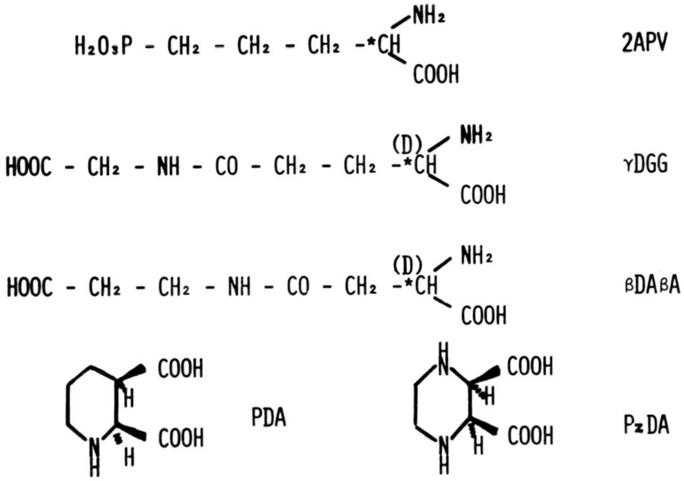

FIG.2.   Structures of 2-amino-5-phosphonovaleric acid (2APV), γ-D-glutamylglycine (γDGG), β-D-aspartyl-β-alanine (βDAβA), *cis*-2,3-piperidine dicarboxylic acid (PDA) and *cis*-2,3-piperazine dicarboxylic acid (PzDA).

TABLE 2.   Apparent dissociation constants for NMDA
receptor-antagonist complex[a]

Antagonist	App K_D (μM)
(±)-2-amino-5-phosphonovalerate (2APV)	2.4
D-α-aminosuberate (DαAS)	15.9
γ-D-glutamylglycine (γDGG)	21.4
β-D-aspartyl-β-alanine	21.7
D-α-aminoadipate (DαAA)	42.4
(±)-cis-2,3-piperidine dicarboxylate (PDA)	53.8
(±)-cis-2,3-piperazine dicarboxylate	104
(±)-α,ε-diaminopimelate (α,ε-DAP)	120
(±)-mono-N-acetyl-α,ε-DAP	120
γ-L-glutamylglycine	147
(±)-2-amino-5-phosphonobutyrate (2APB)	> 200
L-glutamic acid diethyl ester (GDEE)	> 1000

[a]Derived from Gaddum-Schild equation, $K_D = \dfrac{A}{DR-1}$ where K_D is the apparent dissociation constant, A the antagonist concentration and DR the dose-ratio for NMDA antagonism.

NEW ANTAGONISTS

Recently we have found a diversity of new antagonists that, while preserving specificity for excitatory amino acid receptors vis à vis receptors activated by other putative transmitter agonists, in some cases show a somewhat different spectrum of activity compared with monoamino and diamino dicarboxylic acids (7,8,10,11, 40). These new antagonists comprise three main groups: 1) phosphonic acid analogues of monoamino dicarboxylic acids, 2) ω-linked dipeptides of either glutamic or aspartic acids with neutral amino acids, such that the distribution of free carboxyl and amino groups resembles those in monoamino dicarboxylic acids, and 3) conformationally restricted cyclic analogues of aspartate in which the two carboxyl groups are *cis*-related to each other (the *trans* orientation leading to agonist activity as described above). The structures of representatives of these groups are shown in Fig. 2.

All of these compounds block NMDA receptors. The most potent and selective NMDA antagonist yet tested is 2-amino-5-phosphono-valerate (2APV)(7,11), which is the phosphonic acid analogue of α-aminoadipate. An example of the action of this substance in the frog spinal cord is shown in Fig. 3. Based on apparent K_D values for the NMDA receptor-antagonist complex (Table 1), the phosphono analogue (even as the racemate) has approximately 17 times the affinity of DαAA for NMDA receptors in the frog spinal cord. It is likely that the D form of this compound carries the antagonist activity, as has been shown (40) to be the case with the lower homologue, 2-amino-4-phosphonobutyrate (2APB), which is a relatively weak and less selective antagonist (7,13,16,40).

The two dipeptides, α-D-glutamylglycine and β-D-aspartyl-β-alanine (7,10,40) have similar affinities for the NMDA receptor to that of D-α-aminosuberic acid (HOOC-CH$_2$-CH$_2$-CH$_2$-CH$_2$-CH$_2$-CH(NH$_2$)-COOH) (13,16) which they resemble in structure; all are more potent as depressants of NMDA-induced and synaptic excitation in the frog spinal cord than the shorter chain D-α-aminoadipic acid (HOOC-CH$_2$-CH$_2$-CH$_2$-CH(NH$_2$)-COOH) (Table 2).

Of the cyclic compounds, the partial agonist (±)-*cis*-2,3-piperidine dicarboxylate (PDA) is the most potent (7,8,40). The (-) form appears to carry the predominant part of the pharmacological activity of this substance (8,40). A purer though weaker NMDA antagonist activity is shown by the piperazine analogue (Table 2)(8,40).

Unlike 2APV, which is highly selective for NMDA receptors, γDGG and PDA also have actions at non-NMDA receptors (7). Thus, both in the amphibian spinal cord *in vitro* and the cat spinal cord *in vivo*, PDA blocks kainate- and quisqualate- in addition to NMDA-induced excitation. A somewhat similar pattern of activity is shown by γDGG in the frog spinal cord (10), but in the cat spinal cord (7,10) this dipeptide distinguishes clearly between kainate- and quisqualate-induced responses, selectively depressing responses to the former amino acid. This observation supports the evidence previously obtained from studies with DαAA and L-glutamic acid diethyl ester (GDEE) that NMDA, kainate and quisqualate act

TABLE 3.   Effects of excitatory amino acid antagonists
           on responses of cat Renshaw cells[a]

| | ANTAGONIST | | | | |
AGONIST	2APV	GDEE	DγGG	2APB	PDA
NMDA	↓↓↓↓↓	o	↓↓↓	↓↓	↓↓↓
KAINATE	o	o	↓↓(↓)	↓↓	↓↓↓
QUISQUALATE	o	↓↓	(↓)	↓(↓)	↓↓↓
ACh	o	↓(↓)	o	o	o(↑)
L-ASP	↓↓↓	↓(↓)	↓↓	↓(↓)	↓↓↓
L-GLU	↓(↓)	↓↓	(↓)	↓(↓)	↓↓↓
DR-EVOKED	↓↓↓	o	↓↓	↓	↓↓

[a]The number of downward pointing arrows represents the degree of depression, brackets indicating a lower value.

at different receptors (7,13,24,30,31). A summary of the effects
of a range of antagonists on responses of cat Renshaw cells to
various excitants and synaptic activation is given in Table 3.

DO KAINATE OR QUISQUALATE RECEPTORS MEDIATE SYNAPTIC EXCITATION?

The depression of dorsal root-evoked synaptic excitation of
frog motoneurones (DR-VRPs) by a range of excitatory amino acid
antagonists is predominantly related to NMDA receptor blockade
(16). However, not all the DR-VRP is mediated by NMDA receptors.
When these receptors are completely blocked by 2APV a resistant
component of the DR-VRP can be detected (Fig.3a). Both γDGG and
PDA depress this component reversibly (Fig.3a), indicating the
possible involvement of kainate and/or quisqualate receptors in
this response. A differentiation between these two types of
receptors may be possible in the mammalian central nervous system
where γDGG effectively depresses kainate-induced responses in the
absence of marked effects on responses to quisqualate (10).
Experiments to determine whether 2APV-resistant synaptic excitation in the mammalian CNS can be blocked by γDGG or PDA are
currently in progress (14).

Whether or not non-NMDA receptors are involved in synaptic
excitation the possibility that kainate receptors are at least
partially extrasynaptic is raised by the finding that this amino
acid depolarizes isolated dorsal root fibres of the neonatal rat
spinal cord (9). Extrajunctional kainate receptors have been
identified in invertebrates (38) and have been postulated to occur
in the goldfish retina (44). Kainate receptors on dorsal root
fibres are effectively antagonized by PDA (Fig.3b)(8) and also
(less effectively) by γDGG (8) and 2APB (9). The D(-) form of
2APB is the active isomer producing this effect, as also in antagonizing NMDA receptors (8,40).

THE TRANSMITTER(S) AT SITES OF AMINO
ACID-MEDIATED SYNAPTIC EXCITATION

Studies with NMDA antagonists in the mammalian central nervous
system have suggested that the following cells may be activated by
an excitatory amino acid transmitter following stimulation of
specific pathways. a) Renshaw cells, and some other spinal
neurones, activated by dorsal root stimulation (2-4,13,28), b)
cortical neurones activated by pyramidal tract stimulation (37),
c) neurones in the cochlear nucleus activated by auditory stimuli
(32,33), d) lateral geniculate neurones activated by visual
stimuli (27), e) neurones in the cuneate nucleus, excited by
cortical stimulation (37), f) caudate nucleus cells, responding
to cortical stimuli (37), g) granule cells in the dentate gyrus
excited by stimulation of the contralateral hippocampus (25), h)
cerebellar Purkinje cells activated by parallel fibre stimulation
(36). Although, in many cases, responses to L-aspartate were more
sensitive to the antagonists used in these experiments than were

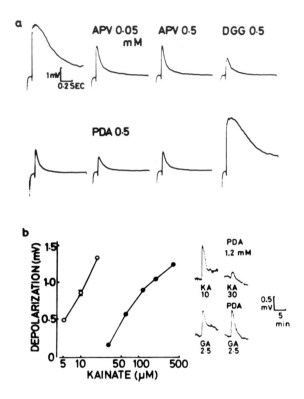

FIG. 3.   a. Action of 2-amino-5-phosphonovalerate (APV), γ-D-
glutamylglycine (DGG) and *cis*-2,3-piperidine dicarboxylate (PDA)
on dorsal root-evoked ventral root potential in frog spinal cord.
From left (uppermost series): control; potential recorded in
presence of 0.05 mM APV showing marked depression; potential
recorded after raising APV concentration to 0.5 mM (no further
effect); with APV (0.5 mM) still present, DGG (0.5 mM) depresses
the APV-resistant potential.   In lower series, from left: with
APV (0.5 mM) still present, recovery from DGG; PDA (0.5 mM)
depresses the APV-resistant response; recovery from PDA; recovery
from APV.   b. Depression of non synaptic kainate receptors by PDA.
Graph shows responses of fibres in isolated dorsal roots of baby
rats to kainate in absence (O) and presence (●) of PDA (1.2 mM).
Traces to the right show (upper series) control response to 10 μM
kainate (KA) and depressed response to 30 μM kainate in presence
of PDA.   Lower series shows that responses induced by GABA (GA),
2.5 μM, are not depressed by PDA.

responses to L-glutamate, responses to both amino acids were often depressed at antagonist doses required to block synaptic excitation. In these cases clearly no conclusions can be drawn as to which (if either) of these two amino acids might be acting as the transmitter at a particular population of synapses. However, in other cases, depression of synaptic excitation has been observed at antagonist concentrations that depress L-aspartate- but not L-glutamate-induced excitation. Such effects have been observed with Renshaw cells in which dorsal root-evoked and L-aspartate-induced excitation were antagonized by low concentrations of 2APV and γDGG that did not affect L-glutamate-induced excitation of the same cells (14). Under these circumstances L-aspartate must be favoured as the likely transmitter. On the other hand, L-glutamate may be the transmitter at 2APV-resistant, PDA-sensitive sites of synaptic excitation, involving kainate and/or quisqualate receptors. Preliminary evidence for the existence of such sites has been obtained in the mammalian (14) as well as the amphibian spinal cord (Fig.3a, above). However, no specific pathways involving these receptors have yet been identified.

While the results described are encouraging, pharmacological studies alone are unlikely to lead to absolute identification of transmitters acting at specific populations of synapses. This will require a correlation of pharmacological and neurochemical data. Recent studies in the hippocampus (25,35,43) and cochlear nucleus (32,33,42) offer promise in this respect, though the possibility cannot be excluded that the transmitter acting at the antagonist-sensitive sites is neither L-glutamate nor L-aspartate but some like substance as yet unidentified (39).

REFERENCES

1. Ault, B., Evans, R.H., Francis, A.A., Oakes, D.J. and Watkins, J.C. (1980): J. Physiol. (Lond.) (in press).
2. Biscoe, T.J., Davies, J., Dray, A., Evans, R.H., Martin, M.R. and Watkins, J.C. (1977): Eur. J. Pharmac., 45:315-316.
3. Biscoe, T.J., Davies, J., Dray, A., Evans, R.H., Martin, M.R. and Watkins, J.C. (1978): Brain Res., 148:543-548.
4. Biscoe, T.J., Evans, R.H., Francis, A.A., Martin, M.R., Watkins, J.C., Davies, J. and Dray, A. (1977): Nature (Lond.), 270:743-745.
5. Collingridge, G.L. and Davies, J. (1979): Neuropharmacology, 18:193-199.
6. Davies, J. and Dray, A. (1979): Experientia (Basel), 35:353-354.
7. Davies, J., Evans, R.H., Francis, A.A., Jones, A.W. and Watkins, J.C. (1980): In: EMBO Workshop on Drug Receptors in the Central Nervous System, edited by M. Balaban, International Science Services, Jerusalem (in press).
8. Davies, J., Evans, R.H., Francis, A.A., Jones, A.W. and Watkins, J.C., unpublished observations.

9. Davies, J., Evans, R.H., Francis, A.A. and Watkins, J.C. (1979): J. Physiol. (Paris), 75:641-645.
10. Davies, J., Francis, A.A., Jones, A.W. and Watkins, J.C. (1980): J. Physiol. (Lond.) (in press).
11. Davies, J., Francis, A.A., Jones, A.W. and Watkins, J.C. (1980): Br. J. Pharmacol. (in press).
12. Davies, J. and Watkins, J.C. (1977): Brain Res., 130:364-368.
13. Davies, J. and Watkins, J.C. (1979): J. Physiol. (Lond.), 297:621-635.
14. Davies, J. and Watkins, J.C. (1980): In: GABA and Glutamate as Transmitters (this symposium). Raven Press, New York.
15. Del Castillo, J. and Engbaek, L. (1955): J. Physiol. (Lond.) 124:370-384.
16. Evans, R.H., Francis, A.A., Hunt, K., Oakes, D.J. and Watkins, J.C. (1979): Br. J. Pharmacol., 67:591-603.
17. Evans, R.H., Francis, A.A. and Watkins, J.C. (1977): Experientia (Basel), 33:489-491.
18. Evans, R.H. and Watkins, J.C. (1978): Eur. J. Pharmac., 50:123-129.
19. Evans, R.H. and Watkins, J.C. (1978): J. Physiol. (Lond.) 277:57P.
20. Evans, R.H. and Watkins, J.C. (1981): Ann. Rev. Pharmacol. Toxicol. (in press).
21. Hall, J.G., Hicks, T.P. and McLennan, H. (1978): Neurosci. Lett., 8:171-175.
22. Hall, J.G., Hicks, T.P., McLennan, H., Richardson, T.L. and Wheal, H.V. (1979): J. Physiol. (Lond.), 286:29-39.
23. Hall, J.G., McLennan, H. and Wheal, H.V. (1977): J. Physiol. (Lond.), 272:52-53P.
24. Hicks, T.P., Hall, J.G. and McLennan, H. (1978): Can. J. Physiol. Pharmacol., 56:901-906.
25. Hicks, T.P. and McLennan, H. (1979): Can. J. Physiol. Pharmacol., 57:973-978.
26. Johnston, G.A.R., Curtis, D.R., Davies, J. and McCulloch, R.M. (1974): Nature (Lond.), 248:804-805.
27. Kemp, J.A. and Sillito, A.M. (1979): J. Physiol. (Lond.), 292:46P.
28. Lodge, D., Headley, P.M. and Curtis, D.R. (1978): Brain Res. 152:603-608.
29. McCulloch, R.M., Johnston, G.A.R., Game, C.J.A. and Curtis, D.R. (1974): Exp. Brain Res., 21:515-518.
30. McLennan, H. and Hall, J.G. (1978): Brain Res., 149:541-545.
31. McLennan, H. and Lodge, D. (1979): Brain Res., 169:83-90.
32. Martin, M.R. (1980): Neuropharmacology (in press).
33. Martin, M.R. and Adams, J.C. (1980): Neuroscience, 4:1097-1105.
34. Meiri, U. and Rahaminoff, R. (1972): Science, 176:308-309.
35. Nadler, J.V., White, W.F., Vaca, K.W., Perry, B.W. and Cotman, C.W. (1978): J. Neurochem., 31:147-155.
36. Stone, T.W. (1979): Br. J. Pharmacol., 66:291-296.
37. Stone, T.W. (1979): Br. J. Pharmacol., 67:545-551.

38. Takeuchi, A. and Onodera, K. (1975): Neuropharmacology, 14:619-625.

39. Watkins, J.C. (1978): In: Kainic Acid as a Tool in Neurobiology, edited by E.G. McGeer, J.W. Olney and P.L. McGeer, pp.37-69. Raven Press, New York.

40. Watkins, J.C. (1980): In: Glutamate: Transmitter in the Central Nervous System, edited by P.J. Roberts, J. Storm-Mathisen and G.A.R. Johnston. John Wiley and Sons, Chichester, England (in press).

41. Weakley, J.N. (1973): J. Physiol. (Lond.), 234:597-612.

42. Wenthold, R.J. and Gulley, R.L. (1977): Brain Res., 138: 111-123.

43. White, W.F., Nadler, J.V., Hamberger, A., Cotman, C.W. and Cummins, J.T. (1977): Nature (Lond.), 270:356-357.

44. Yazulla, S. and Kleinschmidt, J. (1980): Brain Res., 182: 282-301.

Glutamate as a Neurotransmitter,
edited by G. Di Chiara and G. L. Gessa
Raven Press, New York © 1981.

Pharmacology of Glutamate and Aspartate Antagonists on Cat Spinal Neurones

J. Davies and *J. C. Watkins

*Department of Pharmacology, The School of Pharmacy, University of London,
London WC1N 1AX, England; and *Department of Physiology, The Medical School,
Bristol BS8 1TD, England*

INTRODUCTION

Determination of the possibility that the excitatory amino acids, L-glutamate and L-aspartate, function as synaptic transmitters in the mammalian central nervous system (CNS) has been handicapped by the absence of suitable antagonists for either amino acid-induced or synaptically evoked excitation. A number of substances have been proposed as antagonists of excitatory amino acids on CNS neurones (4,13) but the specificity of many of these is questionable as they do not distinguish between amino acid- and non amino acid-induced excitation (1,5,6,19). However, recent studies demonstrate that certain monoamino and diamino dicarboxylic acids antagonize the excitatory actions of amino acids with some degree of selectivity (2,3,13,17). For instance, D-α-aminoadipate (DαAA) and D-α-aminosuberate (DαAS) depress responses to L-aspartate more than responses to L-glutamate. The responses to the aspartate analogue, N-methyl-D-aspartate (NMDA) are extremely sensitive to these agents compared with responses to the glutamate analogues, kainate and quisqualate (3,9,13). These substances are also selective antagonists of synaptic excitation, depressing non-cholinergic, but not cholinergic, synaptic responses of spinal Renshaw cells (3,9,13,16). Such observations provide evidence for the existence of different types of excitatory amino acid receptors and for amino acid mediated synaptic

275

excitation in the CNS.

This report concerns the effects of three new potential excitatory amino acid antagonists (FIG. 1), 2-amino-5-phosphonovaleric acid (2APV) which is the phosphonic acid analogue of α-aminoadipic acid, a dipeptide, ɣ-D-glutamylglycine (ɣDGG) (structurally related to DαAS) and cis-2,3-piperidine dicarboxylate (PDA) (a rigid analogue of aspartic acid). The actions of these substances have been examined on responses of spinal neurones to acetylcholine (Renshaw cells) and a range of amino acid excitants (Renshaw cells and dorsal horn neurones) including, in particular, NMDA, kainate and quisqualate in view of the suggestion that these agents act on different receptors (10,18). Their effects have also been determined on synaptically evoked excitation of spinal neurones. Some of these results have been briefly reported. (11,12)

FIG. 1.

Structure of Excitatory Amino Acid Antagonists

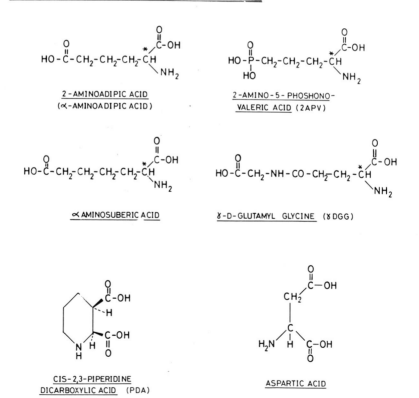

2-AMINOADIPIC ACID
(α-AMINOADIPIC ACID)

2-AMINO-5-PHOSHONO-
VALERIC ACID (2APV)

α AMINOSUBERIC ACID

ɣ-D-GLUTAMYL GLYCINE (ɣDGG)

CIS-2,3-PIPERIDINE
DICARBOXYLIC ACID (PDA)

ASPARTIC ACID

METHODS

Potential antagonists and agonists were administered microiontophoretically near neurones in the lumbar spinal cord of pentobarbitone or α-chloralose anaesthetized cats using conventional techniques (13).

RESULTS AND DISCUSSION

Differentiation Of Antagonist Effects

The effects of the three potential antagonists on neuronal responses to various excitants are summarised in table 1. None of the agents depressed responses of Renshaw cells to acetylcholine while they all depressed responses to excitatory amino acids to varying degrees. The effects of 2APV ejected from dilute solutions (50 mM in NaCl) were similar to those previously reported with DαAA and DαAS (9,13) in that responses to NMDA were reduced with little or no effect on responses to kainate or quisqualate on the same neurones (Table 1). However, 2APV was approximately 15 times more potent

TABLE 1   Selective antagonism of amino acid-induced-excitation of cat spinal neurones

Agonist	No. neurones depressed/No. tested (Mean $\pm$ S.E.% depressed)		
	2APV (16 $\pm$ 3nA)*	γDGG (17 $\pm$ 1nA)*	PDA* (32 $\pm$ 3nA)
NMDA	$12/12$ (90 $\pm$ 4)	$14/14$ (77 $\pm$ 5)	$12/12$ (68 $\pm$ 7)
L-aspartate	$8/10$ (58 $\pm$ 5)	$4/5$ (61 $\pm$ 6)	$11/11$ (71 $\pm$ 6)
L-glutamate	$2/9$ (60 $\pm$ 28)	$1/7$ (40)	$12/12$ (64 $\pm$ 5)
kainate	$2/12$ (20)	$24/24$ (68 $\pm$ 4)	$11/12$ (55 $\pm$ 6)
quisqualate	$0/9$ (0)	$6/17$ (42 $\pm$ 10)	$7/8$ (54 $\pm$ 6)
acetylcholine	$0/7$** (0)	$0/9$ (0)	$0/8$** (0)

*   Mean $\pm$ S.E. ejecting currents (nA). 2APV was ejected as an anion from a 50 mM solution in 165 mM NaCl. γDGG and PDA were both ejected as anions from 200 mM aqueous solutions of each.

**   Responses to acetylcholine were enhanced by 2APV (2 cells) and PDA (4 cells)

than DαAA, based on the ejection currents required
to produce equal depression of responses to NMDA
(FIG. 2). Indeed, the potency of 2APV was such
that, without dilution with NaCl, high retaining
currents did not prevent diffusional escape from
200 mM solutions (as used for DαAA and other
antagonists) sufficient to prevent excitation of
cells by NMDA.

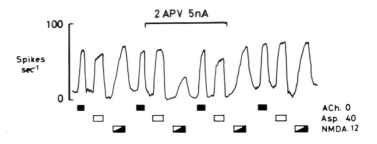

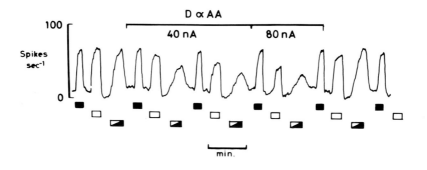

FIG. 2. The effects of 2APV (5 nA) and DαAA (40 and
80 nA) on the firing of the same Renshaw cell by
acetylcholine (0 nA), L-aspartate (40 nA) and NMDA
(12 nA). 2APV and DαAA were ejected from 50 mM
solutions in 165 mM NaCl.

The dipeptide, ɣDGG, also reduced excitatory
responses to NMDA but in addition depressed responses
to kainate while those to quisqualate were
relatively unaffected (Table 1, FIG. 3). The
effects of the L isomer of ɣGG on these amino acid-
induced responses were essentially similar to those
of the D isomer although the latter was approximately
twice as effective (on the basis of equieffective
ejecting currents) as the former in this respect.
Both ɣDGG and 2APV differentiated between responses to
L-aspartate and L-glutamate, preferentially reducing
responses to the former.

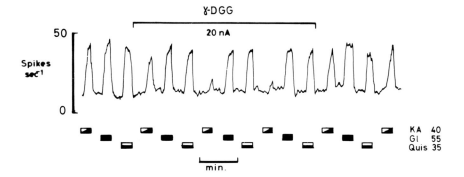

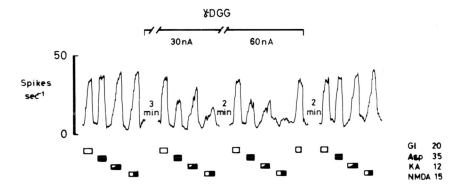

FIG. 3. Upper record: depression of responses of a
dorsal-horn neurone to kainate (KA 40 nA) but not
L-glutamate (Gl 55 nA) or quisqualate (Quis 35 nA)
by ɣDGG 20 nA. Lower record: depression of responses
of a Renshaw cell to L-aspartate (Asp 35 nA), KA
(12 nA) and NMDA (15 nA) but not Gl (20 nA) by ɣDGG
(30-60 nA).

The third potential antagonist, PDA did not
differentiate between the excitatory effects of
NMDA, kainate or quisqualate but depressed
responses to all three agonists. Responses to
L-glutamate and L-aspartate were also generally
reduced in parallel by this agent. However, preceding
antagonism on many occassions excitatory responses
were enhanced, suggesting that this agent has a
partial agonist role. Interestingly, the trans
isomer of PDA was a pure agonist and its effects
were depressed by 2APV and ɣDGG.

The absence of depressant effects of 2APV and
ɣDGG on acetylcholine-induced responses together

with the ability of ϒDGG to differentiate between
responses to kainate and quisqualate, while 2APV
(and such substances as DαAA and DαAS) preferentially
depressed responses to NMDA, provides new evidence
for the existence of separate receptors for these
three excitants. For simplicity, these receptors
will be referred to as NMDA, kainate and quisqualate
receptors. The existence of these receptors has
previously been inferred from iontophoretic studies
with DαAA, DαAS and L-glutamic acid diethyl ester
(GDEE) (10,18). The latter agent is a moderately
effective antagonist of quisqualate-induced responses
but has no effect on kainate- or NMDA-induced
responses (13,18). Unfortunately, GDEE often
depresses excitatory responses to acetylcholine on
spinal Renshaw cells (5,13,18) and hence the value
of this substance as a specific quisqualate-receptor
antagonist is questionable.

The observation that responses to L-aspartate and
L-glutamate were depressed (albeit with varying
degrees of discrimination) by 2APV, ϒDGG and PDA
and by several previously reported amino acid
antagonists, including DαAA, DαAS and GDEE (9,10,13,
18) indicates that these excitants have mixed actions
on different receptors. However, responses induced
by L-aspartate are more susceptible to antagonism by
NMDA receptor antagonists than responses induced by
L-glutamate indicating that L-aspartate mainly acts
on NMDA receptors. On the other hand, responses to
L-glutamate seem to parallel those to quisqualate
with respect to antagonism (e.g. by PDA) or
resistance to antagonism by a range of substances
suggesting that L-glutamate may act predominantly
on quisqualate receptors. An action of L-glutamate
mainly on kainate receptors would seem to be ruled
out by the selective action of ϒDGG.

Effects of antagonists on synaptic excitation.
Synaptic excitatory responses of spinal Renshaw
cells evoked by dorsal root stimulation were reduced
by iontophoretically administered 2APV, ϒDGG and PDA
with currents which depressed responses to
excitatory amino acids but not those to acetylcholine.
Cholinergic excitation of these cells evoked by
ventral root stimulation (7) was unaffected by 2APV
and was either unaffected or enhanced by ϒDGG and PDA.
(Enhancement of cholinergic excitation was the usual
effect observed with PDA and is consistent with the
partial agonist (depolarizing) action of this
compound (Watkins and colleagues, this symposium)).

These effects of 2APV and δDGG were observed with ejecting currents, which, in many instances failed to influence L-glutamate-induced responses while almost abolishing responses to L-aspartate (FIG. 4). Similar observations have been made previously with other NMDA receptor antagonists, DαAA and DαAS, (2,3,13,16) whereas GDEE has little effect on dorsal root evoked responses of Renshaw cells (13). Thus, with the knowledge of the effects of these substances on responses to amino acid, outlined above, L-asparate must be considered the more likely transmitter at this synapse.

Excitation of dorsal horn neurones evoked by stimulation of dorsal roots was also depressed by 2APV, δDGG and PDA. The majority of these neurones were probably activated polysynaptically from dorsal root primary afferents since the central latency for these excitations was invariably greater than 2 m.sec. Neurochemical studies favour L-aspartate as the transmitter released by these spinal neurones on the grounds that reduced levels of this amino acid are correlated with the loss of spinal interneurones produced by temporary hypoxia (8). In keeping with this suggestion, synaptic responses in dorsal horn neurones were reduced by ejecting currents of 2APV which selectively depressed responses to NMDA and L-aspartate.

It has been suggested that L-glutamate may be one of the primary afferent transmitters mainly on the basis of the differential distributions of this amino acid in the spinal cord (14,15). In view of this suggestion the effects of amino acid antagonists have been determined on monosynaptic excitatory responses evoked in dorsal horn neurones by stimulation of low threshold muscle afferents. To date the majority of studies have been made with DαAA. This NMDA receptor antagonist depressed monosynaptically evoked excitation in 3 of 9 dorsal horn neurones but only with high injection currents (>50 nA) which did not clearly differentiate between responses to L-glutamate and L-aspartate. The few preliminary experiments where the effects of 2APV, δDGG and PDA have been compared on the same neurones indicate that monosynaptic responses are generally insensitive to 2APV and δDGG but are reduced by PDA. These observations require confirmation, but suggest the possibility that monosynaptic excitation evoked from low threshold primary afferents is mediated by activation of quisqualate receptors and hence, in view of earlier considerations, implicates L-glutamate as the transmitter released by these primary afferent fibres.

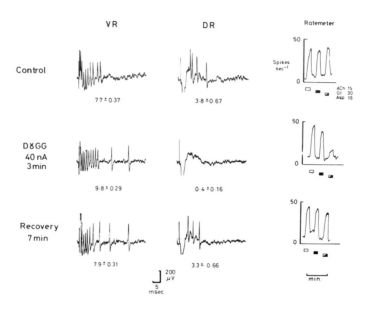

FIG. 4. The records from left to right are from a single Renshaw cell and show representative oscilloscope sweeps of the responses evoked by submaximal ventral root (VR) and dorsal root (DR) stimulation and ratemeter records of responses to acetylcholine (ACh 15 nA) L-glutamate (Gl 30 nA) and L-aspartate (Asp 16 nA). The numbers below the oscilloscope records indicate the mean ± SEM number of spikes in 20 consecutive sweeps. The upper, middle and lower records were obtained before, during and 7 mins after the ejection of 40 nA ƳDGG for 3 mins.

In summary, the present results indicate that 2APV is a highly potent and selective NMDA receptor antagonist and that the depiptide, ƳDGG, is an antagonist at NMDA and kainate receptors but not at quisqualate receptors in the cat spinal cord. In contrast, PDA does not differentiate between receptors for NMDA, kainate or quisqualate. The depression of non-cholinergic, polysynaptic excitation in some neurones by ƳDGG, PDA and, in particular, 2APV, coupled with the selective depression of responses to L-aspartate and NMDA by 2APV, supports other evidence indicating that these responses are mediated by L-aspartate. On the other hand, the relative insensitivity of mono-synaptically evoked excitatory responses in spinal neurones to the NMDA receptor antagonist, DαAA, together with the preliminary observation that these responses are depressed by PDA but not by 2APV or ɣDGG, supports the notion that L-glutamate may be the transmitter mediating such responses. Further investigations will be required to elucidate the function of kainate receptors (and confirm the involvement of quisqualate receptors) in synaptic transmission in the CNS.

REFERENCES

1. Altmann, H., Ten Bruggencate, G., Pickleman, P. and Steinberg, R. (1976): Pflugers Arch. 364 : 249-255.

2. Biscoe, T.J., Davies, J., Dray, A., Evans, R.H., Francis, A.A., Martin, M.R. and Watkins, J.C. (1977) : Eur. J. Pharmac., 45 : 315-316.

3. Biscoe, T.J., Evans, R.H., Francis, A.A., Martin, M.R., Watkins, J.C., Davies, J. and Dray, A. (1977) : Nature 270 : 743-745.

4. Curtis, D.R. (1979) : In : Glutamic Acid: Advances in Biochemistry and Physiology, edited by L.J. Filer, Jr., et al., pp 163-175 Raven Press, New York.

5. Curtis, D.R., Duggan, A.W., Felix, D., Johnston, G.A.R., Tebecis, A.K. and Watkins, J.C. (1972) : Brain Res., 41: 283-301.

6. Curtis, D.R., Johnston, G.A.R., Game, C.J.A. and McCulloch, R.M. (1973) : Brain Res., 49 : 467-470.

7. Curtis, D.R. and Ryall, R.W. (1966) : Expl. Brain Res., 2 : 81-96.

8. Davidoff, R.A., Graham, L.T., Shank, R.P., Werman, R. and Aprison, M.H. (1967) : J. Neuro-chem., 17 : 1205-1208.

9. Davies, J., Evans, R.H., Francis, A.A. and Watkins, J.C. (1978) : In : Advances in pharmacology and therapeutics, vol. 2. Neuro-transmission, pp 161-170 Ed. P. Simon Pergaman Press; Oxford and New York.

10. Davies, J., Evans, R.H., Francis, A.A. and
     Watkins, J.C. (1979) : J. Physiol. (Paris).,
     75 : 641-654.

11. Davies, J., Francis, A.A., Jones, A.W. and
     Watkins, J.C. (1980) : J. Physiol., (in press)

12. Davies, J., Francis, A.A., Jones, A.W. and
     Watkins, J.C. (1980) : Br. J. Pharmac.,
     (in press).

13. Davies, J. and Watkins, J.C. (1979) : J. Physiol.
     297 : 621-635.

14. Duggan, A.W. and Johnston, G.A.R. (1970) :
     J. Neurochem., 17 : 1205-1208.

15. Graham, L.T., Shank, R.P., Werman, R. and
     Aprison, M.H. (1967) : J. Neurochem., 14 :
     465-472.

16. Lodge, D., Headley, P.M. and Curtis, D.R.
     (1978) :Brain Res., 152 : 603-608.

17. McLennan, H. and Hall, J.G. (1978) : Brain Res.,
     149 : 541-545.

18. McLennan, H. and Lodge, D. (1979) : Brain Res.,
     169 : 83-90.

19. Zieglgansberger, W. and Puil, E.A. (1973) :
     Arch. exp. Path. Pharmak., 277 : suppl. R 89.

Glutamate as a Neurotransmitter,
edited by G. Di Chiara and G. L. Gessa
Raven Press, New York © 1981.

Structure-Activity Studies On Ibotenic Acid and Related Muscimol Analogues

P. Krogsgaard-Larsen, T. Honoré, J. J. Hansen, *D. R. Curtis, and *D. Lodge

*Royal Danish School of Pharmacy, Department of Chemistry BC, DK-2100 Copenhagen, Denmark; and *Department of Pharmacology, The Australian National University, Canberra City, A.C.T. 2601, Australia*

There is substantial evidence of the participation of (S)-glutamic acid (GLU) and (S)-aspartic acid (ASP) in excitatory neurotransmission processes in the mammalian central nervous system (CNS) (7,8,28). GLU and ASP presumably have distinct receptors (25,44), which is supported by the findings that various compounds including (S)-glutamic acid diethyl ester (GDEE) and (R)-α-aminoadipic acid (α-AA) (2,3,19,37,43) selectively reduce the excitatory actions of GLU and ASP, respectively. The mechanism of action of α-AA, which is particularly selective towards excitation by the ASP analogue N-methyl aspartic acid (NMDA), and of GDEE is, however, not fully elucidated (44).

Conformational mobility may allow GLU and ASP to adopt shapes which, more or less effectively, interact with the receptors for either amino acid. Consequently, a prerequisite for the identification and pharmacological characterization of these receptors is the development of specific agonists for both receptors. The development of such compounds on a rational basis probably involves incorporation of the parent amino acids into rigid structures, in which they are locked in different conformations.

Some naturally occurring heterocyclic amino acids, including kainic acid, quisqualic acid, and ibotenic acid (IBO), are structural analogues of GLU (Fig. 1). However, the mode of action of these amino acids, all of which are powerful excitants of central neurones, seem to be different. While the excitation by quisqualic acid is sensitive to GDEE (43), that of IBO is fairly resistent to GDEE but readily antagonized by α-AA (43), and kainic acid is relatively insensitive to both antagonists (18,22,43). Thus, quisqualic acid and IBO seem to activate preferentially GLU and ASP receptors, respectively, whereas these receptors apparently only mediate the excitation by kainic acid to a limited extent. None of these heterocyclic GLU analogues interfere with the high-affinity binding sites for GLU on rat brain membranes (4).

The synaptic or extrasynaptic site(s) of action of kainic acid is still unidentified (1,25,38,44,50). Kainic acid has a very high affinity for its binding site *in vitro* (26,34,40,49). Quisqualic acid also binds tightly to this site (26,40,49), whereas GLU and IBO are much weaker as inhibitors of kainic acid binding

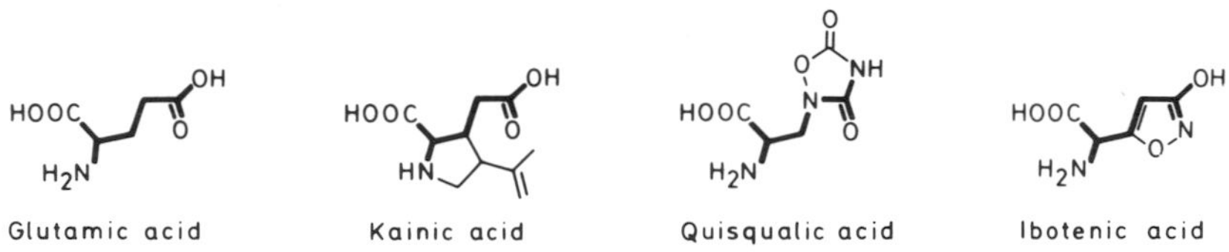

Glutamic acid   Kainic acid   Quisqualic acid   Ibotenic acid

FIG. 1. Structures of GLU and related heterocyclic amino acids.

(26,34,40,49). Since the binding site for kainic acid is not
identical with the physiological postsynaptic GLU receptor (18,
41), kainic acid and perhaps also quisqualic acid appear not to
have sufficient specificity to be useful agonists for studies of
GLU receptors in the mammalian CNS. IBO apparently is a selective ASP agonist, but excitation of neurones by IBO is followed
by a prolonged depression of excitability (10,41), which is sensitive to bicuculline methochloride (10), indicating that IBO
probably is converted by decarboxylation into muscimol (13) during microelectrophoretic ejection near central neurones or at
the synaptic receptor.

MATERIALS AND METHODS

(RS)-α-Amino-3-hydroxy-4-methyl-5-isoxazoleacetic acid (4-me-
thyl-IBO) (20), (RS)-α-amino-3-hydroxy-5-methyl-4-isoxazoleacetic
acid (AMAA) (6), (RS)-α-amino-3-hydroxy-5-methyl-4-isoxazolepro-
pionic acid (AMPA) (20,24), (RS)-α-amino-3-hydroxy-5-isoxazole-
propionic acid (homo-IBO) (20), (RS)-α-amino-3-hydroxy-4-methyl-
5-isoxazolepropionic acid (4-methyl-homo-IBO) (24), (RS)-α-amino-
3-hydroxy-4-bromo-5-isoxazolepropionic acid (4-bromo-homo-IBO)
(20) were prepared by published procedures. The syntheses of
(RS)-α-amino-3-hydroxy-5-isoxazolebutyric acid ((2)homo-IBO) and
(RS)-α-amino-3-hydroxy-5-isoxazolevaleric acid ((3)homo-IBO) (T.
Honoré and J. Lauridsen) will be described elsewhere. The muscimol analogues studied were prepared using published procedures
(5,23,30,32).

Microelectrophoretic experiments were carried out on lumbar
dorsal horn interneurones and Renshaw cells of cats anaesthetized
with pentobarbitone sodium (35 mg per kg body weight intraperitoneally, supplemented when required). Extracellular action potentials were recorded (11) and the approximate potency of each
excitant and depressant assessed relative to those of GLU (34)
and GABA (11), respectively, as described in detail elsewhere.
Antagonism of amino acid excitation by GDEE and α-AA was examined
as described previously (34,37,43).

The ^{3}H-kainic acid (49) and the ^{3}H-GABA (12) binding assays
were performed as described in detail elsewhere, (34) and (33)
respectively, using rat brain membranes isolated and purified by
a published procedure (33). Attempts to reproduce the ^{3}H-GLU
binding procedure of Foster and Roberts (16), in preparation for

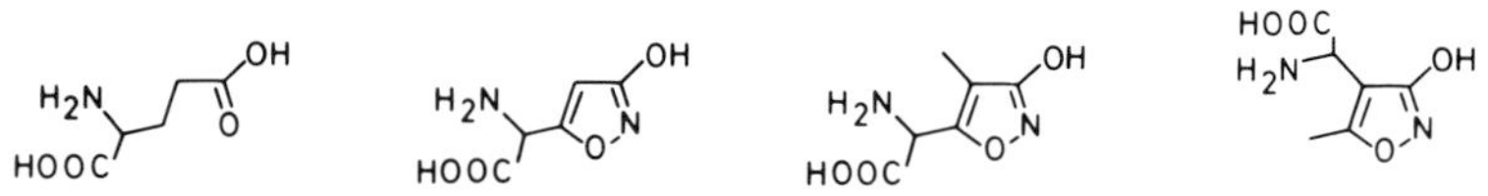

Glutamic acid   Ibotenic acid (IBO)   4-Methyl-IBO   AMAA

Rel. potency
in vivo   + +   + + + +   + + (+)   + +

Antagonism   GDEE : Yes   GDEE : Weak   GDEE : Weak   GDEE : n.s.
    a-AA : Weak   a-AA : Yes   a-AA : Yes   a-AA : Yes

Inh. of kainic acid
binding, IC_{50} 0.4 µM   12 µM   10 µM   >100 µM

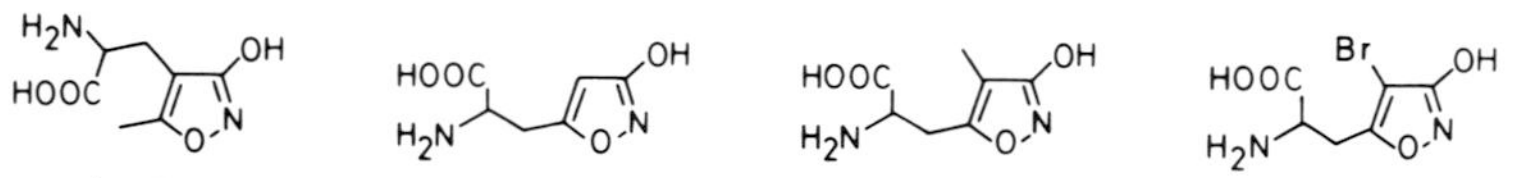

AMPA   Homo-IBO   4-Methyl-homo-IBO   4-Bromo-homo-IBO

Rel. potency
in vivo   + + + + + +   + (+)   + + +   + + + + +

Antagonism   GDEE : Yes   GDEE : Yes   GDEE : Yes   GDEE : Yes
    a-AA : n.s.   a-AA : n.s.   a-AA : n.s.   a-AA : n.s.

Inh. of kainic acid
binding, IC_{50} >100 µM   >100 µM   >100 µM   >100 µM

FIG. 2. The approximate potency of each excitant was assessed relative to that of GLU on the basis of the electrophoretic currents required to produce equal and submaximal excitatory effects on 3-19 neurones. Antagonism of amino acid excitation by GDEE and α-AA was tested in each case on 2-9 neurones as described previously (37,43) using GLU and NMDA as reference excitants. As in these studies antagonism by either GDEE or α-AA was rarely completely specific, and "yes" indicates a consistent and significantly greater reduction of the effects of a particular excitant by one of the antagonists compared with the other. The compounds were tested as inhibitors of the binding of ^{3}H-kainic acid to rat brain membranes (49) as previously described (34).

studies of the interactions of the described IBO analogues with GLU receptors *in vitro*, revealed binding sites with properties different from those published (16).

ANALOGUES AND HOMOLOGUES OF IBOTENIC ACID

It is evident that structural analogues of GLU and ASP are not necessarily pure agonists on the receptors for the respective amino acids. In analogy with the findings for GABA agonists (31), a variety of structural parameters probably have to be considered in designing specific agonists for the central GLU and ASP receptors. In an attempt to develop such compounds IBO has been subjected to systematic structural modifications, including alterations of the structure and placing of the amino acid side chain.

The excitations induced by IBO and 4-methyl-IBO were readily antagonized by α-AA, but only weakly by GDEE, but the latter com-

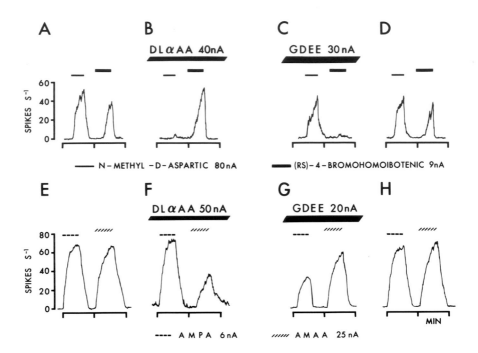

FIG. 3. The effects of GDEE and DL-α-AA on the excitation of two
spinal interneurones by NMDA, (*RS*)-4-bromo-homoibotenic acid
(A-D) and AMPA and AMAA (E-H), all ejected electrophoretically as
indicated by the appropriate horizontal lines. A: NMDA (80 nA,
50 mM in 165 mM NaCl, pH 7), 4-bromo-homoibotenic acid (9 nA,
200 mM, pH 7); B: during GDEE (30 nA, 200 mM, pH 3.5); D: after
GDEE. E: AMPA (6 nA, 200 mM, pH 7), AMAA (25 nA, 200 mM, pH 7);
F: during DL-α-AA (50 nA); G: during GDEE (20 nA); H: after
GDEE. Control responses similar to A and E were recorded between
B and C, and F and G, respectively. Ordinates: firing rate,
spikes s   Abscissae: time, min.

pound was a much weaker excitant than IBO (34) (Fig. 2). In contrast to the excitation by IBO, that induced by 4-methyl-IBO did
not seem to be followed by depression (34). 4-Methyl-IBO probably is just as susceptible to decarboxylation as IBO, but as the
decarboxylation product of the former compound, 4-methylmuscimol,
is a weak neuronal depressant (35) (Table 1), an *in vivo* production of this compound may not have been detectable in these experiments.

    Removal of the side chain of IBO to the 4-position gives AMAA,
which is an analogue of ASP. Accordingly, the excitation of central neurones produced by AMAA was sensitive to α-AA, whereas
GDEE has no significant effect (Fig. 3). Prolongation of the
side chain of AMAA by an additional methylene group converts AMAA

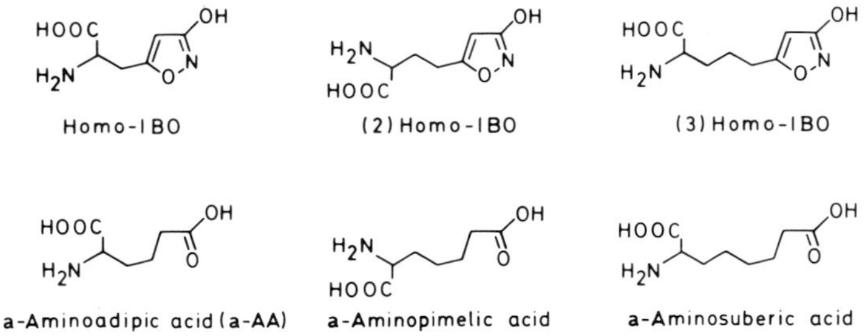

FIG. 4. Structures of homo-IBO, (2)homo-IBO, and (3)homo-IBO and the related aliphatic amino acids.

into AMPA, which is an analogue of GLU and a very powerful, GDEE-sensitive, neuronal excitant (Figs. 2 and 3). The excitations induced by AMAA and AMPA were prolonged compared with that of GLU, suggesting that these isoxazole amino acids are not as effectively removed from the vicinity of the neurones as GLU. In fact AMAA does not interfere significantly with the uptake of GLU and ASP in rat brain slices (P. Krogsgaard-Larsen and G.A.R. Johnston, unpublished).

Homo-IBO is resistent to decarboxylation, and the homologation has converted IBO into a GDEE-sensitive neuronal excitant, slightly weaker than GLU (Fig. 2). However, introductions of substituents into the 4-position of the ring of homo-IBO result in compounds with increased excitatory effects. Thus, 4-methyl- and in particular 4-bromo-homo-IBO are potent neuronal excitants sensitive to GDEE but not significantly to α-AA (Figs. 2 and 3). These substituents in homo-IBO, like the methyl group in AMPA, probably force by steric effects the side chains of the isoxazole amino acids concerned into conformations, similar to the "receptor-active conformation(s)" of GLU.

The binding site for kainic acid and the postsynaptic GLU receptors may be functionally related (39), but they are not identical (18,40,47). In contrast to quisqualic acid and IBO (26,34, 40), AMPA, homo-IBO, and 4-methyl- and 4-bromo-homo-IBO do not affect the binding of kainic acid (Fig. 2), suggesting that the excitatory effects of the latter group of compounds are the results of activation of the GLU receptors.

Like α-AA (2,3,19,37,43) the *R*-isomers of the further homologues of GLU, namely α-aminopimelic and α-aminosuberic acids show excitatory amino acid antagonistic actions (15). These compounds are particularly potent in reducing the frog motoneurone depolarization induced by NMDA. These observations prompted us to develop further homologues of IBO, namely (2)homo-IBO and (3)-homo-IBO (Fig. 4). The effects of the racemic forms of these isoxazole amino acids on GLU- and NMDA-induced excitations of cat spinal neurones have been studied (Fig. 5). In no case did the compounds significantly reduce the excitation by GLU. While homo-IBO potentiated the excitation by NMDA, (2)homo-IBO and (3)-

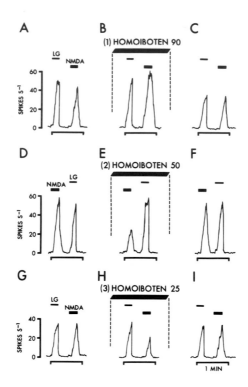

FIG. 5.   The effects of (1)homoibotenate (homo-IBO) (A-C; 90 nA,
100 mM, pH 7), (2)homoibotenate (D-F); 50 nA, 100 mM, pH 7), and
(3)homoibotenate (G-I; 25 nA, 50 mM, pH 7) on the excitation of a
spinal interneurone by GLU (LG; 80 nA, 200 mM, pH 7) and NMDA (30
nA, 50 mM in 150 mM NaCl, pH 7), all ejected electrophoretically
as indicated by the appropriate horizontal lines. While homo-IBO
enhanced the effect of NMDA and possibly also that induced by
GLU, the higher homologues reduced the effectiveness of NMDA as
an excitant (E,H). α-AA had an identical effect (not illustrated) on this neurone. Ordinates: firing rate, spikes s⁻¹. Abscissae: time, min.

homo-IBO showed antagonistic effects against this ASP analogue.
Further studies on the optical antipodes of the compounds concerned are required, before their importance as excitatory amino
acid antagonists can be estimated.

NEUROTOXICITY OF EXCITATORY AMINO ACIDS

    Kainic acid causes degeneration of nerve cells after injection
into various regions of the mammalian brain (42). Similarly,
quisqualic acid, IBO, and also GLU have neurotoxic effects (27,
36, 45, 48). The molecular mechanisms underlying the degenera-

TABLE 1. Comparison of the potencies of some excitants and the corresponding decarboxylated amino acid depressants[a]

ACID AMINO ACID EXCITANT		NEUTRAL AMINO ACID DEPRESSANT		
Compound	Rel. potency in vivo	Compound	Rel. potency in vivo	Inh. of GABA binding $IC_{50}\mu M$
(S)-Glutamic acid	+ +	GABA	− − −	0.033
Ibotenic acid (IBO)	+ + + +	Muscimol	− − − −	0.006
(RS)-4-Methyl-IBO	+ + (+)	4-Methylmuscimol	−	26
AMAA	+ +	4-(2-Aminomethyl)-5-methyl-3-isoxazolol	0	>100
AMPA	+ + + + + +	4-(2-Aminoethyl)-5-methyl-3-isoxazolol	0	>100
(RS)-Homo-IBO	+ (+)	Homomuscimol	− − −	3
(RS)-4-Methyl-homo-IBO	+ + +	4-Methyl-homo-muscimol	0	>100
(RS)-4-Bromo-homo-IBO	+ + + + +	4-Bromo-homo-muscimol	n.t.	75

[a]The approximate potencies of the excitant and depressant amino acids were determined microelectrophoretically and assessed relative to those of GLU (++) (34) and GABA (---) (35), respectively, as described earlier (see also legends for Figs. 2 and 3). The GABA receptor binding studies were performed as described previously (33). n.t., not tested. Data from (33-35).

tion processes are unknown, but the kainic acid binding site is assumed to play a major role (21,39,46,50). However, since AMPA exhibits potent neurotoxic properties after injection into the caudate of rats (G. di Chiara, unpublished), activation of the physiological GLU receptor may be an essential step in the degeneration process.

COMPARATIVE STUDIES ON IBOTENIC ACID AND MUSCIMOL ANALOGUES

Decarboxylation of GLU gives GABA, and the decarboxylated analogues of the excitatory amino acids IBO and homocysteic acid, muscimol (11) and 3-aminopropanesulphonic acid (9) respectively, are potent GABA agonists. Furthermore, quisqualamine, obtained by removal of the carboxyl group from quisqualic acid, has GABA-like actions (14), suggesting that the GLU and GABA receptors have analogous ligand specificities.

In order to test whether this apparent structure-activity analogy is a rule of general application, the order of potency as excitants of the IBO analogues listed in Table 1 was compared with that of the corresponding decarboxylated compounds as neuronal depressants. As exemplified in Table 1 there is generally a close correlation between the potency of muscimol analogues as neuronal depressants and as inhibitors of GABA binding (29). However, a correlation between the activities of these GABA agonists and the ability of the corresponding carboxylated compounds to excite central neurones seems to be an exception rather than a rule. This is clearly illustrated by the total lack of GABA agonist activity of the decarboxylated analogues of AMPA and 4-methyl-homo-IBO (35). These results demonstrate that the mapping of the structural parameters of importance for the design of GABA agonists (31) is of little utility for the development of specific GLU agonists.

ACKNOWLEDGEMENTS

This work was supported by the Danish Medical Research Council. The collaboration of Dr. J.C. Bornstein, Mr. J. Lauridsen, and Mr. H. Mikkelsen is gratefully acknowledged. We wish to thank Mrs. B. Hare for secretarial and Mrs. P. Searle and Mr. S. Stilling for technical assistance.

REFERENCES

1. Bird, S.J. and Gulley, R.L. (1979): Neurosci. Lett., 15:55-60.
2. Biscoe, T.J., Davies, J., Dray, A., Evans, R.H., Francis, A.A., Martin, M.R., and Watkins, J.C. (1977): Eur. J. Pharmacol., 45: 315-316.
3. Biscoe, T.J., Davies, J., Dray, A., Evans, R.H., Martin, M.R., and Watkins, J.C. (1978): Brain Res., 148: 543-548.
4. Biziere, K., Thompson, H., and Coyle, J.T. (1980): Brain Res., 183: 421-433.

5. Brehm, L., Krogsgaard-Larsen, P., and Hjeds, H. (1974): <u>Acta Chem. Scand.[B]</u>, 28: 308-316.
6. Christensen, S.B. and Krogsgaard-Larsen, P. (1978): <u>Acta Chem. Scand.[B]</u>, 32: 27-30.
7. Curtis, D.R. (1979): In: <u>Glutamic Acid: Advances in Biochemistry and Physiology</u>, edited by L.J. Filer, Jr., S. Garattini, M.R. Kare, W.A. Reynolds, and R.J. Wurtman, pp. 163-175. Raven Press, New York.
8. Curtis, D.R. and Johnston, G.A.R. (1974): <u>Ergeb. Physiol.</u>, 69: 97-188.
9. Curtis, D.R. and Watkins, J.C. (1965): <u>Pharmacol. Rev.</u>, 17: 347-391.
10. Curtis, D.R., Lodge, D., and McLennan, H. (1979): <u>J. Physiol. (Lond.)</u> 291: 19-28.
11. Curtis, D.R., Duggan, A.W., Felix, D., and Johnston, G.A.R. (1971): <u>Brain Res.</u>, 32: 69-96.
12. Enna, S.J. and Snyder, S.H. (1975): <u>Brain Res.</u>, 100: 81-97.
13. Eugster, C.H. (1969): <u>Fortschr. Chem. Org. Naturst.</u>, 27: 261-321.
14. Evans, R.H., Francis, A.A., Hunt, K., Martin, M.R., and Watkins, J.C. (1978). <u>J. Pharm. Pharmacol.</u>, 30: 364-367.
15. Evans, R.H., Francis, A.A., Hunt, K., Oakes, D.J., and Watkins, J.C. (1979): <u>Br. J. Pharmacol.</u>, 67: 591-603.
16. Foster, A.C. and Roberts, P.J. (1978): <u>J. Neurochem.</u>, 31: 1467-1477.
17. Haldeman, S. and McLennan, H. (1972): <u>Brain Res.</u>, 45: 393-400.
18. Hall, J.G., Hicks, T.P., and McLennan, H. (1978): <u>Neurosci. Lett.</u>, 8: 171-175.
19. Hall, J.G., Hicks, T.P., McLennan, H., Richardson, T.L., and Wheal, H.V. (1979): <u>J. Physiol. (Lond.)</u>, 286: 29-39.
20. Hansen, J.J. and Krogsgaard-Larsen, P. (1980): <u>J. Chem. Soc. [Perkin I]</u>, (in press).
21. Henke, H. (1979): <u>Neurosci. Lett.</u>, 14: 247-251.
22. Hicks, T.P., Hall, J.G., and McLennan, H. (1978): <u>Can. J. Physiol. Pharmacol.</u>, 56: 901-907.
23. Hjeds, H. and Krogsgaard-Larsen, P. (1976): <u>Acta Chem. Scand.[B]</u>, 30: 567-573.
24. Honoré, T. and Lauridsen, J. (1980): <u>Acta Chem. Scand.[B]</u>, (in press).
25. Johnston, G.A.R. (1979): In: <u>Glutamic Acid: Advances in Biochemistry and Physiology</u>, edited by L.J. Filer, Jr., S. Garattini, M.R. Kare, W.A. Reynolds, and R.J. Wurtman, pp. 177-185. Raven Press, New York.
26. Johnston, G.A.R., Kennedy, S.M.E., and Twitchin, B. (1979): <u>J. Neurochem.</u>, 32: 121-127.
27. Kizer, J.S., Nemeroff, C.B., and Young Blood, W.W. (1978): <u>Pharmacol. Rev.</u>, 29: 301-318.
28. Krnjević, K. (1974) <u>Physiol. Rev.</u>, 54: 419-540.
29. Krogsgaard-Larsen, P. and Arnt, J. (1979): In: <u>GABA-Biochemistry and CNS Functions</u>, edited by P. Mandel and F.V. DeFeudis, pp. 303-321. Plenum Press, New York.

30. Krogsgaard-Larsen, P. and Christensen, S.B. (1976): Acta Chem. Scand.[B], 30: 281-282.
31. Krogsgaard-Larsen, P., Honoré, T., and Thyssen, K. (1979): In: GABA-Neurotransmitters. Pharmacochemical, Biochemical and Pharmacological Aspects, edited by P. Krogsgaard-Larsen, J. Scheel-Krüger, and H. Kofod, pp. 201-216. Munksgaard, Copenhagen.
32. Krogsgaard-Larsen, P., Larsen, A.L.N., and Thyssen, K. (1978): Acta Chem. Scand.[B], 32: 469-477.
33. Krogsgaard-Larsen, P., Hjeds, H., Curtis, D.R., Lodge, D., and Johnston, G.A.R. (1979): J. Neurochem., 32: 1717-1724.
34. Krogsgaard-Larsen, P., Honoré, T., Hansen, J.J., Curtis, D.R., and Lodge, D. (1980): Nature, 284: 64-66.
35. Krogsgaard-Larsen, P., Johnston, G.A.R., Curtis, D.R., Game, C.J.A., and McCulloch, R.M. (1975): J. Neurochem., 25: 803-809.
36. Köhler, C., Schwarcz, R., and Fuxe, K. (1979): Neurosci. Lett., 15: 223-228.
37. Lodge, D., Headley, P.M., and Curtis, D.R. (1978): Brain Res., 153: 603-608.
38. Lodge, D., Johnston, G.A.R., Curtis, D.R., and Bornstein, J.C. (1979): Neurosci. Lett., 14: 343-348.
39. London, E.D. and Coyle, J.T. (1979): Eur. J. Pharmacol., 56: 287-290.
40. London, E.D. and Coyle, J.T. (1979): Mol. Pharmacol., 15: 492-505.
41. MacDonald, J.F. and Nistri, A. (1978): J. Physiol. (Lond.), 275: 449-465.
42. McGeer, E.G., Olney, J.W., and McGeer, P.L., editors (1978): Kainic Acid as a Tool in Neurobiology. Raven Press, New York.
43. McLennan, H. and Lodge, D. (1979): Brain Res., 169: 83-90.
44. Nistri, A. and Constanti, A. (1979): Prog. Neurobiol., 13: 117-235.
45. Olney, J.W. and De Gubareff, T. (1978): Nature, 271: 557-559.
46. Schwarcz, R. and Fuxe, K. (1979): Life Sci., 24: 1471-1480.
47. Schwarcz, R., Scholz, D., and Coyle, J.T. (1978): Neuro-pharmacology, 17: 145-151.
48. Schwarcz, R., Hökfelt, T., Fuxe, K., Jonsson, G., Goldstein, M., and Terenius, L. (1979): Exp. Brain Res., 37: 199-216.
49. Simon, J.R., Contrera, J.F., and Kuhar, M.J. (1976): J. Neurochem., 26: 141-147.
50. Vincent, S.R. and McGeer, E.G. (1979): Life Sci., 24: 265-270.

Glutamate as a Neurotransmitter,
edited by G. Di Chiara and G. L. Gessa
Raven Press, New York © 1981.

Radioreceptor Binding Studies with Glutamate and Aspartate

P. J. Roberts and N. A. Sharif

Department of Physiology and Pharmacology, School of Biochemical and Physiological Sciences, University of Southampton, Southampton SO9 3TU, United Kingdom

L-glutamate and L-aspartate are powerful excitants of almost all neurons in the mammalian central nervous system (14). For a considerable time they have been considered as strong neurotransmitter candidates; for example, glutamate may be the transmitter of a number of descending cortical projections, such as those directed to the striatum (7,17) and nucleus accumbens (28). In the cerebellum, glutamate appears to be associated with parallel fibre terminals (13), and aspartate possibly with the climbing fibres (19).

With the application of ligand-binding techniques to the investigation of receptors for a variety of hormones and neurotransmitters, it is not surprising that glutamate, aspartate, and related excitants have attracted some attention. However, these studies are still at a very rudimentary stage, and the presence of multiple types of receptor, or other sites which may bind both L-asp and L-glu, complicates the issue.

BINDING OF L-GLUTAMATE

Roberts (20) and Michaelis et al (18) were the first workers independently to describe the specific sodium-independent binding of L-glutamate to whole brain or cerebral cortex crude synaptic membranes. An alternative approach was followed by DeRobertis and Fiszer de Plazas (6) who isolated proteolipids by chromatography of chloroform-methanol brain extracts, and found that these specifically bound L-glutamate in a sodium-independent manner.

Kinetic Characteristics

Roberts (20) detected a single population of sites

295

(K_d=8uM and B_{max}=0.03 nmol/mg protein), while for whole brain membranes, Michaelis et al (18) found the binding to be biphasic (K_d's = 0.2 and 4.4 uM and B_{max}'s of 1.8 and 8.8 nmol/mg protein). The proteo-lipid fractions purified from rat cerebral cortex apparently possessed three binding sites for glutamate (6): high-affinity, K_d =.3 uM, B_{max} = 0.53 nmol/mg; medium affinity, K_d = 5 uM, B_{max} = 32 nmol/mg, and low affinity, K_d = 55 uM, B_{max} = 166 nmol/mg protein. It would seem unlikely on the basis of binding site densities that the medium or low affinity proteolipid sites have any relevance to a physiological glutamate receptor. While the pharmacological specificity in each of these studies was qualitatively similar, there were major anomalies, primarily when comparison was made with electrophysiological data. Also, in each of these studies, ^{14}C-labelled L-glutamate was employed, which inevitably imposed a severe restraint on the concentration range of ligand over which binding could be investigated.

More recently, Foster and Roberts (10) reported the binding of highly-labelled L-^{3}H-glutamate to a single population of sites on freshly-prepared, purif-ied cerebellar synaptic membranes, with a K_d = 744 nM and a capacity of 73 pmol/mg protein. Further modific-ations to the preparative method (22) which included washing, sonication, and preincubation of membranes, yielded figures of K_d = 359 nM and B_{max} = 117 pmol/mg protein. The binding of L-glutamate to whole washed homogenates prepared from frozen tissue has also been reported by Biziere et al (3), where saturation iso-therms revealed anomalous binding kinetics. While two sites were identified, with K_d's of 11 and 80 nM respectively, Scatchard analysis yielded V-shaped plots in contrast to other studies. However, we also have identified multiple binding components in striatal synaptic membranes. One component was of very high affinity, with a K_d = 16 nM and B_{max} = 400fmol/mg protein, and at least two other components with K_d's in the upper nanomolar/lower micromolar range were detected (Roberts, unpublished). Although we have no firm evidence, this ultra-high affinity site may correspond to the 11 nM site described by Biziere et al (3).

General Properties of Glutamate Binding

The time course of specific glutamate binding to cerebellar synaptic membranes is relatively slow, attaining complete equilibrium after approx 10 min., whereas non-specific binding was instantaneous and

linear with time. Specific binding was linear with
tissue concentration and had a pH optimum at neutral-
ity. Binding was confined to the CNS and in subcellular fractionation experiments, was found to be enriched some 12 fold in the synaptic membrane fraction
by comparison with crude membranes. Negligible binding was associated with nuclear, mitochondrial or
purified myelin fractions. No glutamate decarboxylase,
glutamate dehydrogenase or glutamine synthetase activity was detectable in the assay system.

Stability of Glutamate Binding Sites

It is worth noting that the majority of receptor
binding studies have been carried out upon previously
frozen membrane preparations. With the exception of
GABA (8), little attention has been paid to the possible deleterious effects upon receptors, of freezing.
We have found that the binding of L-^{3}H-glutamate
is extremely sensitive to denaturation by low temperature (10,22). Specific binding was reduced by at
least 90 percent in membranes that had been frozen
(either in liquid nitrogen, or at -30°C), while the
nonspecific component was not affected. It does appear
however, that the freezing process per se, is not
necessarily the causal factor, since storage of the
membranes at +4°C for 20h, effectively abolished the
^{3}H-glutamate binding activity. Use of cryoprotectants
afforded no protection against this denaturation.
Clearly, these very major effects need to be given
proper consideration when carrying out binding assays
with glutamate, and possibly other transmitters. The
data of Biziere et al (3) were for example, obtained
using previously frozen tissue.
We have found that lyophilisation of membranes
immediately after preparation, not only conferred
stability to the binding sites, but also resulted in
a substantial enhancement, with the binding remaining
stable for at least one month. Detailed kinetic
analysis of binding has revealed that while the K_d
was unchanged at approx 300nM, the B_{max} was increased
from 117 to 277 pmol/mg protein.
Recently, Chang and Michaelis (4) have reported
that synaptic membranes which previously had been
frozen rapidly at -80°C, retained their binding
activity when thawed in a controlled manner, according to the method of Rudnick (21) for platelet
membrane vesicles.

Inhibition of Specific ^{3}H-Glutamate Binding

A large number of glutamate analogues and other neuroactive substances have been investigated for their ability to compete with L-^{3}H-glutamate for the binding site on cerebellar membranes (Table 1).

Table 1   Inhibition of specific ^{3}H-glutamate binding
By various neuroexcitants[a]

Compound	IC_{50} (uM)
Neuroexcitant amino acid:	
L-glutamic acid	4.8
DL-homocysteic acid	10.8
L-cysteic acid	18.2
D-glutamic acid	28.8
L-aspartic acid	42.1
D-aspartic acid	138.0
N-methyl-D-aspartic acid	Inactive
Cyclic derivatives:	
(±)-ibotenic acid	8.1
DL-quisqualic acid	8.4
cis-cyclopentane glutamate	18.5
kainic acid	Inactive
dihydrokainic acid	Inactive
Putative antagonists:	
DL-2-amino-4-phosphonobutyrate	25.6
DL-α-aminoadipic acid	26.3
L-glutamate diethylester	Inactive
HA-966	Inactive

[a]Cerebellar synaptic membranes were incubated with L-^{3}H-glutamate at a final concentration of 0.8uM in the presence of varying concentrations of compounds investigated. IC_{50} values were determined from log dose/percent inhibition plots. Inactive compounds showed less than 10 percent inhibition of binding at 1 mM.

L-glutamate itself was the most potent inhibitor, followed by three compounds which are potent neuroexcitants when applied iontophoretically: (±)-ibotenate, DL-quisqualic acid and DL-homocysteic acid. 1-amino-1,3-dicarboxycyclopentane was also active, although some 3.5 times less potent than L-glutamate. In general, recent data by Biziere et al (3) using

forebrain membranes, concur with our own findings in
the cerebellum. However, the latter workers found in
contrast to our own results, that (±)-ibotenate and
quisqualate were inactive. In both, binding was
markedly stereoselective (as in previous studies),
with the D-isomer being much less active. This is
interesting since the two isomers possess similar
potencies in vivo (5). This might be explicable in
terms of the avid high-affinity uptake system for the
L-isomer, thus potentiating the effects of D-glutamate.

Antagonists of amino acid excitation such as DL-
α-aminoadipate and 2-amino-4-phosphonobutyrate were
effective antagonists, while a variety of other neurotransmitters such as GABA, glycine, 5-HT, dopamine
and noradrenaline, and non neuroactive amino acids,
did not inhibit the specific binding of L-^{3}H-glutam-
ate.

Effects of Protein and Membrane-modifying Agents and Guanine Nucleotides on Specific Glutamate Binding

Digestion of synaptic membranes with either trypsin or phospholipase A (20 ug/ml) produced a moderate
(25%) decrease in specific glutamate binding. In
contrast, phospholipases C and D were unable to alter
glutamate binding (24).

Non-degradative lipid perturbants such as ampho-
tericin B or nystatin, which interact with the lipid
matrix of biomembranes by preferential penetration of
the cholesterol-containing regions, produced a marked
inhibition of specific binding, and membrane lipid
extraction with 0.5% Triton X-100, similarly reduced
the specific binding. The non-specific component was
not altered by treatment with any of the above reagents.

The effects of trypsin indicate that protein
components are necessary for the integrity of the
glutamate binding sites, and concanavalin A also
interfered with binding, suggesting that a membrane
glycoprotein may be involved. The data from experiments with phospholipase and the lipid perturbants,
imply that membrane lipids are crucially involved in
the maintenance of the glutamate receptor conformation.

A number of protein reagents had pronounced
effects on specific L-^{3}H-glutamate binding. For example, reduction of disulphide bonds by dithiothreitol
(DTT) resulted in a 40 percent decrease in binding,
whereas N-ethylmaleimide (NEM) which reacts specifically with exposed thiol groups, produced a 2 fold

increase in binding. Preincubation with DTT followed by NEM resulted in a reversal of the effects of DTT, with no overall change in binding, thus indicating a common site of action. Cd^{2+} and iodoacetamide, which interact with highly reactive -SH groups, in contrast to NEM, produced a 23% decrease in binding. It therefore appears likely that these thiol reagents may have different loci of action.

The water-soluble carbodiimide derivative, 3-(3-dimethylaminopropyl)-1-ethyl carbodiimide, which interferes selectively with carboxyl groups, increased binding by about 200 percent.

In a recent series of experiments (23) where the binding of 25 nM L-^{3}H-glutamate to cerebellar synaptic membranes was investigated, guanine nucleotides at micromolar concentrations produced a substantial inhibition of binding. This effect was not observed with the adenine nucleotides. Although we have no conclusive information as to the mechanism by which guanine nucleotides produce this effect, it is of interest that at least some of the actions of glutamate in the cerebellum may be mediated through the formation of cyclic GMP (11,12). This therefore raises the possibility of a regulatory control mechanism at the glutamate receptor site.

BINDING OF L-ASPARTATE

To date, little attention has been paid to the binding of L-aspartate in the mammalian CNS. Fiszer de Plazas and DeRobertis (9) have investigated binding to proteolipid fractions, and detected 3 kinetically distinct sites of K_d's = 0.2, 10 and 50 uM respectively, and B_{max}'s of 3, 132, and 617 nmol/mg. For the high-affinity site, L-aspartate and N-methyl-D-aspartate (NMDA) were effective inhibitors of binding, while L-glutamate and D-aspartate were of low activity.

We have investigated the binding of L-^{3}H-aspartate to freshly-prepared, sonicated, and extensively-washed cerebellar synaptic membranes (25, and in preparation). Binding was optimal under physiological conditions of temperature and pH, attained equilibrium within 10 min, and exhibited saturability. Kinetic analysis revealed homogeneity of sites with a K_d = 874 nM and a B_{max} = 44 pmol/mg protein, and which exhibited no cooperativity (Hill coefficient = 1.2). A similar lack of cooperativity has also been found for the glutamate binding site (unpublished). A preliminary investigation of the pharmacological specificity of the aspartate binding site has revealed a number of differences from the glutamate system (Table 2).

TABLE 2. Inhibition of specific ^{3}H-aspartate binding[a]

Compound	IC_{50} (uM)
L-glutamic acid	2.0
L-aspartic acid	5.0
(±)-ibotenate	10.0
DL-α-aminosuberate	10.0
HA-966	10.5
L-cysteine sulfinate	125
D-aspartate	457
DL-α-aminoadipate	360

[a]Specific binding of 25 nM L-^{3}H-aspartate was determined in the presence of various concentrations of the agents. IC_{50} values were determined from log dose/ percent inhibition plots.

The binding of L-aspartate was inhibited only by a very restricted range of compounds, as compared with the binding of glutamate. L-glutamate and L-aspartate were of similar potency as inhibitors of binding, while quisqualate, 4-fluoroglutamate and 2-amino-4-phosphonobutyrate, which were good inhibitors of glutamate binding, were only weakly active on the aspartate system. Binding was displaced by DL-α-aminoadipate, DL-α-aminosuberate and HA-966, but not by the proposed aspartate receptor-preferring agonist, NMDA. The potent uptake inhibitor, DL-threo-3-hydroxyaspartate was devoid of any inhibitory activity, in common with kainic acid, which exhibited negligible affinity for both the aspartate and glutamate binding sites.

    As we have reported for the glutamate system (22), the L-^{3}H-aspartate binding was almost abolished following freezing of membranes. Lyophilisation has similarly been found to preserve binding, however, in this case, a marked change in the affinity of the binding sites was observed, indicating a differential effect on the glutamate and aspartate systems. In both the aspartate and glutamate systems, the binding sites exhibited the same specificity of inhibition as observed in fresh membranes. They were however more sensitive to the effects of the various inhibitors by a factor of approx two.

    Several cations have been tested for their ability to modify specific aspartate binding to cerebellar membranes (Fig 1).

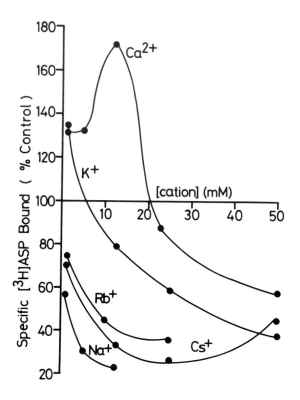

FIG. 1. Effects of various cations
on L-^{3}H-aspartate binding (25 nM).
Each point is mean of at least 3
experiments.

The monovalent ions, Na^+, Rb^+, K^+, and Cs^+, all
produced a marked dose-dependent inhibition of aspartate binding. There was no effect on the nonspecific
binding. The rank order of potency was 1) Na^+, 2) Cs^+
3) Rb^+ and 4) K^+. Strikingly, divalent cations such
as Ca^{2+} and Mn^{2+} (latter, not shown) produced a
marked enhancement of binding at concentrations up to
20 mM, above which, an inhibition was observed. These
ionic effects are strikingly similar to those observed
for glutamate binding in the hippocampus (2) and also
in the cerebellum (Roberts, unpublished), where we
have previously reported that Na^+ caused a marked
inhibition of L-^{3}H-glutamate binding (10).
    At the present time, the physiological significan-
ce of these observations is not clear. Roberts (20)

suggested that binding in the presence of Na$^+$ might represent an interaction with uptake sites. This hypothesis has recently received some support from the observed specificity of various compounds for the inhibition of uptake as compared with inhibition of Na$^+$-dependent binding (1,27); however, a number of anomalies were seen (27) indicating that this view is probably an over simplification.

CONCLUSIONS

L-glutamate and L-aspartate exhibit specific, saturable and reversible binding to distinct sites on synaptic membranes. In our own investigations we have utilised cerebellar preparations, and have identified apparently single homogeneous populations of binding sites for each of these two amino acids, with similar affinities, although the density of sites for L-glutamate was approximately 3 times that for aspartate. The pharmacological specificity of the two sites was qualitatively different, again indicating separate binding sites. This is further supported by the differential effects of lyophilisation on the two systems.

At present, it is difficult to say with certainty whether the binding sites for L-glutamate and L-aspartate are synonymous with their physiological receptor(s). Certainly, they do not appear to be associated either with enzymes, or the recognition sites for either neuronal or glial transport mechanisms (except perhaps when studied in the presence of Na$^+$). All the effective inhibitors of either L-glutamate or L-aspartate binding were either neuroexcitatory amino acids, or were purported antagonists, such as alpha-aminoadipate or 2-amino-4-phosphonobutyric acid. It is especially interesting that kainic·acid, which possesses the glutamate skeleton and is up to 80x as active as glutamate as an excitant and NMDA, which is widely considered to be a selective ligand for aspartate receptors (16) were virtually inactive. It appears extremely likely that these agents may act at different, or sub-populations of excitatory amino acid receptors. For kainic acid in particular, since the original report by Simon et al (26), considerable attention has been directed to its binding site. It is clear that although kainic acid binding is effectively inhibited by glutamate, this binding represents only a very minor proportion of the bulk of L-glutamate binding – perhaps to extrajunctional, or even to presynaptic, receptors.

As mentioned at the outset of this chapter, the

characterisation of the binding sites for glutamate
and aspartate are still at a rudimentary stage by
comparison with many other neurotransmitters.
Johnston (14) has proposed the existence of at least
four separate binding sites in order to accommodate
the various observations that have been made. It is
likely that further investigations with other ligands,
such as the antagonists 2-amino-4-phosphonobutyrate,
α-aminoadipate, and GDEE, and with the agonists NMDA,
ibotenate and quisqualate, will facilitate this
characterisation.

 With the considerable attention now being directed
towards glutamate as a CNS transmitter, and to a
lesser extent, L-aspartate, in addition to the
measurement of presynaptic parameters such as amino
acid concentrations and uptake and release mechanisms,
these binding assays may serve as useful approaches
for the investigation of both normal and altered
glutamatergic function.

REFERENCES

1.   Baudry. M., and Lynch, G. (1979): Eur. J. Pharma-
     col., 57: 283-284.
2.   Baudry, M., and Lynch, G. (1979): Nature, Lond.,
     282: 748-750.
3.   Biziere, K., Thompson, H., and Coyle, J.T. (1980):
     Brain Res., 183: 421-433.
4.   Chang, H.H., and Michaelis, E.K. (1980): J. biol.
     Chem., (in press).
5.   Cox, D.W.G., Headley, P.M., and Watkins, J.C.
     (1977): J. Neurochem., 29: 570-588.
6.   DeRobertis, E., and Fiszer de Plazas, S. (1976):
     J. Neurochem., 26: 1237-1243.
7.   Divac, I., Fonnum, F. and Storm-Mathisen, J.
     (1977): Nature, Lond., 266: 377-378.
8.   Enna, S.J., and Snyder, S.H. (1975): Brain Res.,
     100: 81-97.
9.   Fiszer de Plazas, S., and DeRobertis, E. (1976):
     J. Neurochem., 27: 889-894.
10. Foster, A.C., and Roberts, P.J. (1978):
     J. Neurochem., 31: 1467-1477.
11. Foster, G.A., and Roberts, P.J. (1980): Life Sci.
     (in press).
12. Garthwaite, J., and Balázs, R. (1978): Nature,
     Lond., 275: 328-329.
13. Hudson, D.B., Valcana, T., Bean, G., and Timiras,
     P.S. (1976): Neurochem. Res., 1: 83-92.
14. Johnston, G.A.R. (1978): In: Receptors in Pharm-
     acology, edited by J.R. Smythies and

and R.J. Bradley pp 295-333, Marcel Dekker, New York.

15. Johnston, G.A.R. (1979): In: Glutamic acid: Advances in Biochemistry and Physiology, edited by L.J. Filer, Jr., S. Garattini, M.R. Kare, W.A. Reynolds, and R.J. Wurtman, pp 177-185, Raven Press, New York.

16. McCulloch, R.M., Johnston, G.A.R., Game, C.J.A., and Curtis, D.R. (1974): Exp. Brain Res., 21: 515-518.

17. McGeer, P.L., McGeer, E.G., Scherer. U., and Singh, K. (1977): Brain Res., 128: 369-373.

18. Michaelis, E.K., Michaelis, M.L., and Boyarsky, L.L. (1974): Biochim. biophys. Acta., 367: 338-348.

19. Nadi, N.S., McBride, W.J., and Aprison, M.H. (1977): J. Neurochem., 28: 453-455.

20. Roberts, P.J. (1974): Nature, Lond., 252: 399-401.

21. Rudnick, G. (1977): J. biol. Chem., 252: 2170-2172.

22. Sharif, N.A., and Roberts, P.J. (1980): J. Neurochem., 34: 779-784.

23. Sharif, N.A., and Roberts, P.J. (1980): Eur. J. Pharmacol., 61: 213-214.

24. Sharif, N.A., and Roberts, P.J. (1980): Brain Res., (in press).

25. Sharif, N.A., and Roberts, P.J. (1980): Br. J. Pharmacol., (in press).

26. Simon, J.R., Contrera, J.F., and Kuhar, M.J. (1976): J. Neurochem., 26: 141-147.

27. Vincent, S.R., and McGeer, E.G. (1980): Brain Res., 184: 99-108.

28. Walaas, I., and Fonnum, F. (1979): Neuroscience, 4: 209-216.

Glutamate as a Neurotransmitter,
edited by G. Di Chiara and G. L. Gessa
Raven Press, New York © 1981.

Regulation of Hippocampal Glutamate Receptors: Role of a Calcium-dependent Cystein Proteinase

Froylan Vargas and Erminio Costa

Laboratory of Preclinical Pharmacology, National Institute of Mental Health, Saint Elizabeths Hospital, Washington, D.C. 20032

INTRODUCTION

Neurophysiological and biochemical data suggest that L-glutamate stimulates a number of excitable membranes (4,8,9). Additional evidence indicates that in several brain areas there are nerve terminals which have a specific Na^+-dependent uptake for glutamate, hence the presence of glutamatergic pathways could be considered. However since the uptake for glutamate and aspartate cannot be differentiated, readily, with uptake studies, it is difficult to conclude that a given area contain glutamatergic or aspartergic neurons. Accordingly the conclusion made by Cotman et al. (9) based on uptake and release studies that in vertebrates, glutamate is likely to be the excitatory neurotransmitter of the perforant pathway innervating the dentate gyrus of the hippocampus (16) has been questioned by lesion studies (5). This and other discrepancies prompted studies directed to characterize specific recognition sites for glutamate and aspartate in hippocampus. Michaelis and coworkers (11) have suggested that the postsynaptic recognition site for L-glutamate is a glycoprotein with a molecular weight of 14,000 dalton. In an earlier report (12) they showed that calcium facilitates L-[^{3}H] glutamate binding to crude synaptic membranes (CSM). Efforts by two other groups of investigators (1,7) have resulted in the identification of a temperature-dependent, high affinity (K_D 650-744 nM) recognition site for L-glutamate in cerebellar and hippocampal membranes from rat brain.

Previous communications (2,15) have reported that the expression of glutamate receptors located in CSM prepared from hippocampus of rat brain, is facilitated by a calcium dependent protease. The present report updates this line of investigation focussing on the basic characteristics of the glutamate binding to CSM prepared from rat hippocampus and showing the possibility that the binding of glutamate to CSM can be differentiated from that of aspartate.

Preparation of CSM

CSM from rat hippocampus were obtained as described in Scheme 1.

Scheme 1
Crude Synaptic Membrane (CSM) Preparation

Homogenate (0.32M sucrose)
↓ 1000 x g x 12 min
↓ 15000 x g x 12 min
P_2 pellet

1. P_2 pellet is resuspended in cold distilled water (20 ml/g of fresh tissue) and placed on ice for 10 min.

2. Incubation of disrupted P_2 fraction at 37° for 30 min in Tris-Cl, 50 mM (pH 7.2) and EGTA, 2 mM. Final volume of this suspension is 40 ml/g fresh tissues.

3. The suspension is chilled and membranes are collected by centrifugation at 30,000 x g for 15 min.

4. Membranes are resuspended in 50 volumes of cold Tris-Cl, 50 mM (pH 7.4) with ultraturrax and centrifuged at 30,000 x g for 15 min. This procedure is repeated 3 times. The final pellet (CSM) is resuspended in Tris-Cl, 50 mM (pH 7.4) and ready for binding assay.

Glutamate binding was assessed as described in Scheme 2. Under standard assay conditions, non specific binding represented less than 5% of the total binding, which was substrated from all values.

Scheme 2
Binding Assay

1. Binding was measured in 1 ml of a medium containing (mmoles/liter): KCl, 5.0; KH_2PO_4, 1.2; $MgSO_4$, 1.2; Tris-Cl (pH 7.4), 50; $CaCl_2$, 2.6; sucrose, 230 mM (when calcium was omitted, EGTA was included at a concentration of 0.4 mM); and 100-200 µg of fresh membrane protein.

2. Membranes were preincubated for 3 min and the reaction was initiated by the addition of the labeled aminoacid. The incubation was continued for 30 min at 30°C.

3. L-[^{3}H] Glutamate bound to the membranes was determined by filtration (Whatman GF/C filters). Filters were washed 3 times (4 ml/each) with cold incubation buffer. Radioactivity on the filters was determined by liquid scintillation spectrometry.

4. Specific binding is defined as the difference between total counts minus the counts remaining in the presence of 50 µM of non-labeled glutamate.

Characteristics of the Glutamate Binding

Since glutamate decarboxylase has been shown to bind to membranes in a calcium dependent manner (6), and it may function as an extra "recognition site", we were extra careful in ruling out glutamate decarboxylase as a possible cause for error in glutamate binding studies. Several procedures to study glutamate binding to CSM were tested. Figure 1 shows that EGTA (2 mM) and preincubation at 37°C facilitates glutamate binding. When CSM were incubated in presence of EGTA (2 mM) at 0°C the glutamate binding was slightly increased. However, when CSM were incubated at 37°C for 30 min in presence of EGTA (Step 2, Scheme 1), a larger amount of glutamate binds to the CSM. This increase in glutamate binding was not observed if EGTA was omitted from the incubation medium.

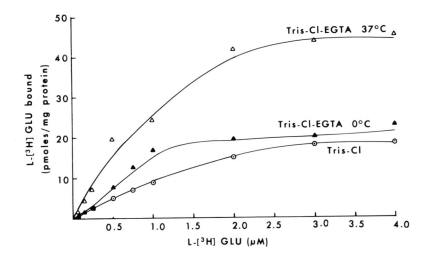

FIG. 1. Binding of L-[^{3}H]glutamate to CSM as a function of ligand concentration. Hippocampal membranes were obtained as described in Scheme 1, with slight variations in Step 2.

Figure 2 shows that the glutamate binding is a temperature-dependent process, at 3°C the amount of ^{3}H-L-glutamate bound to CSM is about one tenth of that measured at 30°C (optimal temperature). Calcium stimulates the binding of ^{3}H-L-glutamate at all concentrations of ^{3}H-L-glutamate studied (1-1000 μM) with a K_A of 25 μM (data not shown). Using ^{3}H-L-glutamate concentration between 20 and 250 nM a typical saturation curve for a specific binding was generated. Scatchard analysis of these data reveals

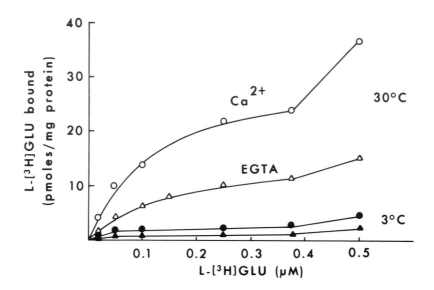

FIG. 2. Binding of L-[³H]glutamic acid to hippocampal CSM
as a function of ligand concentration and in presence and
absence of calcium. Membranes were obtained as described in
Scheme 1 and L-[³H]glutamate binding measured as described
in Scheme 2.

the presence of a high affinity population of recognition sites
(Fig. 3) with a K_D of 110 nM; the number of such binding sites is
14 pmoles/mg protein in absence of calcium. The addition of calcium doubles the number of binding sites, up to 31 pmoles/mg
protein, with no significant change in the K_D (Fig. 3).
     Sodium chloride inhibits the binding in a concentration-depen-
dent manner; its maximal effect is attained at 10 mM (manuscript
in preparation). Figure 4 shows that glutamate bound to CSM is
readily displaced by non-labelled L-glutamate. D-Glutamate is
less active (not shown); sodium chloride (20 mM) is almost as
effective as glutamate in displacing the labelled amino acid bound
to CSM. It is tempting to speculate that the ability of sodium
ions to remove the glutamate from the receptor site may represent
a primary regulatory mechanism through which the action of glutamate operating as a transmitter is silenced.

Role of a Cystein Ca^{2+}-Dependent Protease in the Regulation of Glutamate Receptors

     It has been reported (15) that the time-course of the [³H]-L-
glutamate binding to CSM is a biphasic process which depends on

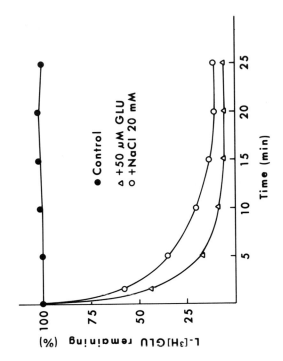

FIG. 3. Scatchard plot of specific binding
of L-[3H]glutamate to CSM from hippocampus.
Membranes were incubated with L-[3H]glutamate
varying in concentrations (20-250 nM) in
presence or absence of Ca2+ (Scheme 2).

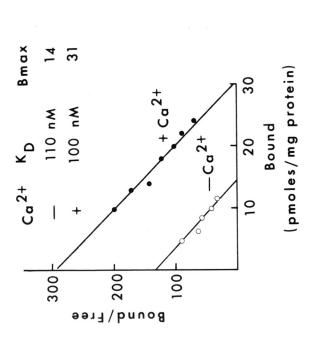

FIG. 4. Displacement of bound L-[3H]glutamate
by unlabeled glutamate and sodium. Membranes
were incubated for 25 min at 30°C in presence
of L-[3H]glutamate and glutamate or NaCl were
added to different sets. L-[3H]glutamate
bound was then determined at different periods
of time as described (Scheme 2).

the presence of calcium. Calcium appears to facilitate glutamate
binding by stimulating a cystein protease (1,2,15) which either
may destroy an inhibitor or by some other mechanism may unmask
some high affinity glutamate recognition sites. By blocking the
protease with leupeptin (15), or with p-chlormercurybenzoicsulpho-
nic acid (PCMBS) a sulphydryl blocker agent (Fig. 5) the calcium
elicited facilitation of glutamate binding is blocked.

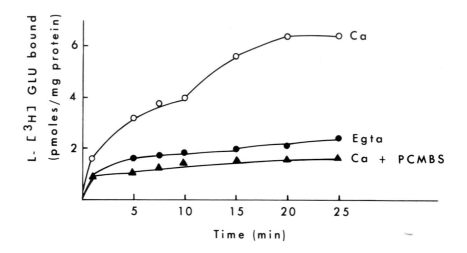

FIG. 5.   Effect of PCMBS (0.1 mM) on the time-course of the L-
[3H]glutamate binding to hippocampal CSM.

    Baudry and Lynch (2) independently have supported a similar
hypothesis on the mode of action of calcium with other evidence.
Moreover they have suggested that this calcium facilitation of
glutamate binding may be operative in the long-term potentiation
of a stimulus linked long lasting potentiation of synaptic events
specific of the hippocampus (1).

Agonist Specificity of ^{3}H-L-Glutamate Displacement

    It is presently very difficult to trace glutamatergic pathways
in the brain, moreover it is particularly problematic to differentiate them from aspartergic pathway. This is because of the
high content of glutamate and aspartate present in brain regions
which are devoid of glutamatergic neurons. An alternative to
solve these problems could be a differentiation of the postsynaptic receptors for the two putative neurotransmitters.

The lack of specific blockers of glutamate receptors able to distinguish between glutamate and aspartate receptor populations has hindered the identification of these receptors. Recently new compounds with potential capabilities to interact with the receptors for these amino acids have been synthesized. Krogsgaard-Larsen et al. (10) have obtained a series of glutamate-rigid analogs derived from ibotenic acid, which are endowed with a glutamate-like action. Two of these compounds, AMPA ((RS)-amino-3-hydroxy-5-methyl-4-isoxyzolepropionic acid) and HIB ((RS)-4-methyl-homo-ibotenic acid) were generously provided to us by Krogsgaard-Larsen. Figure 6 shows that these molecules interact with the glutamate receptor. Glutamate is the most effective displacer

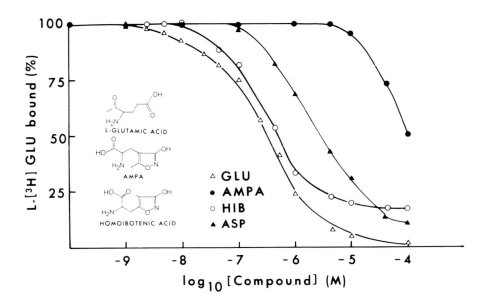

FIG. 6. Inhibition of L-[3H]glutamate binding by unlabeled glutamate and by biologically active rigid glutamate analogues.

agent of ^{3}H glutamate, in our series HIB ranks second, aspartate was about 10 times less effective than glutamate, while AMPA, despite its strong glutamate like excitatory action on motoneurons of the spinal cord of the cat (10) was very weak in displacing the glutamate from the receptor. Another important difference between the binding of aspartate and glutamate is that the binding of aspartate is not facilitated by calcium whereas that of glutamate is facilitated (Fig. 7). Thus by using specific inhibitors of calcium dependent glutamate binding, such as leupeptin, one can probably solve crucial questions in studies of central pathways mediated by glutamate or aspartate.

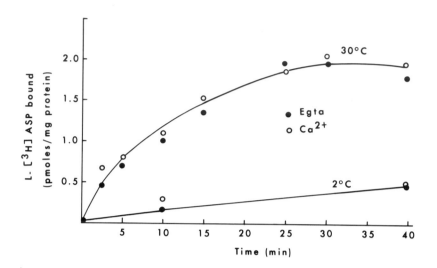

FIG. 7. Time-course of L-[3H]aspartate binding to CSM from
rat cortex. L-[3H]Aspartate binding was measured in the same
conditions as described for L-[3H]glutamate (Schemes 1 and 2).
3H-Aspartate was used at a final concentration of 60 nM.

CONCLUSIONS

The characterization of the glutamate receptors was initiated
by Michaelis et al. (11) with the purification of a 14,000 M.W.
glycoprotein which they proposed to be a recognition site for
glutamate. Despite this early start little or no information was
available until few months ago on the regulatory mechanisms for
glutamate receptors. The results presented herein on the calcium
facilitation of glutamate binding and on the selective inhibition
of this facilitation by leupeptin and PCMBS together with the
findings recently published by Baudry and Lynch (1,2) have shed
some light on one of the most intriguing and exciting areas of
amino acid receptor function. These findings reiterate the view
that the receptors for amino acids have specific regulatory systems, which perhaps protect these receptors from stimulation by
the high content of these amino acids in CSF.

EGTA and preincubation of the membranes at 37°C for 30 min is an
essential procedure to reveal the high affinity binding sites for
3H-L-glutamate. Shariff and Roberts (13) have reported that
sonication, salt treatment or preincubation enhance the binding of
3H-L-glutamate to CSM from cerebellum. The stimulatory effect on
3H-L-glutamate binding by preincubation and that of the chelating
agent might be due to the removal of free endogenous glutamate

and GAD; whether some other factors which modulate the high affinity glutamate binding are being removed is presently under investigation.

Biziere et al. (3) have recently reported the presence of two high affinity binding sites for glutamate (K_Ds of 11 and 80 nM) in CSM from parietal cortex of rat brain. They used membranes washed with distilled water and they assayed the glutamate binding at low temperature in Tris-citrate buffer ($2°C$). A comparison of the binding of glutamate (assessed under our conditions, Scheme 2) to membranes prepared according to Biziere et al. (3) and those treated in the way as described in Scheme 1, shows that the binding of glutamate to these DW-membranes was similar to that observed in our membranes in the absence of calcium (unpublished observations). Additionally, we were able to detect a "super high-affinity" binding site in our membrane preparations with a K_D of 12 nM. In a temperature dependent manner calcium increases also the number of binding sites of this population of super high-affinity receptors (manuscript in preparation). Our results suggests that the selective inhibition of the calcium facilitation of glutamate binding to CSM elicited by leupeptin can be used to differentiate whether a given brain area contains glutamate or aspartate receptors.

REFERENCES

1. Baudry, M., and Lynch, G. (1979): Nature, 282:748-750.
2. Baudry, M., and Lynch, G. (1980): Proc. Natl. Acad. Sci. USA, 77:2298-2302.
3. Biziere, K., Thompson, H., and Coyle, J.T. (1980): Brain Res., 183:421-433.
4. Clark, R.B., Gration, K.A.F., and Usherwood, P.N.R. (1979): J. Physiol., 290:551-568.
5. Di Lauro, A., and Meek, J.L. (1980): Soc. Neurosci. Abst.
6. Fonnum, F. (1968): Biochem. J., 106:401-402.
7. Foster, A.C. and Roberts, P.J. (1978): J. Neurochem., 31:1467-1477.
8. Hamberger, A., Han-Chiang, G., Sandoval, E., and Cotman, C.W. (1979): Brain Res., 168:531-541.
9. Johnson, J.L. (1978): Prog. in Neurobiol., 10:155-202.
10. Krogsgaard-Larsen, P., Honore, T., Hansen, J.J., Curtis, D.R., and Lodge, D. (1980): Nature, 284:64-66.
11. Michaelis, E.K. (1979): Biochem. Bicphys. Res. Commun., 87:106-113.
12. Michaelis, E.K., Michaelis, M.L., and Boyarsky, L.L. (1974): Biochim. Biophys. Acta, 367:338-348.
13. Shariff, N.A., and Roberts, P.J. (1980): J. Neurochem., 34:779-784.
14. Toyo-Oka, T., Shimizu, T., and Masaki, T. (1978): Biochem. Biophys. Res. Commun., 82:484-491.
15. Vargas, F.M., Greenbaum, L.M., and Costa, E. (1980): Neuropharmacology, in press.

16. White, W.F., Nadler, J.V., Hamberger, A., and Cotman, C.W. (1977): <u>Nature</u>, 270:356-357.

Glutamate as a Neurotransmitter,
edited by G. Di Chiara and G. L. Gessa
Raven Press, New York © 1981.

Excitatory Amino Acid–induced Changes in Cyclic GMP Levels in Slices and Cell Suspensions from the Cerebellum

J. Garthwaite and R. Balazs

*MRC Developmental Neurobiology Unit, Institute of Neurology,
London WC1N 2NS, England*

INTRODUCTION

Glutamate is currently thought to serve as the transmitter for the granule cell parallel fibres in the cerebellum (24, 29, 33) while aspartate may be associated with the climbing fibres (20). When these pathways are stimulated or depressed in vivo, cyclic GMP (cGMP) levels in the cerebellum are correspondingly increased or reduced (3, 19, 23). Administration of glutamate in vivo (3) or to cerebellar slices (11, 13) leads to marked increases in cGMP levels. Particularly large increases (200-fold) occur in slices of rat cerebellum during development (8-15 days after birth), the responses being associated with the cells undergoing maturation rather than cell division (12).

This article describes some recent experiments designed to further understand the relationships between excitatory amino acids and cGMP. First, in view of the likelihood of there being multiple excitatory amino acid receptors with overlapping agonist specificities (31), the effectiveness of some amino acids which might act more selectively on certain of the receptor classes, together with the effects of some antagonists, were measured using slices of immature and adult rat cerebellum. Secondly, the potencies of some excitants were compared in slices and in a suspension of cells derived from the cerebellum. In principle, a suspension of viable neural cells provides unique opportunities for studying certain actions of transmitters relatively uncomplicated by diffusional barriers and by the complex electrical, chemical and anatomical relationships present in the intact tissue. In adopting this approach it was hoped, in the first instance, to gain information on the extent to which cellular transport might influence the potencies of excitatory amino acids when applied to intact tissue.

RESULTS

Cyclic GMP Responses in Immature and Adult Cerebellar Slices

Four excitatory amino acids, namely L-glutamate, L-aspartate, N-methyl-D-aspartate (NMDA) and kainate, were tested for their ability to increase cGMP levels.

Immature cerebellum.

Cerebellar slices from 8 day old animals were used in these experiments. The slices were prepared using a tissue chopper, a technique which in young animals ($\leq$ 14 days) yields morphologically well preserved slices (14).

Unstimulated levels of cGMP averaged 0.8 pmol/mg protein after the 1 to 1.5 h incubation required for the levels to stabilize (cf. 10, 25). All four agonists induced dose-dependent increases in cGMP (Fig. 1a). NMDA was clearly the most potent agonist (ED_{50} = 40 μM) followed by L-aspartate and L-glutamate (ED_{50} = 300 - 500 μM). The curves for these three compounds were approximately parallel and attained the same maximum, about 160 pmols/mg protein. This represents a 200-fold increase from basal levels. Kainate differed from the other agonists in that the maximal response was lower (70 pmols/mg protein) although its effective concentrations were in the same range as those of glutamate (ED_{50} = 400 μM).

Accompanying these large changes in cGMP were small changes in the levels of cAMP (not shown). These followed the same concentration dependence as the cGMP responses but maximal changes were only about 2-fold and are probably secondary responses mediated through release of adenosine (22, 26, 27).

Adult cerebellum.

In contrast to the immature tissue, mechanical chopping is not a suitable technique for obtaining morphologically well preserved slices from the adult cerebellum. Slices prepared using a conventional guide and bow cutter are much superior, both morphologically and with respect to cyclic nucleotide responses (13).

Unstimulated levels of cGMP in surface slices prepared in this way from adult cerebella were higher than at 8 days, as found in vivo (28), averaging 6.5 pmols/mg protein. Dose-response curves for the agonists on cGMP levels (Fig. 1b) differed both qualitatively and quantitatively from those found using immature cerebellum. Kainate elicited responses of up to 280 pmols/mg protein (i.e. 4-fold higher than in the immature cerebellum) and was here the most potent agent: the half-maximally effective concentration was about 20 μM, representing an increase in apparent potency of 20-fold compared with the immature cerebellum. NMDA, L-aspartate and L-glutamate, on the other hand, were all less effective in the adult tissue. Full dose-response curves for these compounds were not obtained because of the high concentrations required, but the decrease in potency was at least 5 to

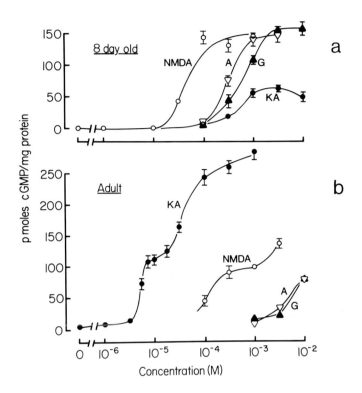

FIG. 1. Dose-response curves for cGMP accumulation in (a) immature and (b) adult rat cerebellar slices exposed to NMDA (O),
kainate (KA; ●), L-glutamate (G; ▲) and L-aspartate (A; ▽). The
slices were inactivated at the peak of the responses (2-5 min in
the immature slices, 5-10 min in the adult) and cGMP levels
measured by radioimmunoassay as described previously (12).

10-fold, the rank order (NMDA > Asp~Glu) remaining the same.
    Effect of antagonists.
    Recently a group of compounds exemplified by D-α-aminoadipate
(DαAA) has been suggested to act as specific excitatory amino
acid antagonists. DαAA, together with the inorganic antagonist
Mg^{2+}, appear to selectively antagonize responses at receptors on
which NMDA preferentially acts while leaving kainate responses
relatively unaffected (4, 8, 9, 16, 21).
    As shown in Fig. 2a, DαAA (250 µM) inhibited cGMP responses to
both NMDA and kainate in the immature cerebellar slices. While
an approximately parallel shift about 3-fold occurred in the dose-
response curve for NMDA, responses to all doses of kainate were
inhibited to a similar extent. In the adult, DαAA retained its
inhibitory action against NMDA but, unlike in the immature tissue,
was ineffective against kainate. In addition, removal of Mg^{2+}

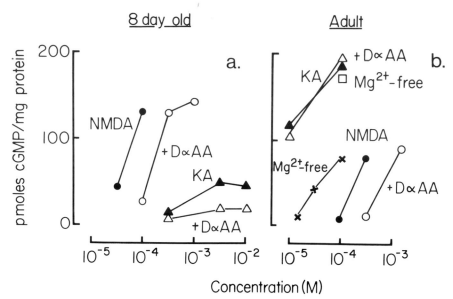

FIG. 2. Effect of antagonists on cGMP responses to NMDA (circles) and kainate (KA; triangles) in a (a) immature and (b) adult cerebellar slices. The slices were exposed to D-α-aminoadipate (DαAA; 250 μM;○ △) or Mg^{2+}-free medium (□,**X**) for 5 and 10 min respectively before addition of the excitants.

(normally 1.2 mM) from the bathing medium enhanced the potency of NMDA while having no demonstrable influence on responses to kainate (Fig. 2b). In both the immature and adult slices, responses to L-glutamate and L-aspartate were resistant to DαAA and were unchanged on removal of Mg^{2+}.

These results indicate that, in the adult cerebellum, activation of several types of excitatory amino acid receptors results in elevation of cGMP levels: those stimulated by NMDA and inhibited by DαAA and by low concentrations of Mg^{2+}, and those that are stimulated by kainate but resistant to the antagonists; receptors responding to L-glutamate and L-aspartate probably comprise a third group (Garthwaite, in preparation). Both in terms of the relative effectiveness of the excitants and their selective blockade, the receptors associated with these cGMP responses show many similarities to those monitored by electrophysiological methods in other areas of the central nervous system (15, 31).

In the immature cerebellum, the low relative potency of kainate and its blockade by DαAA suggest that the receptors on which kainate primarily acts in the adult cerebellum (DαAA-resistant) are either poorly represented in the immature tissue, as seems to be the case in the striatum to judge from binding experiments (5), or that their activation is not associated with cGMP generation.

The decline in potency of NMDA, L-glutamate and L-aspartate

with age might have several explanations, such as changes in the kinetic properties of the receptors, changes in the coupling between receptor activation and cGMP generation or, more simply, a more restricted access of these compounds to receptor sites due, for example, to the smaller extracellular spaces in the adult tissue (14).

Cyclic GMP Responses in Suspensions of Cerebellar Cells

Several amino acids, including L-glutamate and L-aspartate, are rapidly removed from the extracellular space in intact nervous tissue by cellular uptake systems (2). Experimental evidence indicates that this hampers the access of exogenously-applied excitatory amino acids to their receptors such that the observed potencies of transported compounds are likely to be erroneously low (6, 7, 18).

The use of a cell suspension, where compounds can be applied to the cells directly, rapidly and in uniform concentrations should therefore offer many advantages. It has recently become possible to isolate cell bodies in high yield from the developing cerebellum which seem to fulfill the necessary morphological and biochemical criteria of competence (32). In the experiments described below, the potencies of L-glutamate, L-aspartate and NMDA have been compared in slices and cells from the developing (8-day-old) cerebellum. In both cases, the non-responsive dividing cells were deleted by pretreating the animals with an inhibitor of DNA synthesis (hydroxyurea), thereby enhancing the responses (12) without affecting dose-response relationships (compare Figs. 1a and 3a).

Although the cell dissociation procedure involves treating tissue slices with trypsin, this did not markedly affect their responses: both L-glutamate and L-aspartate induced slightly higher increases in cGMP, with no change in apparent potency, in trypsinized slices while the potency of NMDA was somewhat reduced (ED_{50} values in untreated and tryspin-treated slices were 30 µM and 56 µM respectively) with no change in the maximum response (Fig. 3a).

When tested on the dissociated cells, striking differences both in the absolute potencies and the relative potencies of the amino acids emerged (Fig. 3b). L-glutamate was almost 100-times more effective in the cell suspension (ED_{50} = 5 µM) than in slices (ED_{50} = 480 µM); the potency of L-aspartate was also much higher in the cells (ED_{50} = 20 µM) but the change (20-fold) was less than found with L-glutamate. By contrast, the dose response curve for NMDA was very similar to that obtained using slices (ED_{50} = 30 µM).

Other features of the responses in the cell suspension are worthy of note: (a) they occurred more rapidly than in slices (15 sec - 1 min compared with 2 - 5 min); (b) peak elevations of cGMP were about 80% higher than in slices when compared on a protein basis (2×10^7 cells contain approx. 1 mg protein), although basal levels were similar; (c) D-glutamate was about

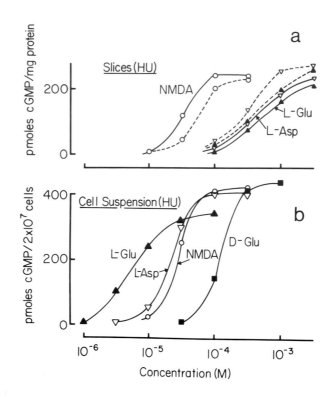

FIG. 3. Comparison of dose-response curves in (a) slices and (b)
cell suspensions from the immature (8 day old) cerebellum.
Broken lines in (a) show responses in slices which had been taken
through the cell dissociation procedure (including trypsin
treatment) up to the point of dispersion. Solid lines in (a)
represent control slices treated in the same way but with ommis-
sion of trypsin. In (b) dissociated cells were incubated at
about 2 x 10⁷ cells/ml. For both slices and cell suspension, the
animals were pretreated with hydroxyurea (HU) to delete dividing
cells from the tissue. Responses in slices and dissociated cells
can be compared quantitatively (2 x 10⁷ cells contain about 1 mg
protein).

25-fold less potent than L-glutamate (Fig. 3) while D-aspartate
(not shown) was equipotent with L-aspartate.
    The simplest explanation of these findings is that, when
applied to the intact tissue, cellular uptake of L-glutamate and
L-aspartate reduces the concentrations of these amino acids in
the vicinity of the receptors to levels well below those in the
bathing medium, thus giving rise to erroneously low estimates of
their potency. The principal site of uptake of exogenous
glutamate and aspartate in morphologically intact slices of both
immature and adult cerebellum (Wilkin et al, in preparation) and

in the cell suspensions (Gordon et al, in preparation) is the glial cells: little or no labelling of neuronal structures, including synaptic terminals could be detected autoradiographically.

The implication from the difference in relative potency of L-glutamate and L-aspartate in slices and in the cell suspension is that L-glutamate is cleared more effectively than L-aspartate in the slices: this is supported by recent preliminary studies showing that the maximum rate of uptake (V_{max}) for L-glutamate into cerebellar cells is 3-fold higher than the V_{max} for uptake of L-aspartate (Gordon et al, in preparation). NMDA, which is unlikely to be significantly accumulated by nerve tissue (2, 9, 17) showed the same potency in the cell suspension as in slices.

It should be added that the potency of L-glutamate observed in the cell suspensions may well be an underestimate. For reasons not fully understood at present, it is necessary to incubate the cells at relatively high concentrations ($> 15 \times 10^6$/ml) in order to attain optimal responses. At these cell concentrations quite a rapid depletion of L-glutamate from the medium by cellular transport occurs (e.g. at $3\mu M$ initial concentration and 20×10^6 cells/ml the rate of uptake is about 5 nmoles/min; Gordon et al, in preparation), and so its observed potency ($ED_{50} = 5\mu M$) can be considered a minimum value.

GENERAL DISCUSSION AND CONCLUSIONS

It is clear from the experiments carried out using slices that the ability of cerebellar cells to increase massively their content of cGMP in response to excitatory amino acids and their analogues is not a feature confined to the immature cerebellum (c.f. 12). The previous failure to record large responses in slices of the adult cerebellum (25, 26) and perhaps in other regions of the brain, can be attributed to the poor structural preservation of the tissue because of inappropriate methods, mechanical chopping, used in preparing the slices (13, 14). Indeed, the maximum levels attained in the adult slices (280 pmoles/mg protein) even exceeded those in the immature tissue (160 pmoles/mg protein, or 240 pmols/mg protein after deletion of the dividing cells, Fig. 3).

As regards the excitatory amino acid-cGMP association in the cerebellum, the responses appear to be mediated by receptors which show many similarities to those mediating electrical responses in other areas of the central nervous system (31). The mechanism by which cGMP is elevated, however, is presently unclear but the responses are probably not peculiar to the action of excitatory amino acids in the cerebellum as both veratridine and increased K^+ concentration induce increases in cGMP of comparable magnitude, both in slices and isolated cells (Garthwaite, in preparation), supporting previous suggestions (1, 10, 30) that it is an event associated with neuronal depolarisation (e.g. Ca^{2+}-influx) which triggers the accumulation of cGMP.

The greatly increased potencies of L-glutamate and L-aspartate when applied to cells in suspension compared to intact tissue slices might have more general implications. The results strongly indicate that the observed relative potencies of excitants in intact systems may be related more to their rates of inactivation (uptake) than to their affinity for receptor sites. Thus, in the present study, the observed relative potencies in the immature slices (i.e. NMDA >Asp~Glu) appear to stem from (i) NMDA not being a substrate for active uptake processes and (ii) L-glutamate being transported more rapidly than L-aspartate, rather than from differences in intrinsic potency. These experiments thus provide evidence that NMDA is not a more potent excitant than the naturally-occuring amino acids, a possibility which has been raised previously (6, 7, 17); the same may also be true for kainate (compare L-glutamate, Fig. 3b with kainate, Fig. 1b). In view of these findings, it will be important to determine whether the apparent selectivity of antagonists towards different agonists differs in cell suspensions and slices.

REFERENCES

1. Ahnert, G., Glossmann, H., and Habermann, E. (1979): Naunyn-Schmiedeberg's Arch. Pharmacol., 307: 159-166.

2. Balcar, V.J., and Johnston, G.A.R. (1972): J. Neurochem., 19: 2657-2666.

3. Biggio, G., and Guidotti, A. (1976): Brain Res., 107: 365-373.

4. Biscoe, T.J., Evans, R.H., Francis, A.A., Martin, M.R., Watkins, J.C., Davies, J., and Dray, A. (1977): Nature (Lond.), 270: 743-745.

5. Campochiaro, P., and Coyle, J.T. (1978): Proc. natl. Acad. Sci. U.S.A. 75: 2025-2029.

6. Cox, D.W.G., Headley, M.H., and Watkins J.C. (1977): J. Neurochem., 29: 579-588.

7. Curtis, D.R., Duggan, A.W., and Johnston, G.A.R. (1970): Exp. Brain Res., 10: 447-462.

8. Davies, J., and Watkins, J.C. (1979): J. Physiol., 297: 621-635.

9. Evans, R.H., Francis, A.A., Hunt, K., Oakes, D.J., and Watkins, J.C. (1979): Br. J. Pharmac., 67: 591-603.

10. Ferrendelli, J.A., Kinscherf, D.A., and Chang, M.M. (1973): Molec. Pharmacol., 9: 445-454.

11. Ferrendelli, J.A., Chang, M.M., and Kinscherf, D.A. (1974): J. Neurochem., 22: 535-540.

12. Garthwaite, J., and Balazs, R. (1978): Nature (Lond.), 275: 328-329.

13. Garthwaite, J., Woodhams, P.L., Collins, M.J., and Balazs, R. (1979): Brain Res., 173: 373-377.

14. Garthwaite, J., Woodhams, P.L., Collins, M.J., and Balazs, R. (1980): Devel. Neurosci., 3: 90-99.

15. Hall, J.G., Hicks, T.P., McLennan, H., Richardson, T.L., and Wheal, H.V. (1979): J. Physiol., 286: 29-39.

16. Hicks, T.P., Hall, J.G., and McLennan, H. (1978): Can. J. Physiol. Pharmacol., 56: 901-907.

17. Johnston, G.A.R., Kennedy, S.M.E., and Twitchin, B. (1979): J. Neurochem., 32: 121-127.

18. Johnston, G.A.R., Lodge, D., Bornstein, J.C., and Curtis, D.R. (1980): J. Neurochem., 34: 241-243.

19. Lundberg, D.B.A., Breese, G.R., Mailman, R.B., Frye, G.D., and Mueller, R.A. (1979): Molec. Pharmacol., 15: 246-256.

20. McBride, W.J., Rea, M.A., and Nadi, N.S. (1978): Neurochem. Res., 3: 793-801.

21. McLennan, H., and Lodge, D. (1979): Brain Res., 169: 83-90.

22. Newman, M., and McIlwain, H. (1977): Biochem. J., 164: 131-137.

23. Rubin, E.H., and Ferrendelli, J.A. (1977): J. Neurochem., 29: 43-51.

24. Sandoval, M.E., and Cotman, C.W. (1978): Neuroscience, 3: 199-206.

25. Schmidt, M.J., Ryan, J.J., and Molloy, B.B. (1976): Brain Res., 112: 113-126.

26. Schmidt, M.J., Thornberry, J.F., and Molloy, B.B. (1977):
     Brain Res., 121: 182-189.

27. Shimizu, H., and Yamamura, Y. (1977): J. Neurochem., 28:
     383-388.

28. Steiner, A.L., Ferrendelli, J.A., and Kipnis, D.M. (1972):
     J. Biol. Chem., 247: 1121-1124.

29. Stone, T.W. (1979): Br. J. Pharmac., 66: 291-296.

30. Study, R.E., Breakefield, X.O., Bartfai, T., and
     Greengard, P. (1978): Proc. natl. Acad. Sci. U.S.A., 75:
     6295-6299.

31. Watkins, J.C. (1978): In: Kainic Acid as a Tool in
     Neurobiology, edited by E.G. McGeer, J.W. Olney, and
     P.L. McGeer, pp. 37-69. Raven Press, New York.

32. Wilkin, G.P., Wilson, J.E., Balazs, R., Cohen, J., and
     Dutton, G.R. (1976): Brain Res., 115: 181-199.

33. Young, A., Oster-Granite, M., Herndon, R., and Snyder, S.H.
     (1974): Brain Res., 73: 1-13.

Glutamate as a Neurotransmitter,
edited by G. Di Chiara and G. L. Gessa
Raven Press, New York © 1981.

Electrophysiological Studies of Kainate, Quisqualate, and Ibotenate Action on the Crayfish Neuromuscular Junction

H. Shinozaki and Michiko Ishida

The Tokyo Metropolitan Institute, Bunkyo-ku, Tokyo 113, Japan

Ibotenic acid (7,20), quisqualic acid (21) and kainic acid (20,22) are heterocyclic amino acids which are comformationally restricted analogs of glutamate. Although their action has considerable analogy with the glutamate action, there are some differences in their action between species remaining without reasonable explanations. At the neuromuscular junction of the crayfish opener muscle, glutamate is an excitatory transmitter candidate and has a powerful depolarizing action (23). The crayfish neuromuscular system is suitable for the study on precise mechanism of drug action on the glutamate receptor (8). Furthermore, it is expected that the study of the system will give suggestion on the mode of drug action on synaptic transmission in the mammalian central nervous system. However, pharmacological studies of the glutamate receptor in the crayfish neuromuscular junction are too limited to allow extrapolation of data obtained to the mammalian central nervous system. In the present paper we describe further studies of electrophysiological actions of ibotenate, quisqualate and kainate on the glutamate receptor in the crayfish opener muscle and discuss the mode of action of these amino acids.

METHODS

The methods used were similar to those reported previously (6,21). In some experiments, the membrane potential of muscle fibers was clamped with intra-cellular micropipettes (12).

RESULTS

Ibotenic Acid

The resting membrane potential of the muscle fiber was hardly affected by ibotenate, but a very slight depolarization was sometimes observed when higher concentrations of ibotenate (i.e.

1 mM) were applied. Glutamate responses were not much affected
by relatively low concentrations of ibotenate (0.1 mM).
Ibotenate dose-dependently reduced the amplitude of excitatory
junctional potentials (EJPs) (19) (see FIG.1.). To determine
whether ibotenate acts pre- or post-synaptically at the neuromuscular junction, a quantum analysis of extracellularly recorded
EJPs was performed (4). When ibotenate (0.2 mM) was added, the
number of failures of extracellular EJPs was substantially
increased. The mean quantum content was reduced to 47 + 5 %
(mean + S.E., n = 7) of the control level. The amplitude of
intracellular EJPs was reduced to about half. These observations
demonstrate that the decrease in EJP amplitude caused by
ibotenate is mainly due to the presynaptic action of ibotenate.
The size of the average unit potential was not much affected by
ibotenate or slightly reduced. It was reported that picrotoxin
blocked the ibotenate action in the locust muscle fiber (2,10).
In the crayfish muscle, the depolarization caused by ibotenic
acid was blocked by 0.01 mM picrotoxin. Picrotoxin (0.01 mM)
almost completely blocked the decrease in amplitude of intracellular EJPs caused by ibotenate (FIG.1.). Even in a concentration
of 1 µM picrotoxin blocked much of the ibotenate action. These
concentrations of picrotoxin are comparable to that expected to
completely block the junctional response to GABA in the crayfish
muscle.

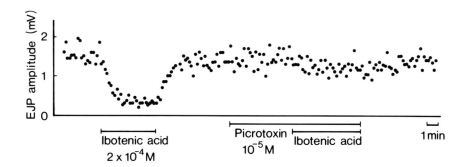

FIG.1.   Effect of ibotenic acid on the EJP amplitude and antagonistic action of picrotoxin. EJPs were elicited by a train of 10
stimuli (100/sec) which was repeated every 10 sec. Ibotenic acid
(0.2 mM) remarkably reduced the EJP amplitude, but picrotoxin
(0.01 mM) almost completely blocked the decrease in the EJP
amplitude caused by ibotenic acid. Oridnate, amplitude of intracellularly recorded EJPs. Abscissa, time.

    Ibotenate produced a decrease in electrotonic potential
induced by current pulses. The minimum effective concentration
of ibotenic acid to decrease the membrane resistance was 0.1 mM.
The decrease in electrotonic potential caused by ibotenic acid
was almost completely blocked by 0.01 mM picrotoxin. The

decrease in electrotonic potential caused by 1 mM ibotenate was similar to that by 0.02 mM GABA, which was about 1/3 of the maximal conductance change caused by GABA. The potency of ibotenate to change the membrane conductance was less than 1/50 of that of GABA on a molar basis. The ibotenate concentration to change the membrane resistance is appreciably higher than that required to reduce the EJP amplitude. For instance, ibotenic acid (0.2 mM) caused a very slight change of the membrane resistance, while it reduced the EJP amplitude to less than 50 % of the control level.

For the lack of a specific antagonist for glutamate actions, only cross desensitization between glutamate and a compound has been an effective means to determine whether the compound acts on the same receptor as glutamate (3,23). When 1 mM ibotenate was added after the glutamate receptor was almost completely desensitized, ibotenic acid produced the same change of the electrotonic potential as in the normal control solution. Therefore, it seems unlikely that ibotenate acts on the glutamate receptor on the crayfish opener muscle.

The increase in chloride permeability at inhibitory synapses of lobster, crayfish and locust is depressed by picrotoxin (5,24, 25). The blockade of the ibotenate action by picrotoxin does not necessarily follow that ibotenate acts on the GABA receptor. Only it can be suggested that ibotenate action is Cl^--mediated in the crayfish muscle. Therefore, the possibility that ibotenic acid acts on the GABA receptor was examined by an analysis of the dose-response curve for GABA in the presence and in the absence of 1 mM ibotenic acid. Various amounts of GABA were concurrently applied with fixed amounts of ibotenic acid, and the membrane conductance change was measured. As the GABA concentration increases the magnitude of the response to GABA plus ibotenate approaches that to GABA alone, even if the current intensity of concurrently applied ibotenate is changed. If ibotenate acts on a receptor other than the GABA receptor, the maximum responses should vary. This result strongly suggests a possibility that, in the crayfish opener muscle, ibotenate acts on the same receptor on the post-junctional membrane as GABA (19). By the analogy with the post-synaptic action, probably ibotenate acts on the presynaptic GABA receptor.

Quisqualic Acid

When the potencies were compared in terms of amplitude of the depolarization produced by bath application, quisqualic acid was several hundred times more powerful than glutamate on a molar basis (21). The depolarization produced by quisqualic acid is not due to the release of the natural transmitter from the presynaptic terminals but to a direct action on the postsynaptic membrane (21). The possibility that quisqualic acid may well act on the same receptor as glutamate in the crayfish opener muscle was confirmed by the following experiments. In the first experiment, it was showed that quisqualic acid did not produce further depolarization when the glutamate receptor was desensitized (21). In the second one, brief application of quisqualic acid to the most sensitive spot, where momentary application of glutamate caused a large response, produced a large depolarization (21). In the third one, an analysis of dose-response curves of glutamate and quisqualate in the voltage-clamped muscle was performed. When the glutamate and quisqualate currents, which are induced by the iontophoretic application of glutamate and quisqualate, are plotted against the logarithm of the current intensity of iontophoretically applied drugs, S-shaped curves resulted. To study interactions between glutamate and quisuqalate, glutamate was concurrently applied with fixed amounts of quisqualate. When the amount of quisqualate was increased, the amplitude of the maximum response to glutamate plus quisqualate did not vary much at the top of the curves.

If quisqualic acid acts on the receptor in the same way as glutamate, one would expect the decrease in EJP amplitude by prolonged application of quisqualate. Bath application of quisqualate (1 μM) produced a large depolarization, but this response was maintained after it reached a maximum. In this case the EJP amplitude was hardly affected by quisqualate. When quisqualate in concentrations above 1 μM was applied, the EJP amplitude was gradually decreased, however, the depolarization was not declined but maintained during the application of quisqualate. To explore a possibility that quisqualate may decrease the EJP size by depressing the process of transmitter release from excitatory nerve terminals, a quantum analysis was performed in the voltage-clamped muscle (4). The quantum content was not appreciably changed by quisqualate. On the other hand, the size of the average unit potential was decreased by quisqualate. FIG.2. shows histograms of size distribution of extracellular EJPs. These results show that the decrease in EJP amplitude caused by quisqualic acid is due to the post-synaptic event. As a matter of course, desensitization of the neuroreceptor should be considered, although the membrane depolarization is not decreased.

Since concanavalin A (con A) completely prevents the desensitization development of the glutamate receptor (11,17), we examined the action of con A on EJPs and glutamate potentials which were depressed by prolonged application of glutamate or quisqualate (16,17). When con A was added, the amplitude of the glutamate potential initially increased, whereas that of EJPs gradually decreased. More than 30 min after the start of application of con A, glutamate was once again added to the saline containing con A. The EJP amplitude gradually decreased in the same way as the control experiment, demonstrating that con A could not prevent the decrease in EJP amplitude. On the other hand, the decrease in amplitude of the glutamate potential was completely prevented by previous addition of con A (17). In the case of prolonged bath-application of quisqualic acid in concentrations above 1.5 μM, a quite similar result was obtained. Under the con A action, prolonged application of quisqualic acid reduced the EJP amplitude.

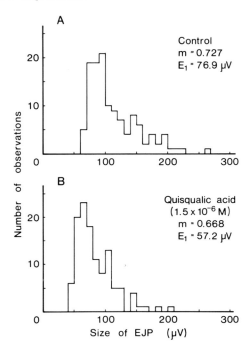

FIG.2.   Histograms of size distribution of extracellularly recorded EJPs from a single junctional area on the voltage-clamped (-85 mV) muscle fiber. Ordinate, number of observations. Abscissa, size of EJPs. EJPs were set up by repetitive pulses (20/sec). Upper graph (A), control; lower graph (B), during application of 1.5 μM quisqualate. In A the number of stimuli was 240, and there were 116 zero potentials (failures). In B, the number of stimuli was 240, and there were 123 failures. m, mean quantum content; E_1, average unit size.

These are puzzling, because the glutamate action on the postsynaptic membrane must be identical with that of the transmitter in every respect if glutamate is an excitatory transmitter. Several possibilities are conceivable to explain the discrepancy between glutamate responses and EJPs. Although these possibilities were discussed elsewhere (17), the possibility that glutamic acid is not an excitatory transmitter at the crayfish neuromuscular junction has to be particularly examined. In our recent paper (6,18), we reported that diltiazem reduced the iontophoretic glutamate potential, whereas it increased the peak amplitude of successive EJPs. The pharmacological discrepancy between glutamate potentials and EJPs revealed by con A and diltiazem was difficult to explain on the glutamate transmitter hypothesis (18).

Kainic Acid

Kainic acid is one of the most potent excitants in the vertebrate neurons (20). Despite its potent anthelmintic properties,
however, kainic acid only weakly excites crayfish muscle fibers
(22). A noticeable electrophysiological action of kainic acid on
the crayfish preparations is its facilitation of glutamate-
induced depolarization (22). The facilitation was conspicuous
particularly when glutamate was applied in a bath. However,
somewhat different results were obtained when glutamate was
applied iontophoretically by brief pulses. Depending on the
experimental conditions, such as the concentrations of kainic
acid, the amount of iontophoretically applied glutamate and the
duration of glutamate pulses, kainic acid caused a slight increase or decrease in amplitude of the glutamate potential. The
glutamate response, as a rule, was enhanced by kainic acid when
the amounts of both glutamate and kainate are small, but it was
reduced in the case of the large amount of them.

Quisqualic acid is closely related to glutamate and produces
similar effects to those of glutamate (21). However, the action
of the former was depressed and that of the latter was facilitated by kainic acid when they were added to the perfusing
solution (15,22). In the case of iontophoretic application, the
depression of the quisqualate response caused by kainic acid was
more remarkable than that of glutamate response. Facilitation of
the quisqualate response was never produced by kainic acid. This
is a difference in pharmacological properties between glutamate
and quisqualate. To explore the feature of this depression of
the quisqualate response by kainic acid, an analysis of the dose-
response curve was performed in the voltage-clamped muscle. The
dose-response curve of quisqualate was shifted by kainic acid in
a parallel fashion. Kainic acid, in relatively high concentrations, inhibited to some extent the response to brief pulses of
glutamate. Therefore, one would expect some influence on the EJP
by kainic acid, if glutamate is in fact the excitatory neurotransmitter at the crayfish neuromuscular junction. It was found
neither the amplitude nor the time course of successive EJPs was
much affected by kainic acid in concentrations lower than 0.1 mM.
At these concentrations the response to bath applied glutamate
was remarkably enhanced by kainic acid. At concentrations above
0.1 mM, however, kainic acid dose-dependently reduced the EJP
amplitude (FIG.3.). The input resistance of the muscle fiber was
increased by kainic acid (above 0.1 mM), therefore, the inhibitory effect of kainic acid on EJPs would be more remarkable than
it looked. A quantum analysis of extracellularly recorded EJPs
showed that the average unit size was decreased during the application of kainic acid without affecting the mean quantum content.

In addition to the decrease in amplitude of the quisqualate
current induced by a short pulse of quisqualate, kainic acid

increased its decay rate.   In a concentration of 0.2 mM, the rate
was approximately doubled.   This is in striking contrast to the
glutamate current.   Kainic acid reduced the decay rate of the
glutamate current.   It is of great interest for examining the
transmitter glutamate hypothesis that slight difference in structure of glutamate agonist causes an opposit response to kainic
acid.   Since glutamate is a putative excitatory transmitter at
the crayfish neruomuscular junction, one would expect that the
excitatory junctional current is prolonged by kainic acid.
However, the half decay time of extracellularly recorded EJPs is
not apparently affected or slightly reduced by kainic acid (1 mM).

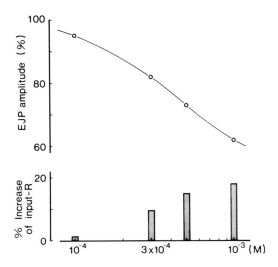

FIG.3.   Effect of kainic acid on the intracellularly recorded
EJP and the input resistance of the crayfish muscle.   Upper
graph: Dose-dependent decrease in the maximal EJP amplitude.
EJPs were set up by trains of pulses at 100 Hz for 90 msec.
Ordinate, percent of maximal response; Abscissa, concentration of
kainic acid on logarithmic scale.   Lower graph: Percent increase
in the input resistance of the crayfish muscle.   EJPs and
electrotonic potentials were alternately evoked at an interval of
5 sec.

   After the glutamate response subsided because of desensitization, kainic acid caused a remarkable depolarization (22),
suggesting that kainic acid inhibits the development of the
desensitization process of the glutamate receptor.   On the other
hand, con A could not restore the desensitized response.   When
con A was added after the glutamate receptor was almost completely desensitized, any further change in the membrane potential was
not observed even though the drugs were applied for a period of
at least 40 min.   After the complete recovery from desensitization, by thoroughly washing the preparation with a solution

containing con A but not glutamate, a very large depolarization
was observed when glutamate in the same concentration was once
again added to the solution (16). These results demonstrate that
there is some differences in mode of action between kainic acid
and con A. Thus, we examined the kainate action on the restoration process of the glutamate response which was reduced due to
desensitization.

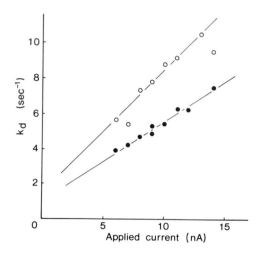

FIG.4.   Relationship between the apparent desensitization rate
constant (k_d) and the intensity of applied currents in the
absence (o) and presence (o) of 0.1 mM kainic acid. K_d was
determined from the slope of the decline (semilogarithmic plots)
of the glutamate response. Ordinate, apparent desensitization
rate constant. Abscissa, intensity of applied currents.

   The prolonged iontophoretic application of glutamate lead to
the rapid development of the glutamate current which then slowly
subsides despite the continued presence of glutamate. The
current declines to a steady plateau level approximately
exponentially. One of the characteristic properties of kainic
acid is the enhancement of the steady plateau level. The plateau
level depends on both the desensitization rate and the speed of
recovery from desensitization. Therefore, we examined the effect
of kainic acid on the desensitization rate. Semilogarithmic
plots of the decline of the glutamate response were nearly linear.
The apparent desensitization rate constant is determined as the
reciprocal of the time constant (6). In the experiment shown in
FIG.4., the apparent rate constants were plotted against the
current intensity of applied glutamate. The slope of the line
drawn through the experimental points decreased by kainic acid,
suggesting that kainic acid depresses the desensitization
development. Next, we examined the effect of kainic acid on the
rate of recovery from desensitization. Double pulses of

glutamate were applied to a glutamate sensitive spot, and the
pulses were adjusted to give equal responses when the interpulse
interval was long enough. As the interpulse interval is
decreased, the depression of the second response is remarkable.
The longer this period, the more complete was the recovery and
eventually the full amplitude of the test response was obtained.
The time course of this restoration apparently reflects the
process of recovery from desensitization. The fractional inhibition of the test response relative to its amplitude in the
absence of a prepulse was plotted on a logarithmic scale against
the interpulse delay. The plot gave a straight line. The rate
of recovery from desensitization was determined from the slope of
the line. The ratio of the rate constant in the absence and
presence of kainic acid was 1.01 ± 0.08 (mean $\pm$ S.E., n = 9).
The results suggest that kainic acid does not affect the recovery
from desensitization.

Concluding Discussion

In this study ibotenic acid was suggested to act on the GABA
receptor. The lack of depolarization of the muscle membrane by
ibotenic acid in the crayfish as well as in the locust is very
interesting in view of the molecular structure of ibotenic acid.
In the locust muscle the site of action of ibotenic acid is the
glutamate receptor. However, since ibotenic acid caused a large
conductance increase when the glutamate receptor was completely
desensitized, it seems unlikely that ibotenate acts on the
glutamate receptor on the crayfish opener muscle. This is
contrary to our expectations, but truly relates to the feature of
the glutamate receptor on the crayfish opener muscle, suggesting
that structural strictness is required to cause a response in the
crayfish muscle rather than in the vertebrate neuron.
The results obtained show that glutamic acid, quisqualic acid
and kainic acid act on the same receptor. The difference in the
kainate action between glutamate and quisqualate responses is of
great interest. Ideas about the mechanism of these actions are
at present bound to remain speculative. Some working hypotheses
have been proposed concerning drug-receptor kinetics (1,9,13).
It is of interest to try certain simple hypotheses and see
whether they can be fitted to the observations. However, the
results obtained are too complicated to suggest a simple working
hypothesis. Kainic acid reduced the apparent desensitization
rate without affecting the rate of recovery from desensitization,
and the decay of the glutamate current is lengthened by kainic
acid. On the other hand, kainic acid shortens the decay of the
quisqualate response. The latter case resembles the barbiturate
action on the ACh response (1,14). Barbiturates produce an
increase in the decay rate of the ACh response at the frog neuromuscular junction (14). In any case, it can be concluded that
kainic acid competes with other glutamate agonists for the
receptive site, however, kainic acid stabilizes the glutamate

depolarizing response but acts as an inactivator of the effective quisqualate-receptor complex. If it is so, one would expect that kainic acid decreases the decay of the excitatory junctional current. However, kainic acid does not so much decrease the decay of the extracellularly recorded EJPs as it slightly increases. Whether this is explained by the sudden release and action of the transmitter or not may be solved by further examinations.

REFERENCES

1. Adams,P.R.(1976): J.Physiol.(Lond).,260:531-552.
2. Cull-Candy,S.G.(1976):In: Moter Innervation of Muscle, edited by S.Thesleff,pp.263-283. Academic Press, London.
3. Dudel,J.(1975): Pfluegers Arch.,356:317-327.
4. Dudel,J. and Kuffler,S.W.(1961): J.Physiol.(Lond),155:514-529.
5. Grundfest,H.,Ruben,J.P. and Rickles Jr.,W.H.(1959): J.Gen. Physiol., 42:1301-1323.
6. Ishida,M. and Shinozaki,H.(1980): J.Physiol.(Lond),298:301-319.
7. Johnston,G.A.R.,Curtis,D.R.,De Groat,W.C. and Duggan,A.W. (1968): Biochem.Pharmacol.,17:2488-2489.
8. Katz,B.(1966): Nerve, Muscle, and Synapse. McGraw-Hill, New York.
9. Katz,B. and Thesleff,S.(1957): J.Physiol.(Lond),138:63-80.
10. Lea,T.J. and Usherwood,P.N.R.(1973): Comp.Gen.Pharmac.,4:333-350.
11, Mathers,D.A. and Usherwood,P.N.R.(1976): Nature,259:409-411.
12. Onodera,K. and Takeuchi,A.(1976): J.Physiol.(Lond),255:669-685.
13. Rang,H.P. and Ritter,J.M.(1970): Mol.Pharmacol.,6:357-382.
14. Seyama,I. and Narahashi,T.(1975): J.Pharmac.Exp.Ther.,192:95-104.
15. Shinozaki,H. and Ishida,M.(1976): Brain Res.,109:435-439.
16. Shinozaki,H. and Ishida,M.(1978): J.Pharm.Dyn.,1:246-250.
17. Shinozaki,H. and Ishida,M.(1979): Brain Res.,161:493-501.
18. Shinozaki,H. and Ishida,M.(1979): J.Physiol.(Paris),75:623-627.
19. Shinozaki,H. and Ishida,M.: Brain Res.,(in press).
20. Shinozaki,H. and Konishi,S.(1970): Brain Res.,24:368-371.
21. Shinozaki,H. and Shibuya,I.(1974): Neuropharmacology,13:665-672.
22. Shinozaki,H. and Shibuya,I.(1974): Neuropharmacology,13:1057-1065.
23. Takeuchi,A. and Takeuchi,N.(1964): J.Physiol.(Lond),170:296-317.
24. Takeuchi,A. and Takeuchi,N.(1969): J.Physiol.(Lond),205:377-391.
25. Usherwood,P.N.R. and Grundfest,H.(1965): J.Neurophysiol.,28:497-518.

Glutamate as a Neurotransmitter,
edited by G. Di Chiara and G. L. Gessa
Raven Press, New York © 1981.

Neuronal Receptor Sites for Kainic Acid: Correlations with Neurotoxicity

J. T. Coyle, R. Zaczek, J. Slevin, and *J. Collins

*Departments of Pharmacology and Experimental Therapeutics, and Psychiatry and the Behavioral Sciences, Johns Hopkins University School of Medicine, Baltimore, Maryland 21205; and *Department of Chemistry, City of London Polytechnic, London EC3N 2EY, England*

To identify specific excitatory amino acid receptors, our group has used ligand-binding techniques. With this method, the topography of the receptor can be inferred from the kinetics of binding inhibition by structurally related compounds. A major limitation of the ligand-binding technique concerns the fact that identification of a binding site does not in itself prove that the site has physiologic relevance. Therefore, it is essential that receptor characteristics be correlated with physiologic responses (7). In our studies, characteristics of the binding site for [3H]KA have been correlated with the acute EEG alterations and pattern of neuronal degeneration resulting from intracerebral injection of excitatory amino acids.

Characteristics of the Specific binding of [3H]-kainic acid. Two Sites. Detailed saturation isotherm of the binding of [3H]-KA (2.1-5.7 Ci/mM) in rat forebrain membranes reveals the presence of at least two sites on Scatchard analysis: one with a K_D of approximately 25-50 nM and a second higher affinity site with a K_D of approximately 3-5 nM. The biphasic binding of [3H]-KA is not an artifact of the radioactive ligand since it could be demonstrated with different batches of [3H]-KA as well as by displacement of one concentration of [3H]-KA with unlabeled KA. Specific binding of [3H]-KA has been found in brain membranes from a variety of vertebrate species and in central ganglia of several invertebrates (16); specific binding does not occur in non-neuronal tissue such as liver and muscle. The higher and lower affinty sites have an uneven and independent distribution in rat brain with high affinity sites contributing up to 30% of total binding in the frontal cortex and striatum but representing 10% or less of the total binding in cerebellum, medulla-pons and retina. In rat, the highest concentrations of sites are found in the corpus striatum followed by cerebral cortex and hippocampus whereas medulla-pons and hypothalamus have low levels. The corpus callosum, a structure enriched with glia but deficient in neuronal perikarya, has negligible levels of specific binding.

Prior KA lesion of the striatum, which causes a virtually complete degeneration of striatal intrinsic neurons (5,6), results in a 50% reduction in [^{3}H]-KA binding within the region. In contrast, decortication, which ablates a major excitatory and presumably glutamatergic input from the cerebral cortex (9), does not produce a sustained reduction in the specific binding of [^{3}H]-KA in the striatum (2). In the chick retina, where the neurons in the inner-nuclear layer are remarkably sensitive to the excitotoxic effects of KA, prior lesion with KA results in a 75% reduction in the specific binding of the [^{3}H]-ligand (3). Thus, in both the retina and the striatum, neuronal cell types vulnerable to the neurotoxic effects of KA appear to be markedly enriched with the receptor.

Receptor Topography. Detailed structural activity analyses have been carried out in the rat cerebellum, which contains only the lower affinty binding site for KA, thus rendering interpretation of the kinetics of inhibition less complicated (15). Kainic acid itself is the most potent inhibitor of specific binding with a K_I of 25 nM, which is consistent with the K_D found with a saturation isotherm of [^{3}H]-KA (Table 1). L-glutamic acid has approximately a 20-fold lower affinity for the site than does KA itself; however, D-glutamic acid, which is virtually equipotent with the L-isomer in exciting neurons in the mammalian CNS, is 100-fold less effective than L-glutamic acid in displacing [^{3}H]-KA. Dihydrokainic acid, in which the double bond in the isopropylene side-chain is reduced, and allo-kainic acid, in which the isopropylene side-chain is oriented in the opposite plane, have negligible affinity for the receptor. Keto-kainic acid, which has a keto group in the place of the methylene group in the isopropylene side-chain, has a 20-fold lower affinity for the receptor; and quisqualic acid (QA) exhibits a K_I of 0.65 μM.

The neuroexcitant ibotenic acid (Ibo) exerts no inhibition at 10 M as is the case for the conformationally restricted analogue of glutamate, cis-cyclopentylglutamate (Cycloglu). Other relevant neuroexcitants with negligible affinity for the [^{3}H]-KA binding site include D,L-homocysteic acid and N-methyl-D,L-aspartic acid. Compounds that antagonize glutamate or N-methyl-aspartate induced neuronal excitation, including L-glutamatic acid diethylester, 2-amino-4-phospho-butyric acid and D-alpha-amino adipic acid, also do not inhibit specific binding at concentrations 200-fold greater than that of the radioligand.

Competitors that bind to some but not all of the attachment sites on the receptor for a radio-ligand can produce shallow displacement curves with Hill coefficients significantly less than one (8). With regard to the effects of inhibitors of the specific binding of [^{3}H]-KA, it is noteworthy that dihydro-kainic acid, L- and D-glutamic acid have Hill coefficients near 0.5. In contrast, KA itself, QA and keto-kainic acid have Hill coefficients of approximately one. These kinetics of inhibition suggest that the Pi electrons in the isopropylene side-chain in

TABLE 1

Inhibition of the Specific Binding of [3H]Kainic Acid
In Cerebellar Membranes

	K_I (µM)	Hill Coefficient	Excitation
Kainic Acid	0.25	0.98	4+
Alpha-Allo- Kainic Acid	>>10.0	ND	±
Dihydrokainic Acid	59.0	0.38	±
Alpha-Keto- Kainic Acid	0.40	0.91	3+
Quisqualic Acid	0.65	0.90	4+
Ibotenic Acid	>>10.0	ND	3+
Cis-cyclopentyl- Glutamic Acid	>>10.0	ND	2+
L-Glutamic Acid	0.44	0.61	1+
D-Glutamic Acid	49.0	0.63	1+
D,L-Homocysteic Acid	>>10.0	ND	2+
N-Methyl-D,L- Aspartic Acid	>>10.0	ND	3+
2-Amino-4-Phos- phonobutyric Acid	>>10.0	ND	I
D-Alpha-Amino- Adipic Acid	>>10.0	ND	I
L-Glutamate Diethylester	>>10.0	ND	I

Receptor binding values are taken from London and Coyle (14)
and Slevin et al. (in preparation). For K_I indicated as >>10.0
µM, no inhibition of the specific binding of 50 nM [3H]-KA was
observed at 10 µM of the drug. Abbreviations: I = reputed
inhibitor of glutamate-induced excitation; ND = not determined.

KA or in the keto groups in QA and keto-kainic acid serve as
essential moieties in binding to the recognition site for [3H]-
KA. Reduction of the isopropylene side-chain, orientation of the
isopropylene side-chain in the opposite plane or absence of Pi
electrons on the appropriate part of the molecule as occurs in D-
and L-glutamic acid, Ibo and Cycloglu result in compounds which
lack an essential component for isographic interaction with the
recognition site for [3H]-KA.

A Glutamate Receptor? These results strongly suggest that the
binding site for KA is unlikely to be the recognition site for
the excitatory effects of glutamic acid. This interpretation is

reinforced by the marked stereoselectivity for the L-form of glutamic acid in contrast to the nearly equipotent excitatory effects of the D- and L-isomers in the mammalian CNS (1). The inability of the reputed glutamate and aspartate excitatory antagonists to inhibit specific binding of [3H]-KA is consistent with the ineffectiveness of these substances in blocking kainate induced neuroexcitation (11). Finally, both Ibo and Cycloglu, which neurophysiologically appear to activate directly a glutamate sensitive site have negligible affinty for the [3H]-KA receptor.

Kainate Receptors and Seizures

Kainic Acid. In the first description of the neurotoxic effects of systemically administered KA, Olney et al. (19) noted that it was a potent convulsant. Subsequent studies revealed that intraventricular (17) or intrahippocampal (21,25) injectionof KA produced a striking seizure disorder that persists for several hours. Abnormal behaviors included dystonic posturing, running fits, wet-dog shakes, proptosis, vibrissae twitching, forelimb clonus and generalized tonic-clonic convulsions. After injection of 2.3 nmoles of KA into the hippocampal formation of rats anaesthetized briefly with ether, profound and generalized disturbances of the cortical EEG develop (18). Within 5 minutes of injection, spiking occurs in the ipsilateral occipital cortex lead overlying the injected hippocampus; by 15 minutes, spikes appear in the contralateral occipital cortex; and by 30 minutes high amplitude spike - waves have spread to all cortical leads (Figure 1). This pattern evolves over the next several hours with recurrent episodes of increasing duration of high amplitudes, synchronous and generalized cortical seizures.

By three hours after injection, striking alterations in neurotransmitter metabolism are observed throughout the cortical regions (18). The concentration of endogenous GABA is significantly elevated in both hippocampi (+ 39%) whereas the concentration of norepinephrine is significantly depressed in the ipsilateral (67%) and contralateral (-33%) hippocampi and the cerebral cortices (-29). There is a temporal correlation between spread of the seizures and regional changes in GABA and norepinephrine levels. Since pretreatment with phenobarbital (100 mg/kg) prevents the development of cortical seizure activity (Figure 1) and blocks the alterations in the GABA and norepinephrine levels, the acute neurotransmitter changes are secondary to the seizures.

Other Excitants. Injection of 55 nmoles of QA in the hippocampus produces cortical seizures of even greater intensity than the 2.3 nmole KA (Figure 1). And 55 nmoles of keto-kainic acid is also a long-acting epileptogenic agent when injected into the hippocampus. Similar to KA, three hours after the injection of the QA, the concentration of norepinephrine is significantly depressed in the ipsilateral (-53%) and contralateral (-29%) hippocampi and cerebral cortices (-26%) whereas GABA is significantly elevated in the hippocampi (+31%). The 20-fold

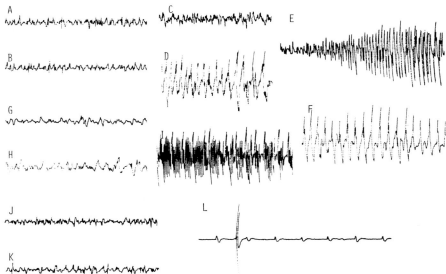

FIG. 1. Electroencephalographic Alterations Produced by Intra-hippocampal Injection of Excitotoxins. Ten days prior to the injections, cortical electrodes were implanted bilaterally in the frontal and occipital cortex with the reference electrode in the olfactory bulb. Agents were injected into the right hippocampus (HIP) in 1 μl of buffered saline while animals were anaesthetized briefly with ether; recordings were obtained with a Grass EEG. A. Frontal cortex, control. B. Occipital cortex, control. C. Frontal cortex, contralateral to HIP KA injection (2.3 nM) five min prior; note increased frequency but absence of spikes in comparison to D Occipital cortex, ipsilateral to HIP KA injection five min prior; note high amplitude spikes. E. Frontal cortex contralateral to HIP KA injection at 90 min with onset of seizure. F. Occipital cortex contralateral to HIP KA injection at 243 min with typical low frequency, high amplitude spike wave. G. Frontal cortex and H Occipital cortex ipsilateral to HIP Ibo injection (55 nM) at 65 min; note slower frequency and absence of seizures. I. Frontal cortex contralateral to HIP QA injection (55 nM) at 84 min; note high frequency seizures. J. Frontal cortex and K Occipital cortex ipsilateral to KA HIP injection at 124 min in a rat pretreated with 100 mg/kg phenobarbital; note absence of seizures. L. Occipital cortex ipsilateral to HIP KA injection at 84 min in rat pretreated with gamma-butyrolactone; note EEG pattern typical for this anaesthetic.

higher doses of QA and keto-kainate required to produce this syndrome correlate with their lower affinity for the KA receptor site. In contrast, Ibo and Cycloglu do not produce cortical seizures following intrahippocampal injection. Furthermore, the concentrations of norepinephrine in the contralateral hippocampus and the cerebral cortices and of GABA in both hippocampi are

unaffected by the Ibo injection. Preliminary results indicate
that allo-kainate and dihydrokainate are also inactive as
convulsants.

Kainate Receptors and Neurotoxicity.

Hippocampus.   Examination of the neurotoxic effects of the
intra-hippocampal injection of KA, QA and Ibo do not reveal a
correlation between neurotoxicity and seizures. In rats
anaesthetized with ether, the 2.3 nmoles of KA, a convulsant
dose, produces a profound degeneration of the pyramidal and
granule cells in the dentate gyrus (Figure 2). QA at 55 nmoles
causes more intense cortical seizures than 2.3 nmoles of KA;
neurochemical and histologic studies reveal only modest damage to
the neurons in the dentate gyrus of the hippocampus. In
contrast, the 55 nmoles of Ibo cause a hippocampal lesion of
comparable severity to QA without any evidence of cortical
seizures. Furthermore, pretreatment with phenobarbital (100
mg/kg) prevents the development of cortical seizures after an
intra-hippocampal injection of 2.3 nmoles of KA but provides only
minimal protection against its neurotoxic effects; in contrast,
anaesthesia for 4-6 hours with pentobarbital-chloral hydrate or
gamma-butyrolactone considerably attenuates its neurotoxicity.

Striatum. Of the analogues examined thus far, KA has proved
to be the most potent, producing lesions nearly 3 mm in diameter
following injection of 2.3 nmoles in ether anaesthetized rats.
The lesion results in greater reductions in the presynaptic
markers for the cholinergic neurons and than the GABAergic
neurons (Table 2). Dihydrokainate and allo-kainate with low
affinity for the KA receptor have negligible neurotoxic effects.
Keto-kainate and QA are neurotoxic in the striatum but with
lesser potencies comparable to their lower affinity for the KA
receptor; like KA, they exhibit greater toxicity at striatal
cholinergic than GABAergic neurons. In contrast, both Ibo and
Cycloglu, while less potent than KA, are nearly equally
neurotoxic to striatal GABAergic and cholinergic neurons.

DISCUSSION

Ligand-binding studies have identified a site with
characteristics that correlate well with the neurophysiologic and
neurotoxicologic effects of KA. The essential role of the Pi
electron group in binding to the receptor has been demonstrated
by the high affinities of QA and keto-kainate (< 1 μM) with Hill
coefficients of 1.0 which contrast with the low affinities ($>> 10$
μM) of dihydrokainate and allo-kainate. Although L-glutamic acid
exhibits a relatively high affinity for the binding site, the low
Hill coefficient suggests that it does not bind isographically to
the receptor. Notably, the excitotoxins, Ibo, Cycloglu and
N-methyl-aspartic acid, have remarkably poor affinity for the
receptor.

Compounds that bind isographically and avidly to the receptor
including KA itself, keto-kainate and QA exhibit potent

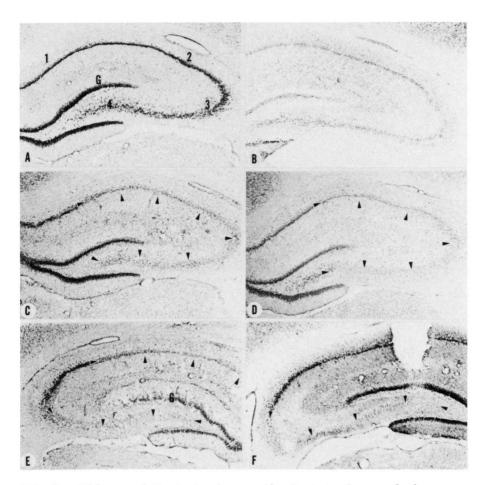

FIG. 2. Effects of Excitotoxins on the Dentate Gyrus of the
Hippocampus. Rats received intrahippocampal injection of agents
in 1 μl of buffered saline 4 days prior to sacrifice; sections
were stained with cresyl violet. A. Control indicating pyramidal
cell subfields CA 1-4 and the granule cells (G). B. KA, 2.3 nM;
note complete degeneration of pyramidal and granule cells. C. QA
- 55 nM, note degeneration of CA 2-4 but intact granule cells.
D. IBO, 55 nM; note degeneration of CA 2-4 but intact granule
cells; more medial injection ablates granule cells. E. KA, 2.3
nM with pretreatment with phenobarbital (100 mg/kg); note spring
of only a portion of CA-2 and degeneration of most of the granule
cells (G). F. KA, 2.3 nM with pretreatment with gamma
butyrolactone (6 hr anaesthesia); note sparing of CA 1-2 and
granule cells.

epileptogenic effects whereas the neuroexcitants with low
affinityfor the kainate receptor such as Ibo and Cycloglu do not
provoke cortical seizures at doses that result in comparable

TABLE 2

Effects of Intra-Striatal Injection of Cyclical Excitants

Drug	Choline Acetylase	Glutamate Decarboxylase
	Percent of Control	
Kainic Acid 2.3 nM	31 + 4**	49 + 3**
Keto-Kainic Acid 90 nM	35 + 8**	59 + 8**
Dihydrokainic Acid 90 nM	101 + 1	105 + 1
Quisqualic Acid 110 nM	73 + 4**	90 + 1*
Ibotenic Acid 80 nM	73 + 4**	74 + 1*
Cis-Cyclopentylglutamic Acid 120 nM	68 + 4**	79 + 6**

Rats anaesthetized briefly with ether received intra-striatal injections of the agents in 0.5-1.0 µl of buffered saline and were sacrificed four days later for measurement of the activities of choline acetylase, glutamate decarboxylase and tyrosine hydroxylase as previously described (21). Results are presented in terms of the percent of uninjected control; there was no significant reduction in the specific activity of tyrosine hydroxylase with any of the treatments (from Zaczek et al. in preparation and 20). N $\geq$ 6.

*p $<$ 0.05; **p $<$ 0.01 versus control by two tailed t-test.

hippocampal lesions. The EEG findings are further supported by the distant effects of the KA receptor agonists on norepinephrine and GABA in hippocampus and cerebral cortex. Taken together, these results indicate that KA is interacting at a specific class of receptors that differ from those mediating the excitatory effects of Ibo, Cycloglu and probably glutamic acid.

Considerable information has accrued that the neurotoxic effects of KA are primarily indirect. Prior destruction of the excitatory, presumably glutamatergic, projections to the corpus striatum (2), dentate gyrus of the hippocampus (12) and the optic tectum (23) markedly attenuate the neurotoxic action of KA. Kainic acid is devoid of neurotoxic effects in the immature rat striatum prior to the development of its receptor and glutamatergic terminal markers within the region (4). These indirect effects of KA should be considered in the context of the neurophysiology of KA at the crustacean neuromuscular junction where it has a weak excitatory effect but potentiates the glutamate induced depolarization (22). In contrast, the uniform sphere of neuronal degeneration observed with intracerebral injection of Ibo and Cycloglu suggests that these agents have direct toxic effects on neuronal perikarya (13).

The neurotoxic effects of the neuroexcitants does not seem directly related to their convulsant action. Doses of anticonvulsants that prevent the cortical seizure activity weakly antagonize the neurotoxic action of KA at the injection site.

Conversely, neuroexcitants that do not interact with the kainate receptor such as Ibo and Cycloglu produce comparable lesions in the hippocampus without precipitating cortical seizures. Decarboxylation of Ibo to form the GABA agonist, muscimol, is an unlikely explanation for this disparity since the decarboxylated product of epileptogenic QA, quisqualamine, is also a potent inhibitor (10). A more parsimonious explanation is that KA receptor agonists diffuse from the injection site, activate KA receptors which enhance neuronal sensitivity to excitatory neurotransmitters, and thus produce generalized seizures. This formulation does not preclude the possibility that increased excitatory neuronal activity, particularly in susceptible areas, contributes to the neurotoxic effects of KA; indeed, such interactions are likely to play an important role since the duration of anaesthesia required for protection against neurotoxicity corresponds with the time when > 75% of the injected KA is cleared from the brain (26).

These results support the existence of a biochemically and neurophysiologically distinct receptor that mediates the effects of KA and related substances. The ionic or metabolic transducers linked to this receptor, which account for its convulsant and indirect neurotoxic effects, remain to be defined. Nevertheless, the KA receptor offers an interesting parallel to the role of the benzodiazepine receptor in GABAergic neurotransmission (24); in an analogous fashion, the KA receptor may serve as a modulatory site which regulates the synaptic action of glutamate and other excitatory neurotransmitters.

REFERENCES

1. Biscoe, T.J., Evans, R.H., Headley, P.M., Martin, M.R. and Watkins, J.C. (1976) Br. J. Pharmacol. 58:373-382.
2. Biziere, K. and Coyle, J.T. (1979) J. Neurosci. Res. 4:383-398.
3. Biziere, K. and Coyle, J.T. (1979) Neuropharmacology 18:409-413.
4. Campochiaro, P. and Coyle, J.T. (1978) Proc. Natl. Acad. Sci. USA 75:2025-2029.
5. Coyle, J.T. and Schwarcz, R. (1976) Nature 263:244-246.
6. Coyle, J.T., Molliver, M.E. and Kuhar, M.J. (1978) J. Comp. Neurol. 180:301-324.
7. Cuatrecasas, P. and Hollenberg, M.D. (1976) Adv. Protein Chem. 30:251-451.
8. DeLean, A., Munson, P.J. and Rodbard, P. (1979) Mol. Pharmacol. 15:60-72.
9. Divak, I., Fonnum, F. and Storm-Mathesin, J. (1977) Nature (Lond.) 266:377-378.
10. Evans, R.H., Francis, A.A., Hunt, K., Martin, M.R. and Watkins, J.C. (1978) J. Pharm. Pharmac. 30:364-367.
11. Hall, J.G., Hicks, T.P., McLennan, H., Richardson, T.L. and Wheal, H.V. (1979) J. Physiol. (Lond) 286:29-39.

12. Kohler, C., Schwarcz, R. and Fuxe, K. (1978) Neurosci. Letts. 10:241-246.
13. Kohler, C., Schwarcz, R. and Fuxe, K. (1979) Brain Res. 175:366-371.
14. London, E.D. and Coyle, J.T. (1979) Molec. Pharmacol. 15:492-505.
15. London, E.D. and Coyle, J.T. (1979) Eur. J. Pharmacol. 56:287-290.
16. London, E.D., Klemm, N. and Coyle, J.T. (1980) Brain Res., in press.
17. Nadler, J.W., Perry, B.W. and Cotman, C.W. (1978) Nature (Lond) 271:676-682.
18. Nelson, M.F., Zaczek, R. and Coyle, J.T. (1980) J. Pharmacol. Exp. Ther., in press.
19. Olney, J.W., Rhee, V. and Ho, O.L. (1974) Brain Res. 77:507-512.
20. Schwarcz, R., Scholz, D. and Coyle, J.T. (1978) Neuropharmacology 17:145-151.
21. Schwarcz, R., Zaczek, R. and Coyle, J.T. (1978) Eur. J. Pharmacol. 50:209-220.
22. Shinozaki, H. (1980) In Kainic Acid as a Tool in Neurobiology (McGeer, E.G., Olney, J.W. and McGeer, P.L., eds.) Raven Press, New York, pp. 17-35.
23. Streit, P., Stella, M. and Cuenod, M. (1980) Brain Res. 187:47-57.
24. Tallman, J.F., Paul, S.M., Skolnick, P. and Gallagen, D.W. (1980) Science 207:274-281.
25. Zaczek, R., Nelson, M.F. and Coyle, J.T. (1978) Eur. J. Pharmacol. 52:323-327.
26. Zaczek, R. Simonton, S. and Coyle, J.T. (1980) J. Neuropath. and exp. Neuro., in press.

Glutamate as a Neurotransmitter,
edited by G. Di Chiara and G. L. Gessa
Raven Press, New York © 1981.

Kainate Effects in Cerebellar Cultures

Fredrick J. Seil, Nathan K. Blank, William R. Woodward, and
*Arnold L. Leiman

*Neurology Research, Veterans Administration Medical Center and Departments
of Neurology, Pathology, and Biochemistry, University of Oregon Health Sciences Center,
Portland, Oregon 97201; and *Department of Psychology, University of California,
Berkeley, California 94720*

On the basis of animal studies of mechanisms of kainic acid neurotoxicity, it has been suggested that kainic acid acted specifically at postsynaptic glutamic acid receptor sites (6,14,15), that it was excitotoxic (15), and that intact glutamatergic fibers were necessary for the manifestation of kainate-induced neuronal destructive effects (2,9,13). Various cell groups studied included striatal, hippocampal and cerebellar cortical neurons, to which kainic acid was generally introduced by direct stereotactic injection.

Another approach to the study of kainic acid neurotoxicity is by use of a well defined in vitro system, as represented by cerebellar tissue cultures derived from newborn mice (18). Such cultures can be uniformly exposed to given concentrations of kainic acid incorporated into the nutrient medium either during development or after maturation.

Structural and functional features of cerebellar cortex in situ have been well established (4,16). Of five neuronal types present, only the granule cells are excitatory, and the neurotransmitter is believed to be glutamic acid (7,12,17,26). Their axons, the parallel fibers, make synaptic contact with all cortical neurons except other granule cells. Such parallel fiber synapses develop after birth in the mouse (10). The remaining cortical neurons, including Purkinje, Golgi, basket and stellate cells, are inhibitory, and are thought to employ transmitters other than glutamic acid (8). Except for Purkinje cells, all cerebellar cortical neurons are interneurons. The primary recipients of the inhibitory output of the cerebellar cortex are the intracerebellar nuclei, whose neurons are the targets of converging Purkinje cell axons. Such neurons are not known to have significant glutamatergic afferent input (3).

Most of the structural and functional features of the cerebellum in situ, including the postnatal development of cortical laminae, are evident in cerebellar tissue cultures (18). Cerebellar explants cut in the parasagittal plane

347

incorporate both cortex and intracerebellar nuclei. All cortical neuronal types are represented, and normal interneuronal relationships are established. A basic difference from the cerebellum in situ is that the cultures are largely devoid of extracerebellar afferents, as the incoming mossy and climbing fibers are transected during explantation. In the absence of excitatory input from mossy and climbing fiber collaterals, the intracerebellar nucleus neurons are not spontaneously electrically active in vitro, in contrast to endogenously discharging cortical neurons, but such subcortical cells remain electrically excitable (20). The in vitro system can be further modified by drastically reducing or eliminating cerebellar granule cells upon exposure to cytosine arabinoside during the first few days after explantation (21). Such granuloprival cultures presumably have very few or no cortical glutamatergic afferent fibers.

This review describes studies of kainic acid neurotoxicity employing the cerebellar tissue culture system (19,22,23). Particularly brought into focus by these investigations are the issues of 1) the specificity of kainic acid action, 2) its postulated excitotoxic mechanism, and 3) the requirement for the presence of presynaptic glutamatergic fibers for its toxic manifestations.

METHODS

Details of the methods employed in these studies have been presented in the original publications (19,22,23). Only a few salient features are repeated here. Parasagittally oriented explants derived from newborn Swiss-Webster mouse cerebellum were placed on collagen-coated coverslips with a drop of nutrient medium, sealed in Maximow chambers and incubated at 35.5 - 36°C. The nutrient medium was changed twice weekly. Kainic acid dissolved in buffered balanced salt solution was incorporated into the nutrient medium to a final concentration of 10^{-4}M and applied to cultures at various ages in vitro and for varying lengths of time. Granuloprival cultures were prepared by exposure of cerebellar explants to 5 μg cytosine arabinoside per ml nutrient medium for the first 5 days in vitro, followed by cultivation in normal medium (21). Cultures were serially observed in the living state and were fixed after varying intervals for thionine (Nissl) or silver staining, or for electron microscopy. Extracellular electrophysiological recordings from mature cerebellar explants were made by established techniques (11,18).

RESULTS

Specificity of Action

Exposure of cerebellar cultures to kainic acid for intervals

ranging from 1-14 days after explantation resulted in a marked
reduction of cortical mass and loss of large cortical neurons
(19) (Figs. 1 and 2). The surviving cortical neuronal elements
consisted of a relatively homogenous population of small
neurons identified as granule cells by light and electron
microscopic examination (Fig. 3). The relative sparing of
cerebellar granule cells from the neurotoxic consequences of
kainic acid was consistent with results obtained from animal
studies (6). However, prolonged exposure (17 days) of
cerebellar cultures to 10^{-4}M kainic acid resulted in a marked
reduction of the granule cell population as well. Neuronal
destructive effects were evident whether kainic acid was
applied to cultures before or after formation of parallel fiber
synapses.

Also notable was a failure of development of cortical
lamination in cerebellar cultures incubated with kainic acid.
Cortical laminae did not develop even in cultures exposed for
brief intervals (24 hours) after explantation, in which there
was incomplete destruction of large cortical neurons. The
mechanism by which kainic acid suppressed cortical laminar
formation was not clear.

Equally sensitive to the toxic effects of kainic acid on
large cortical neurons were the intracerebellar nucleus
neurons. As such neurons are not known to be richly endowed
with glutamic acid receptors, the results of application of
L-glutamic acid to cerebellar cultures was evaluated. Exposure
of cerebellar explants ranging from 19-22 days in vitro to
10^{-4}M L-glutamate produced a transient increase in the rate
of spontaneous cortical discharges, but no activation of
intracerebellar nucleus neurons. Increasing the concentration
of L-glutamic acid to 10^{-3}M resulted in a pronounced increase
in cortical discharge rate followed by a depolarization block,
again without activation of intracerebellar nucleus neurons.
The failure of activation of such neurons by concentrations of
L-glutamate that produced significant electrophysiological
changes in cortical neurons indicated a relative insensitivity
of intracerebellar nucleus neurons to L-glutamic acid, while
these neurons were exquisitely sensitive to the toxic effects
of kainic acid.

Excitotoxic Mechanism

In order to evaluate the possibility that kainic acid
neurotoxic effects might be due to chronic depolarization of
neurons, cerebellar explants were cultivated in medium
incorporating other excitatory amino acids acting at glutamic
acid receptor sites, or to a combination of kainic acid and the
inhibitory compound, gamma-aminobutyric acid (GABA) (23).
Cultures exposed to 10^{-3}M L-glutamic acid or 10^{-3}M
D-glutamic acid, the latter a metabolically inactive isomer of
the former (24), for up to 17 days failed to demonstrate

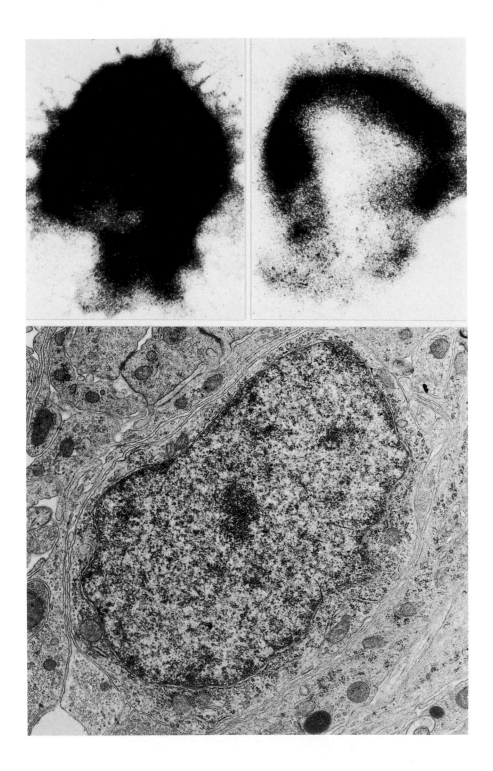

neurotoxic effects like those produced by kainic acid.
Cortical neurons in such cultures appeared normal by light
microscopic and ultrastructural criteria. On the other hand,
explants cultivated in the presence of 10^{-4}M kainic acid plus
either 10^{-3}M or 10^{-2}M GABA, concentrations of GABA known to
produce potent inhibition of glutamate-induced neuronal
discharges in cerebellar cultures (5), were not protected from
the destructive effects of kainic acid. GABA applied by itself
was not toxic to cerebellar explants after prolonged exposure.

In order to assess the approximate excitatory equivalence of
D-glutamic acid, L-glutamic acid and kainic acid, these
compounds were applied successively to a cerebellar explant 20
days *in vitro* while spontaneous cortical activity was
extracellularly recorded. The culture was washed with normal
recording medium between applications of drugs. The increase
produced by each compound on spontaneous cortical discharge
rate was monitored. The results indicated that kainic acid was
not more than 10 times as potent a neuroexcitant in this system
as its glutamic acid analogs. Thus the concentrations of
excitatory amino acids employed appeared valid for purposes of
comparison, and L-glutamic acid and D-glutamic acid with
depolarizing capabilities at least equivalent to neurotoxic
concentrations of kainic acid did not produce neurodestructive
effects.

Requirement for Glutamatergic Afferents

Although the destruction of cortical neurons by exposure to
kainic acid prior to the development of parallel fiber synapses
and the toxic effects upon intracerebellar nucleus neurons (19)
already suggested that presynaptic glutamatergic fibers were

FIG. 1 (Top left, facing page). Normal cerebellar culture, 10
days *in vitro*. Thionine stain. X 30.

FIG. 2 (Top right). Cerebellar culture, 10 days *in vitro*,
exposed to 10^{-4}M kainic acid for 10 days. The cortical
volume is considerably reduced due to loss of all neurons
except granule cells. Thionine stain. X 30.

FIG. 3 (Bottom). Electron micrograph of a granule cell in the
cortex of a cerebellar culture, 14 days *in vitro*, exposed to
10^{-4}M kainic acid for 14 days. A prominent nucleus is
surrounded by a thin shell of cytoplasm containing free
ribosomes, a few mitochondria and scant Nissl substance.
X 17,400.

not necessary for the manifestation of kainate neurotoxicity in
cerebellar cultures, a study was undertaken to specifically
address this question (22). Granuloprival cultures were
exposed beginning at 16 days in vitro to either 10^{-3}M
D-glutamic acid or 10^{-4}M kainic acid for 6 days. The
cortices of granuloprival cerebellar explants incubated with
10^{-3}M D-glutamic acid contained numerous large neurons and
abundant neurites, appearing in every way similar to
granuloprival explants cultivated in normal nutrient medium
(21). Granuloprival cultures incubated with 10^{-4}M kainic
acid contained very few or no large cortical neurons and axonal
processes, and reactive gliosis was prominent. The effects
were similar to those obtained by exposure of normal explants
to kainic acid, and included the destruction of intracerebellar
nucleus neurons. These effects were reproduced upon
application of kainic acid to granuloprival cerebellar explants
cultivated in low-L-glutamate medium.

TABLE 1. Application of amino acids to cerebellar cultures

Amino acid	Excitatory	Glutamatergic afferent fibers present	Neurotoxic
Kainic acid	+	+	+
L-Glutamic acid	+	+	−
D-Glutamic acid	+	+	−
GABA	−	+	−
Kainic acid + GABA	−	+	+
Kainic acid[a]	+	−	+
D-Glutamic acid[a]	+	−	−

[a]Applied to granuloprival cerebellar cultures.

The results of this (22) and the previous study (23) are
summarized in Table 1. It is evident from this table that
kainic acid neurotoxicity in cerebellar cultures can be
dissociated from prolonged neuronal depolarization and from a
requirement for intact glutamatergic afferent innervation.

DISCUSSION

With regard to the first of the described studies (19), the
combination of kainic acid neurotoxic effects on cerebellar
cortical neurons prior to the formation of parallel fiber
synapses, the eventual degeneration of cerebellar granule cells
after prolonged exposure to kainic acid, the inhibition of
cortical laminar formation and particularly the destruction of
intracerebellar nucleus neurons suggested that kainate toxic
effects in cerebellar tissue cultures were not mediated
exclusively by action on glutamic acid receptor sites. In the

second study (23), the failure of depolarizing analogs of kainic acid to reproduce its neurotoxic effects in cerebellar cultures and the failure of the inhibitory amino acid, GABA, to protect cerebellar explants from kainate-induced neuronal destruction suggested that kainic acid did not produce its toxic effects by lethal neuroexcitation. In the final study (22), the neurodestructive properties of kainic acid were seen to persist in cultures without cortical glutamatergic afferent fibers. This result is consistent with an in vivo study in which kainic acid neurotoxic effects on guinea pig cochlear nucleus neurons continued to be expressed after destruction of their glutamatergic afferent innervation (1). Together, these studies suggest that an intact glutamatergic afferent fiber system is not always necessary for the manifestation of kainic acid neurotoxicity. The differences between these studies and in vivo (2,9,13) and tissue culture (25) studies that did demonstrate a requirement for intact glutamatergic afferents might reflect differences in the neuronal populations examined or differences in mechanisms of kainate neurotoxicity in various regions of the nervous system.

In aggregate, the studies of kainate effects in cerebellar cultures have raised questions about 1) the exclusive mediation of kainic acid neurotoxicity by action on postsynaptic glutamic acid receptor sites, 2) excitotoxicity as the mechanism for kainate-induced neuronal destruction, and 3) the requirement for glutamatergic presynaptic fibers for the manifestation of kainate neurotoxicity. In light of these questions, it would appear that some caution is indicated in the interpretation of results of studies with kainic acid.

ACKNOWLEDGEMENTS

Supported by the Veterans Administration (F.J.S. and N.K.B.) and Public Health Service Grant EY02456 (W.R.W.). The technical assistance of Benson Fong, James Jetton, Michele Mass, Joseph Pierce, Jean Quigley and Jan Rising is gratefully acknowledged.

REFERENCES

1. Bird, S.J., and Gulley, R.T. (1979): Neurosci. Lett., 15:55-60.
2. Biziere, N., and Coyle, J.T. (1978): Neurosci. Lett., 8:303-310.
3. Chan-Palay, V. (1977): Cerebellar Dentate Nucleus. Springer, New York.
4. Eccles, J.C., Ito, M., and Szentagothai, J. (1967): The Cerebellum as a Neuronal Machine. Springer, New York.
5. Geller, H.M., and Woodward, D.J. (1974): Brain Res., 74:67-80.
6. Herndon, R.M., and Coyle, J.T. (1977): Science, 198:71-72.

7. Hudson, D.B., Valcana, T., Bean, G., and Timiras, P.S. (1976): Neurochem. Res., 1:73-81.
8. Ito, M. (1978): In: Advances in Neurology, Vol. 21, The Inherited Ataxias, edited by R.A.P. Kark, R.N. Rosenberg, and L.J. Schut, pp. 59-84. Raven Press, New York.
9. Kohler, C., Schwarcz, R., and Fuxe, K. (1978): Neurosci. Lett., 10:241-246.
10. Larramendi, L.M.H. (1969): In: Neurobiology of Cerebellar Evolution and Development, edited by R. Llinas, pp. 803-843. American Medical Association, Chicago.
11. Leiman, A.L., and Seil, F.J. (1973): Exp. Neurol., 40:748-758.
12. McBride, W.J., Nadi, N.S., Altman, J., and Aprison, M.H. (1976): Neurochem. Res., 1:141-152.
13. McGeer, E.G., McGeer, P.L., and Singh, K. (1978): Brain Res., 139:381-383.
14. Olney, J.W., Fuller, T., and De Gubareff, T. (1979): Brain Res., 176:91-100.
15. Olney, J.W., Rhee, V., and Ho, O.L. (1974): Brain Res., 77:507-512.
16. Palay, S.L., and Chan-Palay, V. (1974): Cerebellar Cortex. Springer, New York.
17. Sandoval, M.E., and Cotman, C.W. (1978): Neuroscience, 3:199-206.
18. Seil, F.J. (1979): In: Reviews of Neuroscience, Vol. 4, edited by D.M. Schneider, pp. 105-177. Raven Press, New York.
19. Seil, F.J., Blank, N.K., and Leiman, A.L. (1979): Brain Res., 161:253-265.
20. Seil, F.J., and Leiman, A.L. (1977): Exp. Neurol., 54:110-127.
21. Seil, F.J., Leiman, A.L., and Woodward, W.R. (1980): Brain Res., 186:393-408.
22. Seil, F.J., and Woodward, W.R. (1980): Brain Res., in press.
23. Seil, F.J., Woodward, W.R., Blank, N.K., and Leiman, A.L. (1978): Brain Res., 159:431-435.
24. Takagaki, G. (1976): J. Neurochem., 27:1417-1425.
25. Whetsell, W.O., Jr., Ecob-Johnston, M.S., and Nicklas, W.J. (1979): In: Advances in Neurology, Vol. 23, Huntington's Disease, edited by T.N. Chase, N.S. Wexler, and A. Barbeau, pp. 645-654. Raven Press, New York.
26. Young, A.B., Oster-Granite, M.L., Herndon, R.M., and Snyder, S.H. (1974): Brain Res., 73:1-13.

Glutamate as a Neurotransmitter,
edited by G. Di Chiara and G. L. Gessa
Raven Press, New York © 1981.

Effect of Barbiturates and Benzodiazepines on Local Kainate Toxicity in the Striatum and in the Retina

*G. Di Chiara, *M. Morelli, *A. Imperato, **G. Faa,
†M. Fossarello, and *M. L. Porceddu

*Institutes of *Pharmacology, **Pathological Anatomy, and †Clinical Ophthalmology,
University of Cagliari, 09100 Cagliari, Italy*

Kainic acid, the powerful neuroexcitatory principle extracted from Digenea simplex, is known to be a potent neurotoxin provided of specificity towards neuronal perikarya (9). The intimate mechanism of kainate toxicity is still unknown in spite of many studies addressed to its clarification. A starting point in the understanding of kainate neurotoxicity is the concept that this process is linked in some way to the neuroexcitatory action of kainate (9). Indeed, an axon-sparing type of neurotoxicity, similar to that produced by kainate, seems to be a general property of potent neuroexcitatory compounds locally administered on neural structures (9). Moreover, among structural analogs of dicarboxilic amino acids, there appears to be a relationship between their potency as neuroexcitants and their effectiveness as neurotoxins (9,14). In keeping with such an excitotoxic hypothesis it has been reported that the local neurotoxicity of intra-hippocampal kainate is significantly reduced, although not prevented, by the systemic administration of various anticonvulsants, including diazepam (23).

It has recently become clear that local intracerebral administration of kainate produces damage not only at the

point of injection but also at sites distant from it, particularly at the level of the hyppocampus (3,16,21). Distant
brain damage is most probably related to kainate-induced
status epilepticus and is specifically prevented by the systemic administration of diazepam (2,3). In view of this and
of the fact that intrahippocampal kainate results in status
epilepticus it is conceivable that the local damage produced
by intrahippocampal kainate is not due only to a direct neurotoxic action of kainate in the hyppocampus but also to the
convulsion-related stimulation of hippocampal neurons (Nadler, this volume). In this case the ability of diazepam to
reduce the local neurotoxicity in the hippocampus could be
due to its anti-convulsant action rather than to a blockade
of kainate effects at the site of injection. In order to reexa-
mine the effect of diazepam and of other depressants on local kainate toxicity and to exclude the role of convulsions
we have studied the effect of benzodiazepines and of barbiturates on the local neurotoxicity of kainate on two areas as
the retina and the striatum for which a role of convulsions
can be safely excluded. In fact, kainate, infused in the vitreous humor, fails to produce convulsions even at doses
which are supramaximal for lesioning the retina. Moreover,
the striatum is not a site of seizure-related brain damage
nor of distant damage after intracerebral kainate (3,16).

MATERIALS AND METHODS

Kainic acid was injected under ether or barbiturate or
benzodiazepine anaesthesia in the striatum of 280/300 gr.
Charles River male Sprague-Dawley rats, dissolved in 1.0 ul
of saline at a speed of 1 ul/3 min. or in the vitreous humor
of 200/250 gr. male Charles River Sprague-Dawley rats or
3 days old chicks dissolved in 2.5 ul (rats) or in 5.0 ul
(chicks) at a speed of 1 ul/30 sec.
The neurotoxicity of kainate was estimated by measuring
the loss of neurochemical markers of specific neurons such
as glutamate decarboxilase (GAD) (20) and GABA-uptake (14)
for GABA-neurons, choline acetyltransferase (CAT) (4) and
choline-uptake (14) for cholinergic neurons and dopamine-
sensitive adenylate cyclase (19) as a marker of post-synaptic dopamine (DA) receptors.
Some animals were perfused with formalin and their
brains or eyes included in paraffin and then stained with
hematoxilin .

RESULTS AND DISCUSSION

Intrastriatal Kainic Acid

Neurochemical changes

Since the beginning of our study it became evident that short-lasting anaesthesia by a single administration of depressants such as phenobarbital, pentobarbital, diazepam, clonazepam was without effect on the toxicity of kainate in the striatum as estimated three days later by the loss of neurochemical markers. In contrast, prolonged anaesthesia with phenobarbital effectively reduced the neurotoxicity of kainate. Fig.1 shows the effect of increasing duration of anaesthesia, by phenobarbital, on striatal GAD and CAT loss after intrastriatal infusion of 0.5 ug of kainate. A 4h. anaesthesia with phenobarbital failed to significantly affect the loss of GAD and CAT. Eight hours of anaesthesia significantly reduced only GAD loss, while a 12 h. administration of phenobarbital, which resulted in at least 16 h. of anaesthesia, reduced significantly both GAD and CAT loss; indeed, this schedule protected from kainate toxicity as GAD and CAT activities in the kainate-injected striatum were not significantly different from the values of the intact side.

Administration of phenobarbital protected not only from striatal GAD and CAT loss but also from the loss of other markers of striatal neurons such as striatal DA-sensistive adenylate cyclase as well as nigral GAD and DA sensitive adenylate cyclase, which are known to be localized in striatal interneurons and in terminals of strio-nigral neurons respectively (19) (data not shown).

Another barbiturate, pentobarbital, was tested for its ability to affect kainate-induced neuronal loss in the striatum. As shown in Fig. 2, repeated administration of pentobarbital for 12 h. significantly reduced GAD and CAT loss in the striatum; however, this effect was not as dramatic as after phenobarbital since pentobarbital failed to confer complete protection from GAD and CAT loss. Thus, under pentobarbital, anaesthesia of 0.5 ug of kainate still reduced significantly GAD and CAT activities in respect to the intact side.

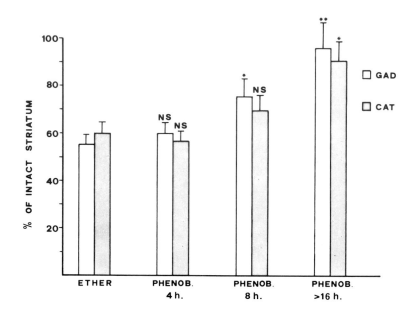

FIG. 1   Effect of phenobarbital anaesthesia on kainate-induced loss of GAD and CAT in the striatum.

Kainic acid (0.5 ug) was injected unilaterally in the stria-tum (A 2.4, L 2.8, V 5.0) (12) of rats. Controls were anaes-thetized with ether only during surgery while the experimen-tal group was anaesthetized with 150 mg/kg of phenobarbital i.p. Phenobarbital administration was repeated at a lower dose (75 mg/kg) at the first sign of recovery of the corneal or righting reflexes. Controls were repeatedly injected i.p. with saline. The time indicated in the figures refers to the duration of deep anaesthesia ±30 min. (4 h.) and ±1h. (8h.). In the case of the longest interval (16h.), rats re-ceived the last injection of the barbiturate 12 h. after intra-striatal kainate and slept for more than 16 h. GAD and CAT were expressed as percent of the values found in the stria-tum not injected with kainate. Values are mean ± s.e. of the results obtained in at least 6 rats per group. The va-lues of GAD and CAT in the intact side were 220 ± 10 and 50.8 ± 4.8 respectively (mean ± s.e. expressed in nmol/h/mg prot.).

*   p<0.05; ** p<0.001 in respect to controls anaesthetized with ether only for the duration of surgery.

Benzodiazepines were also tested for their ability to influence local kainate toxicity in the striatum. As shown in
Fig.2 neither diazepam nor clonazepam, administered at maximally tolerated doses for 12 h. significantly reduced the
kainate-induced GAD and CAT loss in the striatum. Repeated
administration of benzodiazepines for periods longer than 12
h. were attempted but resulted in very high mortality.

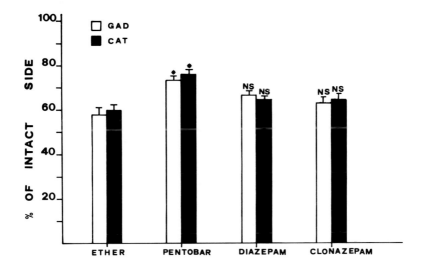

FIG. 2   Effect of a 12 h. treatment with barbiturates or benzodiazepines on kainate-induced loss of striatal GAD and
CAT.
Rats were given 0.5 ug of kainate in the striatum of one
side. Control rats were anaesthetized with ether only for the
duration of surgery. Experimental animals were anaesthetized with repeated injections of maximally tolerated doses of
pentobarbital (first injection 70 mg/kg, subseguent 35
mg/kg), diazepam (first injection 30 mg/kg, subseguent 15
mg/kg), clonazepam (first injection 10 mg/kg, subseguent 5
mg/kg) The last injection of the depressants was given
about 12 h. after the first one.
* $p < 0.05$; ** $p < 0.001$ in respect to the controls (ether).

From these data it appears that, while phenobarbital effectively protects against local kainate toxicity in the striatum, the same does not apply to other related compounds, such as pentobarbital or to potent anticonvulsants such as diazepam or clonazepam administered repeatedly for 12 h. The differences in the efficiency of the various drugs tested in protecting from local kainate toxicity could be due to pharmacodynamic differences in their actions at the neuronal level; however, pharmacokinetic differences might also play a role. In fact, we noticed that about 60% of the rats treated for 12 h. with phenobarbital were still sleeping on the next day, i.e. 24 h. after the beginning of the treatment. In contrast, all the rats treated for 12 h. with pentobarbital or with the benzodiazepines had completely recovered on the next day.

Therefore it appears that in order to protect from kainate-local neurotoxicity, it is necessary to keep neurons under the action of the depressant for at least 16-20 hours.

The reason for this could be a very slow disappearance of kainate from the striatum.

In order to clarify this point we measured the disappearance of ^{3}H-kainate from the striatum after local injection of 0.5 μg of the neurotoxin to control and to phenobarbital-treated rats. As shown in Fig.3 kainate has a bifasic rate of disappearance from the striatum; the first process has a half-life of 2.5 hours in controls and of 3 h. in phenobarbital-treated rats while the second has a half-life of 12.3 hours in controls and of 16.5 hours in the rats treated for 12 h. with phenobarbital.

We do not know the reason for this bifasic disappearance but one can tentatively suggest that the first process is mainly due to diffusion of free kainate from the striatum into the extrastriatal tissue and to its transfer into the plasma compartment. The second process might be due to slow release of kainate from its specific receptors in the caudate.

If this interpretation is correct and if the fraction of kainate bound to its specific receptors is that responsible for its neurotoxicity then it becomes clear why it is necessary such a long treatment with phenobarbital to confer protection against local kainate toxicity or why pentobarbital is much less effective than phenobarbital. In fact, after the first 6 hours of wash-out of the free kainate, the effective fraction of kainate is reduced by 50% after 22 hours and by

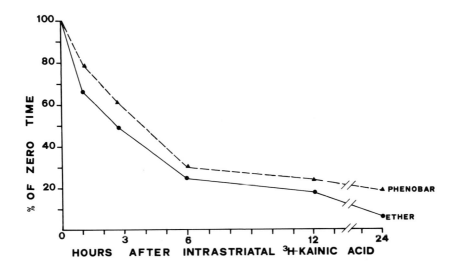

FIG. 3   Time-course of the disappearence of ^{3}H-kainate from the striatum of control and phenobarbital-treated rats. Rats were injected in the striatum of one side with 0.5 ug of cold kainate mixed with labelled ^{3}H-kainic acid. Some rats were treated for 12 h. with repeated injections of phenobarbital. The rats were killed at various time intervals and the caudate of each side was homogenized in 2 ml 90% ethyl alcohol, the homogenate was centrifuged and the supernatant was counted. Thin-layer chromatography of the alcoholic supernatant showed that more than 90% of the label was unchanged ^{3}H kainate. The radioactivity of the caudate of the injected side was always subtracted by that of the non-injected one. At 12 and 24 h. the values of the phenobarbital treated rats are significant different (p<0.05) from those of the controls. Values are the means of 4 rats.

75% after 38 hours from the intrastriatal infusion of kainate
in phenobarbital-treated rats.In this situation protection by
a barbiturate for up to 12 hours has only the effect of post-
poning kainate-neurotoxicity, so that three days thereafter
(the time necessary to allow the loss of striatal enzyme-
markers) no difference will be found between barbiturate
treated and control rats. Therefore, the difference between
phenobarbital and pentobarbital (and possibly benzodiazepines) could be due in part to the fact that only phenobarbital, due to its long half-life and to its tendency to satu-
rate the metabolic disposition processes upon repeated administration, affords protection from kainate-actions for a time
interval long enough to permit the concentrations of bound
kainate to be reduced to values below those effective in producing neurotoxicity.

Morphological changes
     If this hypothesis is correct, barbiturates should afford
protection for the whole duration of their action and therefore should prevent, in animals killed under their action,
the early histological changes of kainate-induced damage
(10).
     In order to investigate this point we injected 0.25 ug of
kainate in the caudate of one side to rats anaesthetized
with ether or phenobarbital (150 mg/kg). Rats were kept
anaesthetized with phenobarbital for 3 hours by repeated administration of the barbiturate and then they were sacrificed.
     In control rats this dose of kainate resulted in histologi-
 cal changes characterized by nuclear picnosis of striatal
neurons, formation of vacuoles of various sizes, enlargement
of capillaries (Fig.4). These changes affected uniformely an
area of about 1.5 mm diameter. Between this core and the
normal tissue, there was an area where nuclear picnosis
did not affect all neurons and the vacuolization appeared
less acute and diffuse.
     In phenobarbital treated rats (Fig.4) the area of diffuse
picnotic changes and of intense vacuolization was much less
extended, being present only around the cannula. In the
rest of the affected tissue the intensity of the changes resembled that typical of the area of incomplete damage produced
by kainate in control rats.
     Thus, from light-microscopic examination it is evident
that phenobarbital drastically reduced the early morphological changes produced by neurotoxic doses of kainate.

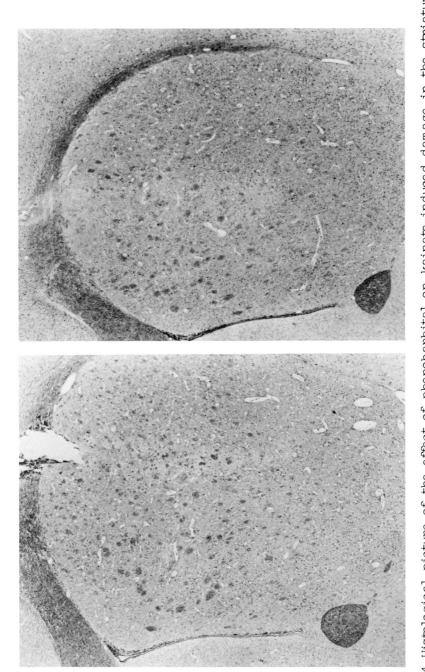

FIG.4 Histological picture of the effect of phenobarbital on kainate-induced damage in the striatum
A: Kainate-injected striatum of control rats (25x); B: idem of phenobarbital-treated rats

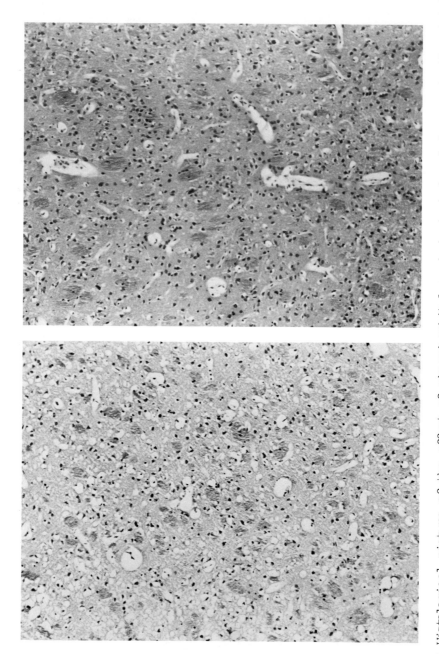

FIG.4 Histological picture of the effect of phenobarbital on kainate-induced damage in the striatum
C: Higher magnification (40x) of A; D: idem of B

Retinal Neurotoxicity

Neurochemical changes

Schwarcz and Coyle (14) reported that intravitreal kainic acid produced a rapid loss of GABA-ergic and cholinergic markers in the retina. As soon as 2 hours after 120 nmol. of kainate, retinal GAD and CAT were reduced by about 50%.

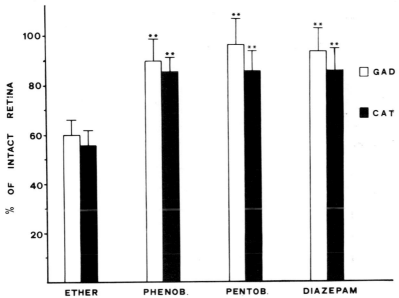

FIG. 5   Effect of barbiturates and benzodiazepines on retinal GAD and CAT loss after intravitreal kainate.
Control rats were anaesthetized with ether and injected intravitreally in one eye with 25 nmol of kainate and in the other one with saline. Other rats were similarly injected with kainate under anaesthesia with phenobarbital (150 mg/kg i.p.), pentobarbital (70 mg/kg i.p.) or with diazepam (30 mg/kg i.p.). In these rats the depressants were repeatedly administered at doses half of the first one in order to keep them deeply anaesthetized for 6 h., at which time they were killed and retina was isolated in order to measure GAD and CAT activity. Values are means ± s.e. of at least 6 determinations performed in triplicate expressed as percent of those in the intact retina. GAD and CAT values in the intact retina were 80±7 and 100±15 respectively (means ± s.e. of 6 determinations, expressed as nmol/mg prot/ hr.).
** p<0.001 in respect to controls (ether).

Such a rapid rate of loss of neurochemical markers in the
retina contrasts with the slowness of the same process in the
caudate, which, after effective doses of kainate, is completed
only after 3 days (6). For these characteristics the retina appears an ideal model to monitor the effect of depressant
drugs on kainate toxicity using neurochemical markers.

As shown in Fig.5, in rats a 6 h. anaesthesia with phenobarbital, pentobarbital or diazepam, significantly reduced,
the kainate-induced loss of GAD and CAT. In chicks, a 6 h.
treatment with diazepam was even more effective than in rats
in reducing the loss of GAD and CAT in the retina after 25
and 50 nmol. of intravitreal kainate. In fact, in chicks diazepam completely prevented the loss of neurochemical markers. In rats, as shown in Fig.6, when the dose of kainate
is increased, diazepam protects more effectively against the
loss of GAD than against the loss of CAT, indicating a certain selectivity of its protective action.

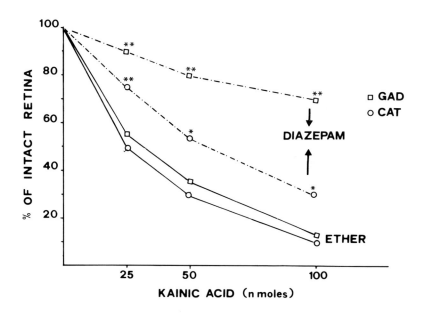

FIG. 6   Effect of diazepam on retinal GAD and CAT loss after increasing doses of intravitreal kainate in rats.
Rats were killed 6 h. after intravitreal kainate. For other
explanations see the legend to FIG.5
* p<0.05; ** p<0.001 in respect to controls (ether).

The ability of diazepam to protect against kainate-toxicity in the retina seems a general property related to excitotoxic processes as it applies also to the retinal neurotoxicity by intravitreal ibotenic acid or by quisqualic acid (data not shown).

Morphological changes

In order to investigate the morphological counterpart of the interaction between benzodiazepines and kainate in the retina, we injected 50 nmol. of kainate in the vitreous humor of chicks and 1 h. later the animals were sacrificed by perfusion with formalin and the eyes processed to be stained with hematoxilin or cresyl-violet. Fig.7 shows representative examples of the histolgical picture obtained. In control chicks injected with kainate intravitreally and anaesthetized with ether only during surgery, the photoreceptors and the outer nuclear layer (ONL) appeared normal, while the outer plexiform layer (OPL) was enlarged and filled up with vacuoles, particularly evident at the phase-contrast examination. The inner nuclear layer (INL) showed diffuse picnosis through all its extent except for a row of neurons adjacent to the OPL (horizontal cells?) which were characteristically spared. The inner plexiform layer (IPL) showed diffuse vacuolization through all its extent. The ganglion cell layer (GL) showed picnosis of only some elements. In rats treated with diazepam (30 mg/kg i.p.) we observed a similar vacuolization at the level of the OPL and IPL but definitely less nuclear picnosis at the level of the INL; in these rats the INL appeared three-layered, consisting of an external row of elements with normal nuclei (horizontal cells?) followed by an intermediate layer of diffuse nuclear picnosis (bipolar cells?) and by an innermost layer with only partial nuclear picnosis (amacrine cells?). Therefore in these conditions diazepam appears to protect from the picnosis of the inner third of the INL, possibly at the level of amacrines.

CONCLUSIONS

Our results demonstrate that in certain conditions barbiturates and benzodiazepines are capable to protect from local kainate toxicity on specific neuronal types as estimated by neurochemical methods. The efficacy of the depressants in protecting from local kainate-toxicity as estimated neurochemically depends from factors which are inherent to the

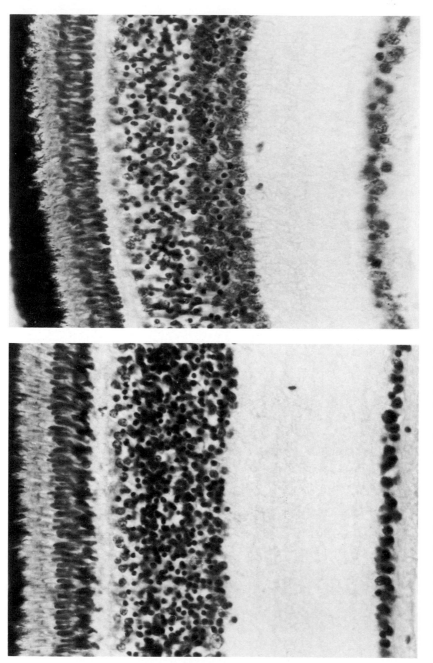

FIG.7 Early histological changes induced by kainate in the chick retina and the effect of diazepam
A: Retina of control chicks injected intravitreally with kainate (40x); B: idem with diazepam

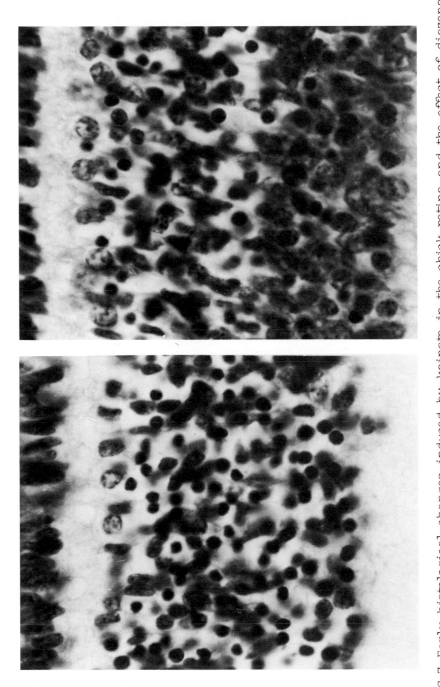

FIG.7 Early histological changes induced by kainate in the chick retina and the effect of diazepam
C: Inner nuclear layer (100x) of A; D: Inner nuclear layer (100x) of B

interaction at the cellular level between the depressants and kainic acid and to the pharmacokinetics of kainate and of the depressants but also to the requirements of the neurochemical technique as a mean to estimate kainate toxicity.

In fact, death of the neuron by kainate takes place within minutes (9) from application of the neurotoxin, while in certain areas, for example in the caudate, the loss of neurochemical markers is complete only after 3 days (6). Therefore, the loss of neurochemical markers after kainate rather than being the reflection of actual damage is the evolution of a process (death of the neuron) happened some time before. In the case of the striatum, the necessity of waiting 3 days before measuring neurochemical markers after local kainate administration coupled to the slow clearance of kainate from the locus of injection makes necessary a very prolonged treatment with the depressants in order to protect from kainate neurotoxicity. In these conditions the most effective depressants are those, like phenobarbital, which are provided with the longest biological half-life and which undergo accumulation after repeated administration.

Failure to undergo accumulation is probably one of the reasons for the failure of a 12 h. treatment with diazepam or clonazepam to reduce kainate-induced damage in the caudate. In contrast, in the retina diazepam and pentobarbital are as effective as phenobarbital in preventing the loss of neurochemical markers after intravitreal kainate. In this case, thanks to the fact that the loss of neurochemical markers in the retina after intravitreal kainate is faster and larger than in the caudate being significant, depending on the dose of kainate used, within 2–6 hours from kainate-application (14), the animals could be sacrificed by 6 hours after intravitreal kainate. With this short survival it was possible to keep the animals under continous treatment with the depressants for the whole period of the survival.

The ability of benzodiazepines and barbiturates to protect from the loss of markers of specific neurons indicates that the depressants protect from the neurotoxicity of kainate on these neurons. However in the retina, the GABA–ergic and cholinergic neurons are most probably only a small proportion of the whole population of neurons which undergo degeneration after intra-vitreal kainate. Therefore the fact that benzodiazepines protect from GAD and CAT loss does not mean that they should protect from the whole pattern of kainate-induced retinal neurotoxicity. This is probably the rea-

son why in spite of the complete protection exerted by diazepam on kainate-induced loss of GABA-ergic and cholinergic
markers, light-microscopic examination shows a reduction of
nuclear picnosis restricted to the inner third of the INL
while the vacuolization in the OPL and IPL appears unaffected. Such protection by benzodiazepines on the kainate-induced damage of neurons located in the INL is however consistent with the evidence that GABA-ergic and cholinergic neurons in the retina have their perikarya in the amacrine cell
layer (1,5,8).

The fact that depressants of neuronal excitability such
as barbiturates and benzodiazepines are capable to protect
from kainate-induced neurotoxicity on certain transmitter-spe-
cific neurons is an important evidence that kainate-induced
toxicity is related to its excitatory actions. Such hypothesis
has been challenged by Seil et al. (17,18 and this volume)
on the basis of two main arguments:
1) Among different classes of cultured cerebellar neurons
there is no relationship between stimulation of firing by kainate and sensitivity to kainate-induced damage.
2) Blockade by GABA of kainate-induced stimulation of firing
fails to protect from kainate-neurotoxicity.
The first argument is not a crucial one since increase in
membrane conductance rather than stimulation of firing might
be directly related to neurotoxicity. In fact, as shown by
Engberg and his collaborators (this volume) kainate, while
produces an irreversible and incommensurable increase of
conductance, is hardly capable of increasing neuronal firing.
Indeed, although both the increase in firing and the neurotoxicity are probably casually related to the conductance changes produced by the drug, one might predict that kainate,
at doses which result in neurotoxicity, produces conductance
changes of such an intensity to be less effective in eliciting
stimulation of firing.

Therefore, since in the studies of Seil et al. (17,18) no
measurements of conductance by intracellular recording were
performed, we cannot exclude the possibility that there is a
strict relationship between the sensitivity of a certain neuronal type to kainate-induced conductance changes and to kainate-induced damage.

On the other hand, the inability of GABA to block kainate toxicity at doses which block kainate-induced stimulation of firing (18) is not valid unless one demonstrates that
the depressant was capable to block kainate excitatory ac-

tions for the entire period of exposure to kainate. This indeed was not tested in the study of Seil et al. (18).

These considerations and our present findings indicate that Olney's original excitotoxic hypothesis of kainate neurotoxicity is still viable and might be even extended to the brain damage related to prolonged seizure activity. In this case, the excitotoxic agents would be some endogenous neurotransmitters like glutamate, aspartate or any other one capable of eliciting an intense and prolonged increase in conductance of neurons eventually provided with a particularly low seizure threshold (e.g. hippocampal pyramidal neurons). Perhaps, in view of the findings by Engberg et al.(this volume) and of the above considerations on the lack of relationship between stimulation of firing and neurotoxicity, one might refine Olney's original hypothesis by suggesting that neurotoxicity by excitatory agents is related rather than to excitation (stimulation of firing) to their ability to produce such a vast increase in conductance to functionally abolish the neuronal membrane. Complete permeabilisation of neuronal membrane and loss of internal milieu would mean, for a specialized element such as the neuron, a complete derangement of its functions and a rapid death.

REFERENCES

1. Baughman, R.W. and Bader, C.R. (1977): Brain Research, 138:469-485.
2. Ben-Ari, Y., Tremblay, E., Ottersen, O.P. and Naquet, R. (1979): Brain Research, 165:362-365.
3. Ben-Ari, Y., Tremblay, E. and Ottersen, O.P. (1980): Neuroscience, 5:515-528.
4. Kobayashi, R.M., Brownstein, M., Saavedra, J.M. and Palkovits, M. (1975): J.Neurochem., 24:637-640.
5. Marshall, J. and Voaden, M. (1976): In: Transmitters in the Visual Process, edited by E.G. McGeer, J.W. Olney and P.L. McGeer, pp. 107-125, Pergamon Press.
6. McGeer, P.L., McGeer, E.G. and Hattori, T. (1978): In: Kainic Acid as a Tool in Neurobiology, edited by E.G. McGeer, J.W. Olney and P.L. McGeer, pp.123-138, Raven Press, New York.
7. Nadler, J.V., Perry, B.W. and Cotman, C.W. (1978): In: Kainic Acid as a Tool in Neurobiology, edited by E.G. McGeer, J.W. Olney and P.L. McGeer, pp. 219-239, Raven Press, New York.

8. Nakamura, Y., McGuire B.A. and Sterling, P. (1980):- Proc. Nat. Acad. Sci. U.S.A., 77, pp.658-661.

9. Olney, J.W. (1978):In :Kainic Acid as a Tool in Neuro-biology, edited by E.G. McGeer, J.W. Olney, P.L. Mc-Geer, pp. 95-121, Raven Press, New York.

10. Olney, J.W., Fuller, T. and DeGubareff, T. (1979):Brain Research, 176:91-100.

11. Olney, J.W., Rhee, V. and Ho, O.L. (1974):Brain Re-search, 77:507-512.

12. Pellegrino, L.J. and Cushman, A.J. (1971): In: A Stereo-taxic Atlas of the Rat Brain, edited by L.J. Pellegrino and A.J. Cushman, Meredith, New York.

13. Ross, C.D. and McDougal Jr., D.B. (1976):J.Neurochem., 26:521-526.

14. Schwarcz, R. and Coyle, J.T. (1977):Invest. Ophthalmol. Visual Sci., 16:141-148.

15. Schwarcz, R., Scholz, D. and Coyle, J.T. (1978):Neuro-pharmacology, 17:145-151.

16. Schwob, J.E., Fuller, T., Price, J.L. and Olney, J.W. (1980): Neuroscience, 5:991-1041.

17. Seil, F.J., Blank, N.K. and Leiman, A.L. (1979):Brain Research, 161:253-265.

18. Seil, F.J., Woodward, W.R., Blank, N.K. and Leiman, A.L. (1978):Brain Research, 159:431-435.

19. Spano, P.F., Trabucchi, M. and Di Chiara, G. (1977):- Science, 196:1343-1344.

20. Tappaz, M.L., Brownstein, M.J. and Palkovits, M. (1976): Brain Research, 108:371-379.

21. Wuerthele, S.M., Lovell, K.L., Jones, M.A. and Moore, K.E. (1978):Brain Research, 149:489-497.

22. Yazulla, S. and Kleinschmidt, J. (1980):Brain Research, 182: 287-301.

23. Zaczek, R., Nelson, M.F. and Coyle, J.T. (1978):Eur. J. Pharmacol., 52:323-327.

Glutamate as a Neurotransmitter,
edited by G. Di Chiara and G. L. Gessa
Raven Press, New York © 1981.

Kainic Acid and Other Excitotoxins: A Comparative Analysis

John W. Olney

*Department of Psychiatry, Washington University School of Medicine,
St. Louis, Missouri 63110*

Kainic acid (KA) is one of the most powerful of a group of analogs of glutamate (Glu) and aspartate (Asp) that have both neuroexcitatory and neurotoxic activities and a parallel order of potencies for the two types of activity. Ultrastructurally, the toxic action of any of these agents appears to involve dendritic and somal membranes, where excitatory post-synaptic receptors are located, but does not involve axons. These were the basic observations that gave rise to the excitotoxic concept - that an excitatory mechanism underlies the neurotoxicity of these agents and that both the excitatory and toxic activities may be mediated through post-synaptic excitatory receptors, possibly receptors specialized for glutamergic or aspartergic transmission. While I have been inclined to stress the similarities among excitotoxins that permit classifying them as a group of like-acting neurotoxic agents, it is quite clear that there are important differences, especially between the heterocyclic newcomer KA and the more traditionally studied straight-chain Glu/Asp analogs. Here I will explore some of the more important similarities and differences between KA and other excitotoxins in an effort to ascertain how well KA fits the "excitotoxic" mold we began cultivating for it some years ago when its potent excitatory and neurotoxic properties first came to light.

SIMILARITIES AMONG EXCITOTOXINS

Molecular Specificities

The structure activity correlations developed initially in the 1960's by Curtis and colleagues (1, 2) pertaining to the excitatory activities of Glu analogs and the observations by my group (3-6) and Coyle and Schwarcz et al. (7, 8) in the 1970's, that parallel structure-activity correlations obtain for the neurotoxic activities of these agents, KA included, have powerfully conditioned my way of thinking about the neuroactive amino acids and,

of course, these correlations were what prompted me to coin the
term "excitotoxin" as a referent for these intriguing compounds
(3-6). These correlations strongly imply, not only that both the
excitatory and neurotoxic phenomena are receptor-mediated processes, but that the same general type of mechanism and class of receptor mediates both phenomena (which does not rule out receptor
subclasses, multiple co-factors and numerous other complicating
variables). My conviction on this theme was most recently reinforced by two simple studies, one pertaining to α-amino adipate
(αAA) and the other to mesencephalic fifth nucleus neurons.

The αAA Story

In 1971, we reported (3) that DL-αAA, when administered sc to
the immature mouse, exerts toxic activity against glia in the arcuate hypothalamic (AH) region but not against AH neurons (Fig.1).
Lack of the Glu-type AH neurotoxicity correlated well with the
earlier observation by Curtis and Watkins that DL-αAA was devoid
of Glu-type neuroexcitatory activity. To explore the stereoselectivity of the gliotoxicity of DL-αAA, we recently administered the
separate D and L isomers to immature mice and found (9) that D-αAA
induces mild gliotoxicity and no neurotoxicity but L-αAA causes a
striking toxic reaction that unequivocally has both gliotoxic *and*
neurotoxic features. In re-testing the DL-racemic preparation,
we again observed that it induces only a gliotoxic reaction without neurotoxic features.

The observation that L-αAA, which McLennan and Hall recently
described as a neuronal excitant (10), has significant neurotoxicity, lends new support for the excitotoxic hypothesis, but more
importantly, the neurotoxicity of the L-isomer and non-neurotoxi-
city of the DL-racemic preparation, signifies that D-αAA is an

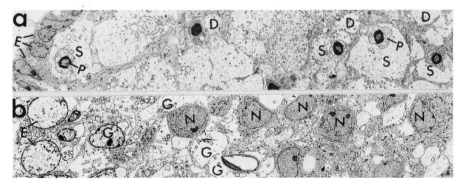

Fig. 1. (a) Glu administered orally (1 mg/g) to infant mouse.
Acute edematous degeneration of dendrosomal (D or S) components
of AH neurons, also nuclear pyknosis (P) while ependymal (E) and
glial elements are unaffected. (b) Administration of DL-αAA
(2 mg/g sc) to infant mouse; ependymal (E) and glial (G) elements
become grossly edematous while adjacent neurons (N) remain normal
(X 900) (modified from Olney et al., Ref. 3).

effective antagonist of the neurotoxicity of L-αAA. In other recent experiments, we demonstrated that DL-αAA
suppresses the AH neurotoxicity and the LH-releasing action of N-
methyl aspartate (NMA), both of which actions we believe are mediated by the depolarizing action of NMA on excitatory receptors
located on the dendrosomal surfaces of AH neurons. In microelectrophoretic studies (reviewed in Ref. 2), others have observed
that D-αAA effectively blocks both NMA-induced excitations and
physiologically stimulated synaptic transmission at certain puta-
tively Asp-preferring synapses. While blockade by D-αAA of both
the neurotoxic and excitatory actions of NMA at its excitatory receptor, as these several findings imply, fulfills the prediction
of the excitotoxic hypothesis in relation to NMA, similar proofs
in relation to KA have not been possible because of the lack of a
suitable antagonist for blocking the action of KA at the subclass
of receptor with which it may preferentially interact.

The Story of Mesencephalic Fifth Nucleus Neurons

One way of testing the hypothesis that Glu-type excitatory receptors mediate KA neurotoxicity would be to search for neurons
that are not sensitive to the toxic wrath of KA and see if they
are responsive to the excitatory actions of Glu. Since it has
been believed for a number of years that most, if not all, central neurons are responsive to the excitatory actions of Glu, and
recent research with KA suggests that the vast majority of central
neurons are also KA-destructible, it would presumably be more
than chance coincidence if a given type of central neuron could be
found which is totally unresponsive to either KA neurotoxicity or
the depolarizing actions of Glu. Colonnier (11), and Lund and
de Montigny (12) recently conducted the relevant experiments,
which began with the observation that mesencephalic fifth nucleus
neurons are insensitive to the toxic action of KA and ended with
the finding that these neurons are totally unresponsive to the
excitatory actions of either KA or Glu. While this does not pin-
point the specific receptor-mediated mechanisms that link KA neurotoxicity and the excitatory action of Glu, it does keep very
much alive the prospect that the link is there awaiting elucidation.

Cellular and Subcellular Specificities

Consistent with the excitotoxic hypothesis, we have observed
(6) that the earliest detectable changes in CNS neurons following
exposure to any excitotoxin, including KA, is acute swelling of
post-synaptic dendrosomal elements in the absence of changes in
the presynaptic axonal bouton (Figs. 2a-g). Another prominent
feature of the early toxic reaction in neurons is in specific
mitochondria located in the affected dendrosomal portions of the
neuron (Fig. 2a,b). These mitochondria undergo transient swelling at the same time that the dendrosomal elements first become
edematous, then their membranes become thickened and the entire
organelle undergoes a condensation and vacuolization reaction

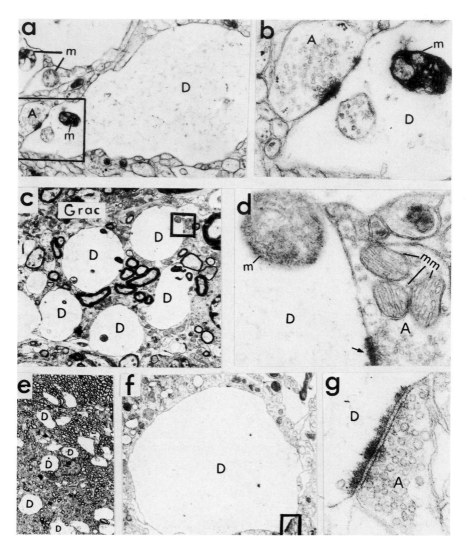

FIG. 2. (a,b) Acute edematous degeneration of dendritic (D) but
not axonal (A) elements in mouse AH 30 min after sc Glu. Note
several stages of pathological changes in dendritic mitochondria
(m). (c,d) Similar dendrotoxic changes with axonal sparing in
nucleus gracilis (Grac) 45 min after intraventricular injection
of KA, 15 nmoles. Note abnormal mitochondrion (m) in degenerating
dendrite (D) and normal mitochondria (mm) in presynaptic axonal
bouton (A); synapse at arrow. (e-g) acute toxic changes in dendrites (D) but not axons (A) in hippocampus (CA-1 basilar dendritic field) 4 hrs after sc injection of KA, 12 mg/kg to adult rat
(a,c,e & f = X500-10,000; b & d = X36,000; g = X50,000). (Modified from Olney et al., Refs. 6, 13 and 15).

that gives its internal content an irregular, smudged and darkened appearance. Mitochondria in nearby axon terminals retain a normal appearance, which suggests the possibility that the drastic changes in dendritic mitochondria reflect an effort on the part of these energy-generating organelles to replenish the energy being spent in the cell's futile attempt to restore ionic balance across its continuously depolarized plasma membrane.

When KA is administered either intraventricularly (Fig. 2c,d) or systemically (Fig. 2e-g), it induces dendrotoxic changes in many CNS regions that are not fundamentally different from the dendrosomal swelling and mitochondrial changes seen in lesions produced by other excitotoxins (4, 6, 13, 14). In addition, there are features of the early pathological reaction to KA, especially in the hippocampal and olfactory cortices, that could possibly be regarded as unique. One of the earliest detectable responses in these cortical areas is massive swelling of specific astroglia that surround the cell bodies of pyramidal neurons (14), and the first detectable changes in the cell bodies of the pyramidal neurons tend to be dark cell changes (condensation of cytoplasmic and nucleoplasmic compartments with loss of cell water). Dark cell changes are a recognized characteristic of any excitotoxin lesion but usually only a small fraction of the neurons at the lesion site respond in this manner. Thus, it is not clear whether the dark cell transformations seen in pyramidal hippocampal and olfactory neurons following KA administration should be considered evidence that KA does or does not behave like other excitotoxins.

Glial swelling is a recognized accompaniment of lesions produced by large doses of the straight-chain excitotoxins. For example, systemic administration of large doses of Glu results in glial swelling as well as neuronal necrosis in the arcuate hypothalamic nucleus (AH)(15). The gliotoxic reaction to Glu, however, is readily dissociable from Glu neurotoxicity since the gliotoxic reaction is only seen following massive doses of Glu; lower doses produce a neurotoxic reaction without gliotoxicity. Moreover, systemic administration of the Glu analog, DL-αAA, causes a gliotoxic AH reaction in the absence of neurotoxic manifestations. Since the AH gliotoxic and neurotoxic reactions can be reproduced independently of one another, neither can be considered causally dependent upon the other. The neurotoxic and gliotoxic reactions in the limbic cortex of KA-treated rats, however, are not readily dissociable phenomena and we suspect that the latter occurs as a result of the former (see below).

DISSIMILARITIES

Regional and Species Specificities

When straight-chain excitotoxins are administered systemically, they all induce lesions which are selective for circumventricular organ (CVO) regions of brain. Lack of blood brain barriers in CVO brain regions seems to be the best explanation for the regional selectivity of excitotoxic lesions for these areas (16,17).

The regional distribution of lesions following systemic KA administration to adult rats is distinctly dissimilar to the above. Initially, we administered KA to mice in an attempt to induce typical CVO lesions, and were able to do so in a few animals, but a lesioning dose was always rapidly lethal (4). Subsequently, we administered KA systemically (10-12 mg/kg sc) to adult rats, and found that it induces a widespread pattern of brain damage that runs rampantly through the entorhinal and pyriform cortices, several amygdaloid nuclei, the hippocampus (Fig. 2), lateral septal nucleus and several thalamic nuclei - but with total sparing of all CVO zones (13, 14). We have reviewed slides from our previous mouse studies and do not find evidence in the mouse for this pattern of brain damage (except for rather atypical hippocampal changes).

Tentatively we interpret the above observations as follows: The heterocyclic structure of KA may confer different properties on this molecule with regard to its penetrability of cerebral vasculature. Thus, it may have general access to both CVO and non-CVO brain regions and the pattern of non-CVO brain damage induced by KA may reflect relative hypersensitivity of certain non-CVO neurons compared to the relative hyposensitivity of CVO neurons to KA. In addition, however, we suspect that an epileptic mechanism mediates much of the brain damage induced by systemic KA (see below), whereas this is not the case for other excitotoxins; if so, differences between mice and rats in limbic circuitry may account for the different responses of these species to systemic KA administration.

Distant Lesions

KA produces "distant" as well as local lesions when introduced by direct injection into the brain (14, 18). Distant lesions probably occur only in association with extensive convulsive activity, although this correlation has not been established by systematic observations. We have administered N-methyl DL-aspartate (NMA), the most potent commercially available straight-chain excitotoxin, directly into various brain regions (Olney, J.W. and Fuller, T.A., unpublished) and find that it faithfully induces an impressive Glu/Asp-type lesion locally wherever it is introduced (Fig. 3), but does not induce distant lesions nor does it produce the temporal lobe status epilepticus associated with KA injection. Regions where we have introduced NMA (pyriform cortex, amygdala, several hippocampal regions and caudate nucleus) are regions in which KA cannot be injected without producing distant lesions and temporal lobe status epilepticus at least some of the time. While these findings certainly suggest that NMA and KA differ in their neurotoxic behaviors, this does not rule out the possibility that an excitatory mechanism underlies the neurotoxicity of both agents. It is entirely possible, for example, that KA acts by an excitotoxic mechanism comparable to that of NMA and, in addition, acts by other mechanisms which merely complicate the excitotoxic picture.

The Role of Convulsions

All excitotoxins induce convulsions (generalized tonic-clonic seizures and sometimes "running fits") if administered in sufficient dosage systemically, but KA induces convulsions which are qualitatively different. KA-type convulsions are referable more specifically to the limbic lobe and eventuate in status epilepticus of the limbic system. Staring and wet-dog shakes typically occur early after sc KA (10-12 mg/kg) and these behaviors correlate with transient seizures (recordable by depth electrodes) within the limbic system (19). In more severe cases, a "rearing, praying, salivating" pattern of behavior occurs repetitively with increasing frequency until there is little or no respite between seizures (status epilepticus); some animals expire during the period of status seizures, which may last several hours, and some survive. In either case, if the brain is examined after such seizure activity there is always a characteristic pattern of damage affecting limbic structures. Diazepam protects against convulsions and much of the brain damage induced by systemic administration of KA (20), just as it protects against both the convulsions and distant lesions following intra-amygdaloid injection of KA (18). Although diazepam also prevents convulsions in rats given massive systemic doses of straight-chain excitotoxins, it does not protect against the CVO brain damage associated with such treatment (Olney, J.W., unpublished); moreover, straight-chain excitotoxins readily produce CVO brain damage at non-convulsive doses, whereas the limbic pattern of brain damage induced by systemic KA does not seem

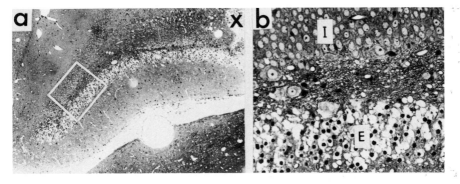

Fig. 3. (a) Forty nmoles of N-methyl-DL-Asp (NMA) in 0.5 µl was injected 4 hrs earlier into the adult rat hippocampus at X, a locus between the CA-3,4 region and external layer of dentate granule (DG) neurons. Some of the CA-3 pyramidal neurons to the right of the injection site degenerated (not shown), but the most dramatic toxic reaction was evident in external DG neurons. (b) Degenerating external (E) but well preserved internal (I) DG neurons from boxed region. This animal did not display any obvious seizuring and distant brain lesions were looked for but not found. (a = X 30; b = X 180).

to occur in the absence of significant seizure activity. These various observations all tend to support the view initially propounded by Nadler et al. (21) and Ben-Ari et al. (18), that seizure activity per se may play a causal role in damage sustained in limbic regions of KA-treated rats.

Recently we observed that diphenylhydantoin does not protect against convulsions or brain damage induced by systemic administration of KA (22). Since diazepam does effectively protect against both KA-induced convulsions and brain damage, it may be of value to explore the possible role of benzodiazepine receptors and perhaps GABAergic transmitter mechanisms in KA neurotoxicity, e.g., could KA be interfering with GABAergic inhibitory circuits at the same time that it hyperexcites glutamergic circuits to give a combined effect that differs from the more simple hyperexcitation mechanism of other excitotoxins? KA may simultaneously hyperexcite and disinhibit limbic circuits causing them to fire continuously in perhaps a self-perpetuating cycle until pathological changes occur in the post-synaptic elements receiving the brunt of the discharge activity. Since the excitatory transmitters being released at many of the synapses in these limbic circuits may be Glu or Asp, this would represent an example of an endogenous excitotoxic brain damage phenomenon being triggered by an exogenous excitotoxin (KA). Conceivably, the various dendrotoxic changes we have described in the hippocampus in the early period following KA administration, and which we have attempted to correlate with the location of glutamergic or aspartergic post-synaptic receptors (13), may be a reflection of these receptors being excessively stimulated by repetitive release of natural transmitter (Glu or Asp) rather than by direct action of KA on these receptors. It seems more likely, however, that it may involve a complex combination of factors: (1) natural transmitters being repetitively released at these receptors; (2) KA blocking their reuptake, thereby causing them to accumulate, with KA, at the receptor; (3) KA acting with natural transmitter to enhance and prolong its depolarizing action on the receptor.

Recently we reported (20) that systemically administered morphine markedly augments the neurotoxicity (both limbic convulsions and brain damage) of KA. One possible interpretation would be that morphine is acting at certain enkephalin receptors in the hippocampus where opiates are thought to block GABAergic transmission. If morphine were to join KA in blocking GABAergic transmission while KA is simultaneously hyperexciting limbic circuits, this would explain why morphine augments KA neurotoxicity.

The glial swelling observed in the hippocampal and olfactory pyramidal layers in KA-treated rats may reflect repetitive depolarization of pyramidal neurons with consequent release of K^+ which, when present in high extracellular concentration, may depolarize and alter the membrane permeability of astrocytes. Thus, this type of glio-toxic reaction may occur secondary to the hyperexcitation/disinhibition neurotoxic process which we postulate as the primary mode of toxic interaction between KA and brain.

Dipiperidinoethane, A Kaino-Mimetic Convulsant and Neurotoxin

Earlier this year, Levine and Sowinski (23) reported that sc administration of dipiperidinoethane (DPE) to adult rats acutely destroys neurons in the amygdala, pyriform cortex, hippocampus and related brain regions. Although these authors did not observe convulsions in their DPE-treated rats, we have now examined the neuroactive properties of DPE and find (24) that a single sc dose (400 mg/kg) reproduces in the adult rat both the limbic status epilepticus syndrome and the limbic pattern of brain damage that characterizes the neurotoxicity of systemically administered KA; moreover, diazepam (20 mg/kg sc) prevents DPE, just as it prevents KA, from inducing either convulsions or limbic brain damage. Paradoxically, when DPE is injected directly into the amygdala in relatively high doses (400 nmoles), it does not cause either convulsions or significant histopathological changes either locally or in distant brain regions. It is of interest that DPE, although not closely related in structure to KA, does resemble tremorine, a putative cholinergic agonist. Since DPE is relatively non-toxic when introduced directly into limbic brain regions, it will be important to explore the possibility that DPE owes its convulsogenic and brain damaging actions to an active metabolite generated peripherally. If such a metabolite exists, will its molecular structure resemble that of KA or will it retain features of the tremorine molecule which presumably confer cholinergic agonist activity? Elucidation of the mechanism of DPE neurotoxicity may yield valuable clues to the mechanism underlying KA-induced status seizures and limbic brain damage. In view of the strong possibility that the brain damage induced by either KA or DPE is a seizure-induced form of brain damage, and since both of these brain damage syndromes are preventable by early treatment with diazepam, KA and DPE are very promising chemical tools for studying mechanisms of epilepsy and epileptic brain damage and for developing therapeutic or prophylactic approaches to these conditions in man.

CONCLUSIONS

I have compared the neurotoxicity of KA with that of other excitatory analogs of Glu. An important feature distinguishing KA from other excitotoxins is its ability to induce sustained limbic seizures and widespread limbic brain damage. Conjecturally, I have proposed an explanation: KA may act by a compound hyperexcitation/disinhibition mechanism, whereas, other excitotoxins act by simple hyperexcitation without disinhibition. A kaino-mimetic agent (DPE), which may shed new light on the mechanism of KA neurotoxicity, is described.

ACKNOWLEDGMENTS

Supported in part by USPHS grants NS-09156, DA-00259, Career Research Scientist Award MH-38894 and a Wills Foundation grant.

REFERENCES

1. Curtis, D.R. and Watkins, J.C. (1960): J. Neurochem., 6:117-141.
2. Watkins, J.C. (1978): In Kainic Acid As A Tool In Neurobiology, edited by E.G. McGeer, J.W. Olney and P.L. McGeer, pp. 37-70. Raven Press, New York.
3. Olney, J.W., Ho, O.L. and Rhee, V. (1971): Exp. Brain Res. 14: 61-76.
4. Olney, J.W., Rhee, V. and Ho, O.L. (1974): Brain Res. 77: 507-512.
5. Olney, J.W., Sharpe, L.G. and de Gubareff, T. (1975): Neurosci. Abstr. 1: 371.
6. Olney, J.W. (1978): In Kainic Acid As A Tool In Neurobiology, edited by E.G. McGeer, J.W. Olney and P.L. McGeer, pp.95-121, Raven Press, New York.
7. Coyle, J.T., Biziere, K. and Schwarcz, R. (1978): In Kainic Acid As A Tool In Neurobiology, edited by E.G. McGeer, J.W. Olney and P.L. McGeer, pp. 177-188, Raven Press, New York.
8. Schwarcz, R., Scholz, D. and Coyle, T.J. (1978): Neuropharmacology 17: 145-151.
9. de Gubareff, T., Olney, J.W., Collins, J.F. (1980): Neurosci. Abstr., in press.
10. McLennan, H. and Hall, J.C. (1978): Brain Res. 149: 541-545.
11. Colonnier, M., Steriade, M. and Landry, P. (1979): Brain Res. 172: 552-556.
12. Lund, J.P. and de Montigny, C. (1979): Neurosci. Abstr. 5: 592.
13. Olney, J.W., Fuller, T., de Gubareff, T. (1979): Brain Res. 176: 91-100.
14. Olney, J.W. and de Gubareff, T. (1978): In Kainic Acid As A Tool In Neurobiology, edited by E.G. McGeer, J.W. Olney and P.L. McGeer, pp. 201-217, Raven Press, New York.
15. Olney, J.W. (1971): J. Neuropath. Exp. Neurol. 30: 75-90.
16. Perez, V.J. and Olney, J.W. (1972): J. Neurochem. 19: 777-1782.
17. Price, M.T., Olney, J.W., Lowry, O.H. and Buchsbaum, S. (1980): Neurosci. Abstr., in press.
18. Ben-Ari, Y., Tremblay, E., Oltersen, D.P. and Noquet, R. (1979): Brain Res. 165: 362-365.
19. Collins, R.C., McLean, M., Lothman, E., Klunk, W., Olney, J. (1980): Epilepsia 21: 186.
20. Fuller, T. and Olney, J.W. (1979): Neurosci. Abstr. 5: 556.
21. Nadler, V., Perez, B.W., Cotman, C.W. (1978): Nature 271: 676-677.
22. Fuller, T. and Olney, J.W. (1980): Neurosci. Abstr., in press.
23. Levine, S. and Sowinski, R.J. (1980): J. Neuropath. Exp. Neurol. 39: 56-64.
24. Olney, J.W., Fuller, T., Collins, R.C. and de Gubareff, T. (1980): Neurosci. Abstr., in press.

Glutamate as a Neurotransmitter,
edited by G. Di Chiara and G. L. Gessa
Raven Press, New York © 1981.

Epilepsy: Changes in Local Glucose Consumption and Brain Pathology Produced by Kainic Acid

Y. Ben-Ari

Laboratoire de Physiologie Nerveuse, Département de Neurophysiologie Appliquée, C.N.R.S. 91190 Gifs/Yvette, France

INTRODUCTION

Limbic structures are highly vulnerable to a variety of deleterious conditions, such as chronic temporal lobe epilepsy and status epilepticus. Thus, in mesial temporal sclerosis -which is the commonest cerebral lesion found in patients with epilepsy in institutions (11), the hippocampal neurons degenerate and are replaced by a proliferation of glial elements (6). Brain damage is also found in other structures which are part of (or strongly connected with) the "limbic" system such as the amygdala, medial thalamus and limbic cortex.

A similar pattern of vulnerability has been observed in experimental animals following systemic, intracerebroventricular or focal intracerebral injections of kainic acid (2,12,15). This pattern could reflect a differential sensitivity to the toxin. However, the administration of the toxin also induces severe epileptiform activity and generalized seizures (see below) ; since there is good clinical experimental correlation between seizure duration and incidence and severity of pathological sequelae (6) the possibility that these discharges themselves provoke the brain damage requires investigation. In the present chapter, the electrographic, clinical and histological sequelae of systemic or intracerebral administration of kainic acid are reviewed with special reference to the pathology of epilepsy. Also, the local glucose utilisation following KA administration is described.

INJECTION OF KAINIC ACID IN THE AMYGDALOID COMPLEX

A. Electrographic and clinical correlates

Injections of KA (usually 1.2 µg in 0.3 µl phosphate buffer)
via a chronically implanted cannula in the unanaesthetized,
unrestrained rat, produces repetitive secondarily generalized
convulsive seizures. 5 to 60 min. after the injection, epileptiform activity accompanied by wet shakes was apparent in the
amygdala ; the sustained epileptiform activity rapidly propagated to the ipsilateral ammon's horn (fig. 1, case EAK 12) and
contralateral amygdala ; after a longer delay it also involved
the cortical EEG. The motor events were similar to those induced
by daily electrical stimulation of the amygdala (i.e. "kindling",
see ref. 9) ; they include head nodding, masticatory movements,
facial myoclonus, forepaw tremor, rearing and falling . These
typical "amygdaloid" seizures were recurrent at a variable
frequency (often one per 2-10 min.) for periods of 1 to 4 hrs.
A longer delays the motor events were more complex and included
circling, barrel rotation and intense agitation.

B. Brain damage

After short survival times (e.g. 1-2 hrs) at the site of
injection, the neuronal somata were shrunken, triangular and
darkly staining. During the subsequent few hours, the neurons
became fragmented and finally disappeared. Depending on the dose
(and volume) of KA injected, these pathological alterations were
confined to a single amygdaloid nucleus whereas the entire complex and adjacent structures were affected in others cases. It
is worth noting that the abundant microglial proliferation which
was apparent already 10-20 hrs after the injection, can be used
to evaluate the extent of diffusion of KA ; in the "remote"
brain damage (see below) the gliosis which was very modest (or
completely absent), was not apparent before several days.
Outside the site of injection, the earliest pathological change
(30 to 90 min. after the injection) were particularly prominent
in the rostral CA3 hippocampal field (see fig. 2A-B-C). These
changes were characterized : a) by an intense argyrophylic color-
ation at the distal segment of the CA3 apical dendrites which
are innervated by the perforant path (10) ; b) by a vacuolization at the level of the proximal segments of the CA3 apical
dendrites which are innervated by the mossy fibers (5) ; c) by
the distortion and shrinking of the pyramidal perikarya (fig.1C).
At longer survival times, the ipsilateral hippocampal lesions
proceeds to a complete necrosis of CA3-CA1 and CA4 ipsilaterally
whereas CA2 and the fascia dentata are usually preserved. In
addition, to pyramidal neurons, degenerated interneurons could
be identified. Pathological alterations were present in other
distant structures in particular after longer survival times ;

these included : the contralateral hippocampus and amygdala,
bilaterally the claustrum, cingulate cortex and neocortex
(layers III, V and VI) adjacent to the rhinal sulcus and midline
thalamic nuclei bilaterally the medio-dorsal, parataenial,
reuniens, postero-median and parafascicular complex).

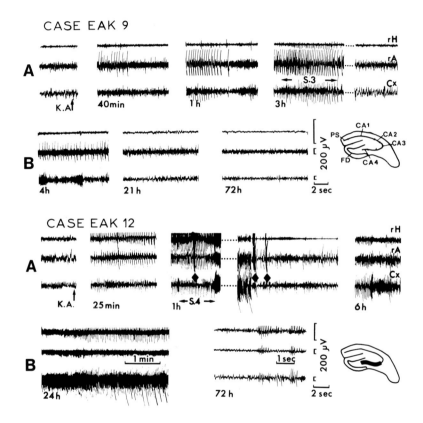

FIG. 1

   Relationship between seizure severity and associated pathology
in the right hippocampus (rH) after KA in the right amygdala (rA).
In case EAK 9 their was little seizure activity in the right
hippocampus and no subsequent hippocampal pathology (schematic
diagram). In case EAK 12 their was a rapid spread (25 min.) of
spike discharges to hippocampus and cortex (cx). Spikes were seen
after 24h and intermittently after 72h. Neuronal loss was conspicuous in CA3-CA4. Survival time 3 days for both cases.
S3 : mouth and facial myoclonus, head nodding, forelimb clonus.
S4 : rearing and forepaw tremor ; lozenge : wet shakes.

C. Relationship between seizure discharge and subsequent hippocampal pathology

As already noted, ammon's horn ipsilateral to the injected amygdala -in particular the CA3 field- was by far the most susceptible to the epileptogenic action of KA. Inspection of the electrographic records revealed a good correlation between the severity of seizure discharge in the hippocampus and the subsequent pathology ; thus : a) in different cases, the more severe the epileptiform discharge in the hippocampus (in terms of postictal depressions or seizure discharge associated with motor activity) the more prominent the subsequent pathology (see fig.1 and ref. 3) ; b) within a given case, the ipsilateral hippocampus displayed more severe seizure discharge than the contralateral one (3) ; c) within the ipsilateral ammon's horn, the epileptiform activity appeared first and was more prominent in CA3 than CA1 or other hippocampal regions (not illustrated). The epileptiform activity was readily blocked by i.p. administration of diazepam. To investigate the relationship between seizure and brain damage, repeated doses of diazepam (3-5 mg/kg i.p.) were administered starting from the onset of epileptiform activity in the injected amygdala. This treatment reduced considerably the electrographic and clinical consequences of intra-amygdaloid injections of KA as well as the distant brain damage. In contrast, the damage at the site of injection was similar to that seen in control cases, in spite of the reduction of the severity

FIG. 2 : Photomicrographs of frontal sections through the hippocampal formation in rats submitted to intra-amygdaloid injections of KA without (A,B,C) and with D,E,F) a preceding transection of the perforant path. A : Early hippocampal lesion in case EAK29 (survival time 7 hrs). The pathological alterations included the stratum lucidum (Lu), lacunosum moleculare (LM) and pyramidale. The stratum lucidum appears spongy or "vacuolated". Fink-Heimer (8). Bar = 250 μm. B : Larger magnification of degenerating pyramidal cells in CA3 at a more caudal level than A (case EAK29). Both apical and basal dendrites show argyrophilia. Fink-Heimer stain, bar 80 μm. C : CA3 pyramidal neurons at a frontal level adjacent to the one shown in A (EAK29). The cells are shrunken and have a triangular shape, compare to F ; Nissl stain, bar = 35 μm. D : Degeneration of axons terminals in the stratum lacunosum moleculare of CA1 and outer twothirds (MP) of the dentate molecular layer due to the interruption of the perforant path (case E1, 4 days survival). Fink-Heimer stain, bar = 240 μm. E : Nissl stained section through the septal one-third of the hippocampus in case EAK20, the area enclosed in the rectangle is shown at higher magnification in F. No pathological changes are present ; compare with C. E : bar : 700 μm, F = same magnification as C. O,P and R indicate the strata oriens, pyramidale and radiatum respectively. G : Granular layer of fascia dentata.

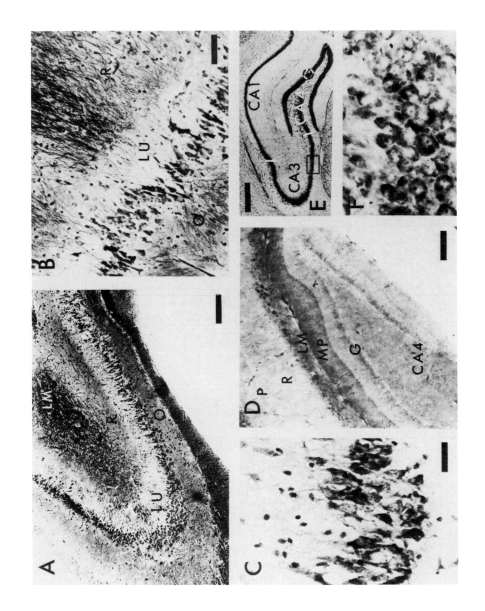

of the epileptiform activity often observed (1,4). In an effort
to investigate the anatomical support of the propagation of the
epileptiform activity to the hippocampus and its subsequent
pathological consequences, the perforant path was unilaterally
transected before the intra-amygdaloid injection of KA. Unilateral perforant path transection was found to both reduce the severity of seizure manifestations and hippocampal brain damage without affecting to toxic action of KA at the site of injection
(see fig. 2 and ref. 4).

INJECTIONS OF KA IN OTHER BRAIN SITES

Injections of KA in other telencephalic structures induced
a different pattern of clinical events and subsequent pathological alteration. Thus, following an injection of KA in the bed
nucleus of the stria terminalis or preoptic region (in similar
doses and conditions as described above), the animal exhibited
wet shakes, circling behavior, exophtalmos, abundant salivation,
lacrimation, tail rigidity and vihissae tremor. Little (or no)
seizure discharge was present in the hippocampus. One week later,
in spite of the severe necrosis present at the site of injection,
hippocampal damage was seldom present. Similar results were
obtained following an injection of the toxin in the septum. In
contrast injections of KA in the caudal caudate putamen or globus
pallidus produced severe motor seizures (including barrel rotation, general agitation and with a longer delay "amygdaloid"
type motor seizures) and pathological alterations in the ipsilateral CA3-CA4 hippocampal fields.

SYSTEMIC ADMINISTRATION OF KA

Systemic administration (i.p.) of the toxin readily produced
motor and EEG seizures similar to those seen after intra-amygdaloid KA. The epileptiform activity appeared first and was more
sustained the entorhinal cortex (20 min. after the injection),
it then propagated to the amygdala and ammon's horn (CA3 field).
After 9 mg/kg (i.p.), the animal displayed numerous wet shakes
(50 to 80 wet shakes 30 to 45 min. after the injection), and the
first "amygdaloid type" seizure (see above) usually 30 min. later.
Similar convulsions were recurrently present during 15-60 min.at
a frequency of one every 5 min. After longer delays more complex
motor events were noted, they often included agitation, circling,
jumps (4). Diazepam administration readily abolished the epileptiform and motor events.
Neuronal necrosis after systemic KA was found bilaterally in
the neocortex (layers III, V and VI), hippocampus (CA4, CA1 and
CA3 fields), the amygdala, medial thalamic structures such as the
medio-dorsal and reuniens) and the pyriform and entorhinal cortices. Damage was also found in the anterior olfactory nucleus
and related structures (also see ref. 15).

LOCAL CONSUMPTION OF GLUCOSE FOLLOWING SYSTEMIC
OR INTRACEREBRAL INJECTIONS OF KA

In an effort to examine the local changes in metabolism in relation to seizure activity and the subsequent brain damage, the (^{14}C) deoxyglucose method developped by Sokoloff (16) was used. Following systemic or intracerebral KA, a rise in local metabolism was found almost exclusively in those limbic structures in which pathological alterations have been found. Thus, as previously reported by Sokoloff (16), in control cases, the radioactive material was concentrated in the inferior colliculi, medial geniculate and neocortex. In contrast, less than 1h after the administration of KA (i.e. before the first seizure, the animal had displayed only wet shakes), the radioactive material was almost exclusively concentrated in the hippocampus and entorhinal cortex and decreased from the neocortex. 1 to 4 hrs after the injection (see fig. 3) labelling was almost exclusively confined to the amygdala, stria terminalis fibers and bed nucleus, limbic

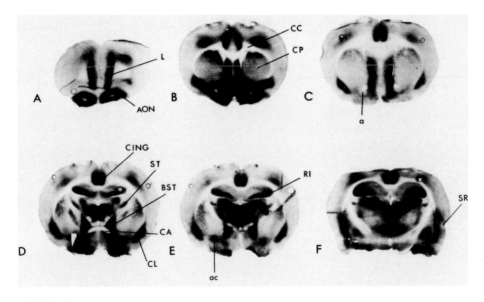

FIG. 3
Changes in local metabolism following systemic (i.p.) administration of KA and 2 hrs of convulsive seizures. Abbreviations : ac : accumbens ; AON : anterior olfactory nucleus ; BST : bed nucleus of the stria terminalis ; CA : anterior commissure ; CING : cingulate cortex ; CC : corpus callosum ; CP : caudate putamen ; CL : claustrum ; L : limbic (frontal) cortex ; RI : regio inferior ; SR : sulcus rhinalis ; ST : stria terminalis.

cortex (infra- and pre-limbic, cingulate and cortex adjacent
to the rhinal fissure), lateral septum, ammon's horn (CA3-CA4
fields) medial thalamus in particular medio-dorsal nucleus) and
the anterior olfactory nucleus (fig. 3 and refs 2 and 7). It is
worth noting the considerable decrease in labelling of neocortex.
2-3 days after the injection of KA, this decrease in labelling
was still present. A bilateral intense labelling was exclusively
present in the lateral or medial amygdala.

Following an intra-amygdaloid injection of the toxin, a rise
in local metabolism was noted at the site of injection 30-60 min.
later. In addition the labelling was increased ipsilaterally in
the adjacent caudate putamen and pyriform cortex, stria terminalis system and frontal limbic cortex, ammon's horn and medial
thalamus. An increase in metabolism was also conspicuous, in
the contralateral claustrum,ammon's horn and amygdala in several
cases (report in preparation).

DISCUSSION

The following observations suggest that the remote brain
damage seen after focal intra-amygdaloid (or intra-striatal)
injections of the toxin cannot be readily attributed to a
diffusion of small amonts of KA to areas of high sensitivity
(1,3,4) : 1. Damage in the medial thalamus contralateral to the
injected site is often larger than the ipsilateral one ; 2. In
ammon's horn, the damage occurs earlier -and often is limited
to- the rostral (septal) pole rather than the caudal region
which is closer to the injected amygdala ; 3. Injections of KA
in the septum or BST-preoptic area do not readily reproduce the
hippocampal pathology, in contrast small injections in the more
distant entorhinal cortex are particularly efficient to elicit
hippocampal damage (15) ; 4. Following injections of ^{3}H-KA
(5 mmol/1 μg) into the striatum, very small amounts of radioactivity are found in areas other than the injection site (14) ;
5. There is a good relationship between the severity of epileptiform discharge in ammon's horn and the subsequent pathological
alterations ; 6. Repeated administration of a potent anticonvul-
sivant reduces or abolishes the epileptiform activity and remote
brain damage without affecting the local lesions (1,4) ; 7.
Important morphological differences between the local and remote
lesions are observed (microglial proliferation), this suggests
that different aetiological factors may be involved ; 8. Destruction of the perforant path abolishes distant but not local
(intra-amygdaloid) damage (4), in contrast a similar procedure
does not abolishe the hippocampal damage following i.c.v. administration of KA (13).

The possibility of uptake and distant release of the toxin
(or its metabolite) is also unlikely since : 1. There are no
direct connections in either direction between central amygdala
and ammon's hors ; 2. There is little (or no) damage in structures strongly interconnected with the central amygdala such as

the BST or the nucleus parabrachialis ; 3. There are important morphological differences between the local and remote damage (see above) ; 4. The onset of pathological alterations in the hippocampus (30 min.) cannot be readily reconciled with a possible uptake and transport of the toxin.

These observations suggest therefore that the intense epileptic activity is responsible for a large part of the remote neuronal loss or necrosis seen after local KA injections. Furthermore, using the deoxyglucose method (16) it has been shown that following systemic (also see ref. 7) or focal intracerebral injection of the toxin, there is an increase in neuronal metabolism in the hippocampus and other limbic structures in which epileptiform activity and lesions are present. This suggests that the pathological alterations are causally related to the excessive increase in neuronal activity and metabolism.

In conclusion, simple clinical observation provides an inadequate indication of the diffuse and sustained nature of the epileptic activity that follows the administration of kainic acid. The absence of EEG recordings in previous studies has led to an underestimation of the role of epileptic activity in the behavioural and structural abnormalities that follow intracerebral injections of KA. As a tool to produce circumscribed brain damages ; the common use of intracerebral injections of KA appears unwarranted. On the other hand, the acute clinical, electrographic, metabolic and pathological sequelae of systemic or intracerebral administration of the toxin constitute a particularly suitable model to investigate the relationship between epilepsy and brain damage.

The author acknowledges financial support from INSERM (CRL) and CNRS (ATP).

REFERENCES

1. Ben-Ari, Y., Tremblay, E., Ottersen, O.P., and Naquet, R. (1979) : Brain Res., 165 : 632-635.

2. Ben-Ari, Y., Riche, D., Tremblay, E. et Charton, G. (1980a) : C.R. Acad. Sci. (Paris), in press.

3. Ben-Ari, Y., Tremblay, E., and Ottersen, O.P. (1980b) : Neuroscience, 5 : 510-528.

4. Ben-Ari, Y., Tremblay, E., Ottersen, O.P., and Meldrum, B.S. (1980c) : Brain Res., 191 : 79-97.

5. Blackstad, T.W., Brink, K., Hem, Y., and Jeune, B. (1970) : J. Comp. Neurol., 138 : 433-400.

6. Blackwood, W., and Corsellis, J.A.N. (Eds) (1976) :
   Greenfield's Neuropathology, Arnold London.

7. Collins, R.C., Mc Lean, M., Lothman, E., Klunk, W., and
   Olney, J.W. (1980) : Epilepsia, 21 : 186p.

8. Fink, R.P., and Heimer, L. (1967) : Brain Res., 4 : 369-374.

9. Goddard, G.V., Mc Intyre, D.C., and Leech, C.K. (1969) :
   Exptl. Neurol., 25 : 295-330.

10. Hjorth-Simonsen, A. (1972) : J. Comp. Neurol., 146 : 219-231.

11. Margerison, J.H., and Corsellis, J.A.N. (1966) : Brain, 89 :
    499-530.

12. Nadler, J.V., Perry, B.W., and Cotman, C.W. (1978) : Nature,
    (Lond.), 676-677.

13. Nadler, J.V., and Cuthbertson, G.J. (1980) : Brain Res., in
    press.

14. Scherer-Singler, U., and Mc Geer, E. (1979) : Life Sciences,
    24 : 1015-1022.

15. Schwob, J.I., Fuller, T., Price, J.L., and Olney, J.W. (1980):
    Neuroscience, in press.

16. Sokoloff, L. (1979) : Brain, 102 : 653-668.

Glutamate as a Neurotransmitter,
edited by G. Di Chiara and G. L. Gessa
Raven Press, New York © 1981.

Role of Excitatory Pathways in the Hippocampal Damage Produced by Kainic Acid

J. Victor Nadler

*Department of Pharmacology, Duke University Medical Center,
Durham, North Carolina 27710*

Injections of the convulsant, kainic acid (KA), are being used by many investigators to make lesions in specific brain loci without directly damaging afferent fibers or fibers of passage. KA preferentially destroys neurons that are also sensitive to prolonged paroxysmal activity, particularly those in the hippocampal formation. Given its extreme potency as a convulsant, both in vivo and in vitro (nanomolar concentrations (23)), it would appear to be a useful tool in studies of epilepsy and especially of epileptic brain damage. Therefore my laboratory has been very much interested in its neurotoxic mechanism.

Because of its structural resemblance to glutamate and its potent neuroexcitatory properties, KA was initially supposed to destroy neurons by interacting with a postsynaptic glutamate receptor, thereby initiating toxic excitatory activity (11,22). However, the ability of KA to destroy striatal neurons has been shown to depend on an intact corticostriatal pathway (4,5,14,15), a finding that is seemingly incompatible with the simple notion of a critical interaction with the postsynaptic receptor. Since the corticostriatal tract is thought to be glutamatergic, it was suggested that, rather than interacting with a postsynaptic glutamate receptor, KA somehow augments the potency of excitatory glutamatergic projections, thus killing through excessive excitation those cells which receive such projections. According to this view, elimination of excitatory glutamatergic pathways should neutralize the neurotoxicity of KA, whereas elimination of excitatory non-glutamatergic pathways should not. We have tested this hypothesis by using rat hippocampal neurons as model targets of KA neurotoxicity (17). The hippocampal formation is particularly useful for this purpose, since its excitatory projections can be readily manipulated and we now have considerable information about their transmitters.

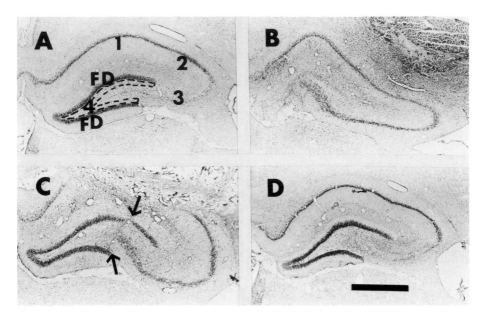

FIG. 1 Hippocampal lesions made by intraventricular KA alone
or 3 days after a prior lesion. (A) Effect of 3.75 nmol of KA
on ipsilateral hippocampal formation. Abbreviations: 1,2, etc.,
hippocampal areas CA1-CA4; FD, fascia dentata. Note loss of
neurons in areas CA3 and CA4. Survival time of 7 days. (B) KA
given 3 days after destruction of mossy fibers with locally-
applied colchicine. Few CA3 pyramidal cells were killed by KA.
Dentate granule cells were killed by the colchicine treatment.
(C) KA given 3 days after mechanical transection of the mossy
fibers. Note survival of CA3 pyramidal cells lateral (right),
but not medial, to the cut (arrows). (D) KA given 3 days after
ablation of ipsilateral entorhinal cortex. Neurotoxicity of KA
was unaffected (c.f. A). Scale bar = 1 mm. Data from Ref. 17.

EFFECTS OF LESIONS MADE 3 DAYS BEFORE KA INJECTION

In one series of studies we injected KA <u>intraventricularly</u> at
a dose (3.75 nmol) that destroys the ipsilateral CA3-CA4 neurons
(FIG. 1A). These studies showed that the presence of the mossy
fibers is crucial for the destruction of CA3 pyramidal cells by
intraventricular KA. Both transection of these fibers and destruction of the dentate granule cells with colchicine (10) markedly reduced the toxicity of KA toward these neurons, when the
toxin was injected about 3 days later (FIG. 1B,C). This interval
allowed sufficient time for terminal degeneration, but not enough
for reinnervation (8). Conversely, removal of entorhinal (FIG.
1D), commissural or septohippocampal fibers did not affect the KA
lesion, nor did removal of entorhinal afferents along with either
of the other two pathways. These findings do not support the

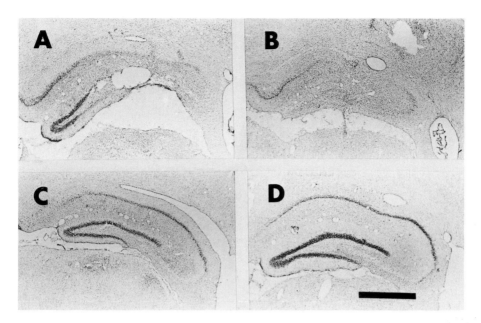

FIG. 2 Hippocampal lesions made by locally-injected KA alone or 3 days after a prior lesion. All sections shown here were taken from the edge of the injection site. (A) Effect of 2.34 nmol of KA injected 7 days previously. Only the most medial dentate granule cells and CA1 pyramidal cells survived. In some cases these cells were killed, but h_2 pyramidal cells (those in area CA2 and adjacent segment of area CA3) survived. (B) KA given 3 days after destruction of the mossy fibers with colchicine. Colchicine treatment did not attenuate neurotoxicity of locally-injected KA, in contrast to its efficacy against intraventricular KA (FIG. 1B). (C) KA given 3 days after ablation of ipsilateral entorhinal cortex. Note preservation of dentate granule cells (see also Ref. 12) and more lateral CA1 pyramidal cells. (D) KA given 3 days after ablation of medial septum. Result was virtually identical to that shown in C. Scale bar = 1 mm. Data from Ref. 17.

view that KA neurotoxicity results from a specific interaction with glutamatergic pathways, since the hippocampal mossy fibers do not appear to use glutamate as their transmitter (21,27), whereas the entorhinal and commissural projections to area CA3 appear to be predominantly glutamatergic (25).

Further evidence against a specific involvement of glutamatergic projections was obtained from studies with locally-injected KA. In this case the dose used (2.34 nmol) destroyed nearly every hippocampal neuron for a distance of several millimeters from the injection site (FIG. 2A). Now destruction of the mossy fibers conferred no protection against KA neurotoxicity (FIG. 2B) nor, as in the case of intraventricular injection, did

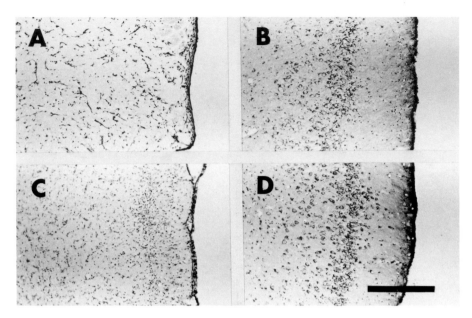

FIG. 3 Ipsilateral pyriform cortex after injection of KA
intraventricularly (A) or directly into the hippocampal formation
(B). A prior medial septal lesion essentially abolished destruction of pyriform cortical (and other extrahippocampal) neurons by either intraventricularly-injected (C) or locally-injected (D) KA. Other prior lesions of excitatory hippocampal
afferent projections had a similar effect. Scale bar = 0.2 mm.
Data from Ref. 17.

a commissurotomy, but ablation of the medial septum (FIG. 2C) or
ipsilateral entorhinal cortex (FIG. 2D) prevented destruction of
the dentate granule cells and all but the most medial CA1 pyramidal cells. A prior lesion of the lateral septum, which interrupted only hippocampal outflow to lower centers of the brain,
had no effect. The protective action of a medial septal or ipsilateral entorhinal lesion was not specifically directed at CA1
pyramidal cells and dentate granule cells, however, since a
combination of the two prior lesions also partially prevented
destruction of CA3 pyramidal cells. It seems likely that the
major effect of these lesions was to reduce the overall toxicity
of KA rather than to protect specific cell types, because all
hippocampal neurons could be protected from locally-injected KA
and neurons relatively less susceptible to KA (such as dentate
granule cells) were more readily protected by deafferentation
than more susceptible neurons (CA3 pyramidal cells). Our results
argue against a specific involvement of glutamatergic pathways
in the neurotoxicity of locally-injected KA, since the septo-
hippocampal fibers are known to be cholinergic (13) and, whereas
the entorhinal projection to the fascia dentata (perforant path)

probably uses glutamate as its transmitter (20,21,25,27), the
entorhinal projection to area CA1 (temporo-ammonic tract) may not
(20,21).

Both intraventricularly-injected and locally-injected KA at
the doses used in these studies destroyed neurons in several
extrahippocampal limbic regions, especially the amygdala, pyriform cortex, claustrum-insula and anterior, mediodorsal and midline thalamus. This phenomenon cannot be attributed primarily to
diffusion of the toxin from the site of injection, because an
intrahippocampal injection of KA killed neurons in regions, such
as the contralateral pyriform cortex and amygdala, that were not
damaged by a higher dose injected into the lateral ventricle.
Interruption of any excitatory projection to the hippocampal formation markedly attenuated the destruction of neurons in other
regions of the brain, regardless of its effect on the hippocampal
lesion (FIG. 3).

These observations emphasize the dependence of KA neurotoxicity on specific excitatory circuitry, but do not suggest a
relationship to any particular excitatory transmitter. They also
cast doubt on the idea, often uncritically accepted, that only
neurons which receive glutamatergic innervation can be killed by
KA. Our studies were not specifically designed to test this
hypothesis, however.

The dependence of KA neurotoxicity on excitatory innervation
suggests an indirect mechanism and is consistent with mounting
evidence that the prolonged seizure activity that KA induces is
intimately linked to the lesion. Epileptic wave forms have been
recorded after intracerebral injections of KA and have been
correlated with the severity of the hippocampal lesion (1,2).
The susceptibility of rat hippocampal neurons to destruction by
KA parallels their sensitivity to its epileptogenic action in
vitro (23). Excitatory input may be necessary for the initiation
of KA-induced seizure activity, as it is for penicillin-induced
seizure activity (24). Anticonvulsants reduce the toxicity of KA
toward hippocampal neurons, whether the toxin is injected at a
distance from the hippocampal formation (3) or directly into this
region (28). Finally, the brain lesions made by intraventricular
KA (18,19) more closely replicate those associated with severe
epilepsy and prolonged status epilepticus than with other deleterious conditions (6,9), and also resemble the lesions made in
experimental animals by other convulsants (7,16).

In accordance with this evidence, we have proposed that it is
primarily the prolonged status epilepticus triggered by KA that
kills neurons, not KA directly (17). The critical pathways are
those along which the seizure activity propagates, and they
differ according to the route by which KA is administered. Extrahippocampal neurons may be more readily protected from KA by
prior lesions than are hippocampal neurons, because they are less
susceptible to epileptic brain damage and thus require only a
slight reduction of seizure activity to survive. Thus, according
to this view, it is not simply excessive neuroexcitation per se

that accounts for the neurotoxicity of KA, but rather the paroxysmal nature of the excitation and its duration and intensity.

EFFECTS OF ACUTE LESIONS

The hypothesis that status epilepticus accounts for the neurotoxicity of KA implies that a prior lesion should immediately
attenuate its toxicity, since all that should be required is
cessation of impulse flow. It should be unnecessary to wait for
terminal degeneration. In fact, transection of the mossy fibers
did confer upon CA3 pyramidal cells immediate protection from
intraventricular KA and all lesions of hippocampal afferent projections immediately prevented damage to most extrahippocampal
regions. These results are entirely consistent with the idea
that KA induces a prolonged status epilepticus that is lethal to
seizure-sensitive neurons. Acute lesions had a somewhat more
complex effect on the neurotoxicity of KA injected directly into
the hippocampal formation, however. Ablation of the medial
septum immediately protected dentate granule cells and h$_2$ pyramidal cells from KA. This lesion did not immediately prevent
destruction of the more lateral CA1 pyramidal cells, however.
Moreover, an acute ipsilateral entorhinal lesion had little or no
effect on the toxicity of locally-injected KA toward hippocampal
neurons, although it did prevent most extrahippocampal damage.
Similarly, McGeer et al. (15) and Biziere and Coyle (5) have reported that decortication does not immediately prevent the destruction of striatal neurons by locally-injected KA, but rather
that protection of these neurons is fully expressed only after an
interval of a few days. An even longer interval seems to be required for ablation of the contralateral retina to spare neurons
in the pigeon optic tectum from destruction by locally-injected
KA (26).

CONCLUSIONS

On the basis of our evidence, it seems likely that KA destroys
neurons in the CNS by at least two mechanisms, both of which depend on specific excitatory circuitry. First, it initiates a
prolonged status epilepticus that travels along particular nerve
pathways and kills any neuron in the seizure circuit that is
vulnerable to intense paroxysmal activity. In this case certain
excitatory pathways probably are required for the full neurotoxicity of KA simply because they are essential components of
the seizure circuit. Lesions of these pathways thus attenuate
such toxicity. This mechanism is especially important when KA
is administered at a distance from the site of neurotoxicity,
but also appears to be involved in the destruction of hippocampal neurons by local administration of KA. Second, locally-
injected KA destroys neurons, in part, by an interaction with
certain excitatory pathways that appears independent of on-going
activity within those pathways. Specific lesions gradually re-

duce this form of KA neurotoxicity as the afferent pathway degenerates. In several cases of delayed protection from locally-injected KA the transmitter of the degenerating pathway appears to be glutamate, and thus it has been suggested that KA kills postsynaptic neurons by interacting with glutamate that is spontaneously released (5,15,26). However, such an interaction could not easily explain our observation that ablation of the medial septum, which deprives the hippocampal formation of cholinergic, not glutamatergic, innervation, also requires some time interval before it can protect lateral CA1 pyramidal cells from locally-injected KA. This result suggests that a specific interaction with glutamatergic pathways probably cannot account for this form of KA neurotoxicity, but rather that a more general interaction with excitatory inputs may be involved. Perhaps the structural resemblance between KA and glutamate has unduly constricted our thinking on this issue.

In particular situations either or both of the proposed mechanisms may be operative. Further studies are needed to determine whether they are entirely independent or whether the second mode of interaction between KA and excitatory innervation indeed leads to a status epilepticus.

ACKNOWLEDGMENTS

I gratefully acknowledge the superior technical assistance of Ms. Debra Evenson, Mr. Gilbert Cuthbertson and Mr. E. Michael Smith and the secretarial assistance of Mrs. Peggy Smith. These studies were supported by research grants BNS 78-13051 from the National Science Foundation and NS 16064 from the National Institutes of Health and by Research Career Development Award NS 00447.

REFERENCES

1. Ben-Ari, Y., Lagowska, J., Tremblay, E., and Le Gal La Salle, G. (1979): Brain Res., 163: 176-179.
2. Ben-Ari, Y., Tremblay, E., and Ottersen, O.P. (1980): Neuroscience, 5: 515-528.
3. Ben-Ari, Y., Tremblay, E., Ottersen, O.P., and Naquet, R. (1979): Brain Res., 165: 362-365.
4. Biziere, K. and Coyle, J.T. (1978): Neurosci. Lett., 8: 303-310.
5. Biziere, K. and Coyle, J.T. (1979): J. Neurosci. Res., 4: 383-398.
6. Blackwood, W. and Corsellis, J.A.N., editors (1976): Greenfield's Neuropathology. Edward Arnold, London.
7. Blennow, G., Brierley, J.B., Meldrum, B.S., and Siesjö, B.K. (1978): Brain, 101: 687-700.
8. Cotman, C.W. and Nadler, J.V. (1978): In: Neuronal Plasticity, edited by C.W. Cotman, pp. 227-271. Raven Press, New York.
9. Gastaut, H., Naquet, R., Meyer, A., Cavanagh, J.B., and Beck,

     E. (1959): J. Neuropathol. Exp. Neurol., 18: 270-293.
10. Goldschmidt, R. and Steward, O. (1978): Soc. Neurosci.
     Abstr., 4: 221.
11. Herndon, R.M. and Coyle, J.T. (1977): Science (N.Y.), 198:
     71-72.
12. Köhler, C., Schwarcz, R., and Fuxe, K. (1978): Neurosci.
     Lett., 10: 241-246.
13. Kuhar, M.J. (1976): In: Biology of Cholinergic Function,
     edited by A.M. Goldberg and I. Hanin, pp. 3-27. Raven
     Press, New York.
14. McGeer, E.G., McGeer, P.L., and Singh, K. (1978): Brain
     Res., 139: 381-383.
15. McGeer, P.L., McGeer, E.G., and Hattori, T. (1978): In:
     Kainic Acid As a Tool in Neurobiology, edited by E.G.
     McGeer, J.W. Olney and P.L. McGeer, pp. 123-138. Raven
     Press, New York.
16. Meldrum, B.S., Horton, R.W., and Brierley, J.B. (1974):
     Brain, 97: 407-418.
17. Nadler, J.V. and Cuthbertson, G.J. (1980): Brain Research,
     in press.
18. Nadler, J.V., Perry, B.W., and Cotman, C.W. (1978): In:
     Kainic Acid As a Tool in Neurobiology, edited by E.G.
     McGeer, J.W. Olney and P.L. McGeer, pp. 219-237. Raven
     Press, New York.
19. Nadler, J.V., Perry, B.W., Gentry, C., and Cotman, C.W.
     (1980): J. Comp. Neurol., in press.
20. Nadler, J.V., Vaca, K.W., White, W.F., Lynch, G.S., and
     Cotman, C.W. (1976): Nature (Lond.), 260: 538-540.
21. Nadler, J.V., White, W.F., Vaca, K.W., Perry, B.W., and
     Cotman, C.W. (1978): J. Neurochem., 31: 147-155.
22. Olney, J.W. (1976): Advanc. Exp. Med. Biol., 69: 497-506.
23. Ryan, J. and Cotman, C.W. (1978): Soc. Neurosci. Abstr.,
     4: 227.
24. Schwartzkroin, P.A. and Prince, D.A. (1978): Brain Res.,
     147: 117-130.
25. Storm-Mathisen, J. (1978): In: Functions of the Septo-
     Hippocampal System, CIBA Foundation Symposium 58, edited
     by K. Elliott and J. Whelan, pp. 5-24. Elsevier, Amsterdam.
26. Streit, P., Stella, M., and Cuenod, M. (1980): Brain Res.,
     187: 47-57.
27. White, W.F., Nadler, J.V., and Cotman, C.W. (1979): Brain
     Res., 164: 177-194.
28. Zaczek, R., Nelson, M.F., and Coyle, J.T. (1978): Eur. J.
     Pharmacol., 52: 323-327.

Glutamate as a Neurotransmitter,
edited by G. Di Chiara and G. L. Gessa
Raven Press, New York © 1981.

Glutamate-induced Neuronal Degeneration: Studies on the Role of Glutamate Re-uptake

Robert Schwarcz, *Christer Köhler, Richard M. Mangano, and **A. N. Neophytides

*Neuroscience Program, Maryland Psychiatric Research Center, Baltimore, Maryland 21228; *Research Laboratories, Astra Läkemedel AB, S-15185 Södertälje, Sweden; and **Department of Neurology, Veterans Administration Hospital, New York, New York 10010*

Over the last few years, much interest has been focussed upon the neurotoxic properties of a number of neuroexcitatory amino acids like kainic acid (KA; 20) and ibotenic acid (IBO; 21). Microinjection of these "excitotoxic" compounds (15) into the striatum of the rat leads to the degeneration of intrinsic nerve cells while leaving fibers of passage or extrinsic neurons unaffected. Thus, they provide an animal model for the neurodegenerative disorder, Huntington's disease (HD; 4, 13). The structural analogy of KA and IBO with the ubiquitous amino acid- and putative neurotransmitter substance- glutamic acid (GLU) has given rise to the hypothesis that irregularities, i.e. increases, in GLU function may be causally related to the nerve cell death observed in the human disorder (Table 1).

There exists some confusion in published literature concerning the neurotoxicity of GLU. More than 20 years ago, subcutaneous injections of monosodium glutamate into infanct mice have been shown to cause damage to retinal neurons (12) and the work of Olney's group has subsequently convincingly confirmed and extended the original observation (18, 19). Reports on GLU-neurotoxicity have been subject to intensive debate over the past decade (see (7) for review). However, while the excitotoxic concept-referring to an excitatory mechanism as the basis of toxic effects (15)- is still controversial, there can be little doubt to date as to the potential of GLU as a neurotoxin.

Intrastriatal injections of high doses of GLU result in only very limited damage to neurons in the area of infusion (13, 17, 23). One possible explanation for the inefficacy of GLU injections into the striatum and into other brain regions could be the

presence of powerful local GLU-uptake mechanisms which rapidly
remove GLU from the synaptic cleft (1,8,11). Conversely, it seems
conceivable that experimentally evoked or genetic defects in
these efficient removal processes may lead to enhanced (toxic)
synaptic accumulations of GLU.

In the present study we first investigated the latter hypothesis in the rat model by applying GLU intracerebrally after
surgical removal of defined GLU-containing neuronal pathways. In
a closely related project we then proceeded to examine the possibility of an etiological role of (a reduction in) GLU-uptake
in HD. For that purpose we employed blood platelets from controls
and HD-patients after having demonstrated that GLU-uptake
mechanisms in platelets closely resemble those of brain tissue.

MATERIALS AND METHODS

Animal studies

Male Sprague-Dawley rats (175-200g) were used for our experiments. The animals were operated in a David Kopf stereotaxic in-
strument under Membumal anesthesia. For perforant path transections, a dura-knife was angled 10^0 to the coronal plane and
introduced into the brain at the level of lambda. A deep cut was
then made extending 5 mm laterally from the midline. Immediately
after the perforant path transections, a commissural cut was performed on the contralateral brain hemisphere (coordinates:
A: 0.0-7.8, L: 0.5, V: 4.0) in view of the fact that sprouting of
the crossed perforant path has been observed after degeneration
of the ipsilateral perforant path (26). Four days after the operation, GLU (300µg/0.5µl), GABA (300µg/0.5µl) or glutamine (35µg/
0.5µl) were infused into the dorsal hippocampus at the following
coordinates: A: 4.6, L: 1.7, V: 3.5. Five days later, the rats
were killed by transcardial perfusion with 100ml Macrodex^R followed by a solution containing 4% paraformaldehyde and 1% glutaraldehyde in 0.1M phosphate buffer, pH 7.4. The brains were
then processed for thionin- or acetylcholinesterase-staining
according to standard procedures.

Fornix-fimbria were transected at A: 7.8. L: 0.0-4.0, V: 5.0.
Intrahippocampal injections of GLU (300µg/µl) were made four days
later and the animals killed and the brains processed after
another five days.

To control for successful knife cuts (N=3 for perforant path-
and fornix-fimbria transections, respectively) extrahippocampal
parts of the brain were cut horizontally through the respective
transection areas at 30µm and the sections stained with thionin.

Human Blood Platelets

Whole blood was collected from drug-free donors or HD-patients
by venipuncture. The samples were immediately transferred to ice
cold polypropylene tubes. Within maximally six hours after blood

Table 1. Irregularities in glutamate function that could con-
          ceivably result in excessive neuroactive glutamate

A) Synaptic processes

    1) Reduced re-uptake into nerve endings and/or glia
       a) Decreased number of uptake sites
       b) Impaired regulation by endogenous inhibitors/activators

    2) Increased neuronal activity (release)
       a) Local defects (e.g. impairment of ion fluxes)
       b) Impaired regulation of feedback loop(s)

    3) Elevated postsynaptic response
       a) Increased sensitivity of receptors
       b) Increase in the number of receptor sites

B) Metabolic processes

    1) Increased anabolism
    2) Decreased catabolism
    3) Increased glia-neuron "shuttle"

---

collection the tubes were centrifuged at 300 x g for 5 min at
4°C. The supernatant platelet-rich plasma (PRP) was carefully removed with a plastic pipet tip and re-centrifuged at 7000 x g for
10 min. The pellet was then resuspended in 2 ml ice cold 0.32 M
sucrose (pH 7.4) so that no visible pellet aggregates remained.
After another centrifugation (7000 x g, 5 min) the resulting
platelet pellet was resuspended in one-fifth of the original PRP-
volume in buffered sucrose. 50µl of the homogenate were added to
430µl of ice cold Tris-citrate buffer (pH 6.5) and the samples
preincubated for 15 min at 37°C. Uptake was started by addition
of 20µl L-^{3}H-GLU (0.4µCi; 10^{-7}M) and incubation continued for
10 min. Uptake was stopped by rapid cooling of the tubes and the
cold suspension centrifuged at 49,500 x g for 10 min. The supernatant was discarded, the platelet pellet washed with cold incubation medium and then solubilized in Protosol and counted by
liquid scintillation spectrometry. Net accumulation of the radio-
label was determined by subtracting no-sodium- (high-affinity
site) or 4°C- (low-affinity site) blanks from the total counts
taken up under regular experimental conditions.
    Drug-free blood donors were recruited from the staff of the
Maryland Psychiatric Research Center (age range: 28-45); drug-
free HD-patients (age range: 31-59) - VA Hospital, New York,
N.Y. - had been diagnosed according to family history and chore-
atic symptomatology and were in the early to medium stages of HD.

RESULTS

Studies on rat hippocampus

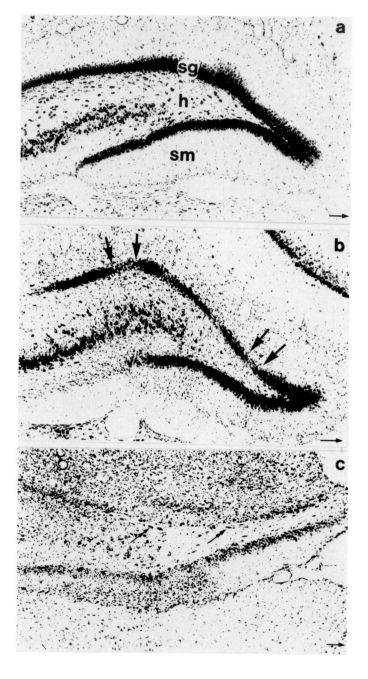

Injections of 300µg/0.5µl GLU into the intact hippocampus resulted in only marginal neuronal degeneration around the site of
infusion. Some brains displayed a patchy pattern of degenerated
cells in both dorsal and ventral blades of the area dentata
(arrows in Fig.1b). Frequent intact and hilar cells could be observed in the immediate vicinity of the needle track (N=15).

Combined transections of the perforant path and commissural
fibers four days prior to the GLU injection significantly increased neurotoxicity (N=15; Fig.1c). The lesion was restricted
to the granule cells of the area dentata and a small population
of pyramidal and bipolar cells in the hilar region. Many intact
hilar cells could be seen in close vicinity of degenerated granule cells. Degeneration extended up to at least 1 mm around the
injection site. The pattern of acetylcholinesterase-staining
in the inner molecular layer of the area dentata showed no difference as compared to an intact GLU-injected hippocampus
(micrographs not shown).

GLU injections into hippocampi where the septal cholinergic
input had been removed through fornix-transections failed to produce the neuronal degeneration seen in perforant path transected
rats (N=10). Also, infusion of GABA (N=5) or glutamine (N=5) in
normal or deafferentated animals did not result in any detectable
degeneration of hippocampal neurons (micrographs not shown).

Glutamate uptake into human blood platelets

GLU uptake could be shown to exist in human blood platelets
and to display remarkable similarities to the corresponding process in rat striatal synaptosomes. Whole blood could be stored
up to six hours at 4°C prior to platelet isolation and assay
without any deleterious effects on the uptake process. Linearity
of the uptake with time, pH-dependency and pharmacological properties of platelet- and synaptosomal preparations show close
resemblance (Table 2).

Figure 1. Photomicrographs of the area dentata of the dorsal
hippocampus. a) Area dentata of an intact rat injected with 0.5µl
NaCl. Abbreviations: sg: stratum granulosum, sm: stratum moleculare, h: hilus. b) Area dentata of an intact rat injected with
GLU (300µg/0.5µl) into the dorsal hippocampus. Large arrows point
to the patches of degenerated granule cells. c) Area dentata of
a deafferentated rat injected with GLU (300µg/0.5µl) four days
after the transections. Note the many intact cells in the hilus
(two cells have been marked by double arrow heads). All sections
were obtained approximately 500µm away from the center of the injection site. Small arrows in the lower right corner indicate
medial direction. Marker bar: 50µm (from Köhler and Schwarcz,
submitted for publication).

Table 2. Characteristics of Glutamate Uptake in Human Platelets and Rat Striatal Synaptosomes

	Platelets	Synaptosomes
Time Curve	Linear up to 10 min	Linear up to 5 min
pH Optimum	6.5	7.2 - 7.4
Temperature Dependence	yes	yes
Sodium Dependence	yes; high-affinity site	yes; high-affinity site
Kinetics		
High affinity	K_m = 3.1 µM V_{max} = 14 pMoles/mg prot x 10 min	K_m = 3.4 µM V_{max} = 325 pMoles/mg w.w. x 10 min
Low affinity	K_m = 88 µM V_{max} = 313 pMoles/mg prot x 10 min	K_m = 357 µM V_{max} = 3759 pMoles/mg w.w. x 10 min
IC_{50} - values (µM)		
L-aspartate	4	2
Threo-3-hydroxy-DL-aspartate	13	2
L-glutamate	19	8
DL-aspartate-β-hydroxamate	156	28
D-glutamate	950	400

Platelet GLU uptake could be demonstrated to consist of two components (Fig.2A): a sodium-dependent high-affinity site (K_m= 3.1μM) and a temperature-dependent low-affinity site (K_m= 88.2μM) Moreover, metabolism of the amino acid could be shown to be negligible during the 10 minute incubation since 90-95% of the radioactivity could be recovered as authentic GLU.

GLU uptake was determined in three consecutive (weekly) blood samples of normal donors to test inter- and intrasubject variation of the method. At 10^{-7}M GLU, uptake ranged from 121.9 to 1270.0 fMoles/mg protein x 10min for individual values (N=12) and from 157.6±26.5 to 955.2±158.4 fMoles/mg protein x 10min (means±S.E.M.) for intrasubject values of the same population. All coefficients of variation (S.E.M./mean) fell within the range of 0.09-0.28.

At 10^{-7}M GLU, parallel measurement of GLU uptake into platelets from normal subjects (N=17) and HD-patients (N=9) did not result in significant differences between the two populations: 768.8±130.0 fMoles/mg protein x 10min for controls vs. 814.1± 159.3 fMoles/mg protein x 10min for HD-patients. However, preliminary kinetic data on platelets from four HD-patients indicate a trend towards lower K_m-values (higher affinity) of the high-affinity uptake site (Fig.2B).

DISCUSSION

The hippocampal formation of the rat lends itself to the study of excitotoxic mechanisms because of its well defined glutamatergic circuitry (27). In particular, the projection from the entorhinal cortex to the granule cells of the dentate gyrus - the perforant path - can be assumed to employ GLU as its neurotransmitter (14,28).

Following similar experiments using the exogenous excitotoxins KA and IBO (9,10,22), we were curious if the neurotoxicity of GLU could be modulated by perforant path transections. As reported here, GLU-toxicity versus the granule cells, only marginal in control animals, was significantly enhanced after deafferentation. Most importantly, this effect could be shown to be specific to GLU and GLU-containing afferents and to save fibers of extrinsic origin - here the septo-hippocampal cholinergic fibers assessed histologically by acetylcholinesterase-staining. Therefore it can be concluded that the degeneration induced by GLU belonged to the axon-sparing type known from KA- and IBO-lesions (4,13,20,21). In a broader perspective, it thus seems conceivable that - under certain experimental conditions in the animal or pathological conditions in man - GLU could cause neuronal damage throughout the adult central nervous system similar to the retinal and hypothalamic lesions observed in infant animals after subcutaneous administration (18,19).

The apparent increase in GLU-neurotoxicity could be due to one or both of the following mechanisms: 1) development of supersensitivity of GLU-receptors after deafferentation and 2) reduction of uptake sites resulting in a decreased rate of clearance of

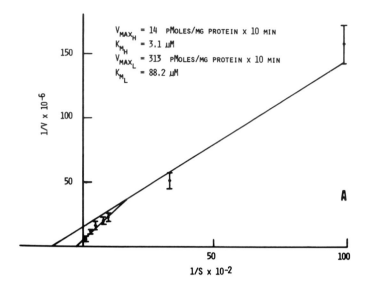

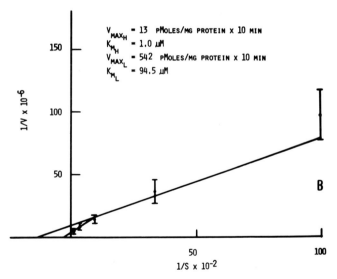

Figure 2. Double reciprocal plot of glutamate uptake by human blood platelets. Points indicate the mean ± S.E.M. of four independent experiments. Solid lines approximate the computed best fit of the two component rate equation to the experimental data. Velocity (V) is expressed as fMoles/mg protein x 10 min and substrate concentration S as μM. A: control subjects; B: Huntington's disease patients.

GLU after its intracerebral infusion. Increased sensitivity of
cholinergic (2,3) or amino acid (24) receptors has been reported
previously in the hippocampal region after removal of the respective afferent fibers. However, out of two circumstantial
reasons, we currently favor the second alternative: a) we could
not demonstrate enhanced sensitivity to IBO in deafferentated
animals (unpublished observation); since IBO is believed to be a
directly acting GLU-receptor agonist - without, however, compe-
ting with the GLU-uptake site (21,22) - enhanced receptor sensitivity after glutamatergic deafferentation should have affected
IBO-toxicity as well; b) as judged from comparable experimental
situations in other neurotransmitter systems the minimal time
necessary after transection to obtain enhancement of GLU-toxicity
(two days) seems too short for the development of receptor-super-
sensitivity.

In the present report we also demonstrated that human blood
platelets display GLU-uptake properties which are highly remi-
niscent of rat brain synaptosomes (Table 2). GLU-uptake was Na^+-
dependent and saturable and kinetics as well as pharmacological
characteristics were shown to be similar to those of brain tissue
Moreover, inter- and intrasubject variability proved satisfactory
for clinical endeavors. We therefore concluded that GLU-uptake
measurements in human platelets, similar to analogous determinations of serotonin-uptake (see (25) for review), may validly reflect experimentally inaccessible glutamatergic processes in the
brain.

We and others (5,6,16) have suggested earlier the possibility
of a primary etiological involvement of (a reduction in) GLU-
uptake in HD. However, our present data on GLU-uptake determinations in platelets from HD-patients did not lend support to
that hypothesis: under high-affinity uptake conditions (10^{-7}M
GLU) no significant decreases could be observed in HD as compared
to control uptake values. Instead, preliminary kinetic data on
platelets isolated from HD-blood indicated a modest trend towards
higher (more efficient) uptake. Thus, it seems quite unlikely
that the - genetically determined - primary defect in HD does
indeed lie in the GLU-uptake process. Further studies will be
necessary in order to evaluate possible causal relationships of
other irregularities in central glutamatergic functions (Table 1)
with the neuronal degeneration observed in HD.

In conclusion, the two sets of experiments reported here tentatively answer two related questions regarding the potential of
GLU as a selective neurotoxin and as a possible etiological factor in HD: 1) our data justify and lend support to further
efforts to elucidate a possible role of GLU in the pathogenesis
of human neurodegenerative disorders like HD (neurotoxicity of
GLU could occur during pathological interference with central
glutamatergic function); 2) testing one of the possibilities for
GLU-dysfunction, our data do not support the hypothesis that an
impairment of GLU-uptake is causally related to the nerve cell
death in HD-patients.

ACKNOWLEDGEMENT

This work was supported by a grant from the Wills Foundation.

REFERENCES

1. Balcar,V.J.,and Johnston,G.A.R.(1972):J.Neurochem.,19:2657-2666.
2. Bird,S.J.,and Aghajanian,G.K.(1975):Brain Res.,100:355-370.
3. Burchfiel,J.L.,Duchowny,M.S.,and Duffy,F.H.(1979):Science, 204:1096-1098.
4. Coyle,J.T.,and Schwarcz,R.(1976):Nature,263:244-246.
5. Coyle,J.T.,Schwarcz,R.,Bennett,J.P.,and Campochiaro,P.(1977): Prog.Neuro-Psychopharmac.,1:13-30.
6. Divac,I.(1977):Acta Neurol.Scand.,56:357-360.
7. Filer,L.J.Jr.,Garattini,S.,Kare,M.R.,Reynolds,W.A.,and Wurtman R.J.,editors(1979):Glutamic Acid:Advances in Biochemistry and Physiology,Raven Press,New York.
8. Johnson,J.L.(1978):Prog.Neurobiol.,10:155-202.
9. Köhler,C.,Schwarcz,R.,and Fuxe,K.(1978):Neurosci.Lett.,10: 241-246.
10. Köhler,C.,Schwarcz,R.,and Fuxe,K.(1979):Brain Res.,175:366-371
11. Logan,W.J.,and Snyder,S.H.(1972):Brain Res.,42:413-431.
12. Lucas,D.R.,and Newhouse,J.P.(1957):AMA Arch.Ophthalmol.,58: 193-201.
13. McGeer,E.G.,and McGeer,P.L.(1976):Nature,263:517-518.
14. Nadler,J.V.,Vaca,K.W.,White,W.F.,Lynch,G.S.,and Cotman,C.W. (1976):Nature,260:538-540.
15. Olney,J.W.(1974):In:Heritable Disorders of Amino Acid Metabolism,edited by W.L.Nyhan,pp.501-512.Wiley,New York.
16. Olney,J.W.(1979):In:Advances in Neurology,Vol.23,edited by T. N.Chase,N.S.Wexler,and A.Barbeau,pp.609-624.Raven Press,New York.
17. Olney,J.W.,and de Gubareff,T.(1978):Nature,271:557-559.
18. Olney,J.W.,Ho,O.L.,and Rhee,V.(1971):Exp.Brain Res.,14:61-76.
19. Olney,J.W.,and Sharpe,L.G.(1969):Science,166:386-388.
20. Schwarcz,R.,and Coyle,J.T.(1977):Brain Res.,127:235-249.
21. Schwarcz,R.,Hökfelt,T.,Fuxe,K.,Jonsson,G.,Goldstein,M.,and Terenius,L.(1979):Exp.Brain Res.,37:199-216.
22. Schwarcz,R.,Köhler,C.,Fuxe,K.,Hökfelt,T.,and Goldstein,M. (1979):In:Advances in Neurology,Vol.23,edited by T.N.Chase, N.S.Wexler,and A.Barbeau,pp.655-668.Raven Press,New York.
23. Schwarcz,R.,Scholz,D.,and Coyle,J.T.(1978):Neuropharmac.,17: 145-151.
24. Segal,M.(1977):Brain Res.,119:476-479.
25. Sneddon,J.M.(1973):Prog.Neurobiol.,1:153-198.
26. Steward,O.,Cotman,C.W.,and Lynch.G.(1976):Brain Res.,114:181-200.
27. Storm-Mathisen,J.(1977):Prog.Neurobiol.,8:119-181.

Glutamate as a Neurotransmitter,
edited by G. Di Chiara and G. L. Gessa
Raven Press, New York © 1981.

Role of Glutamate and Zinc in the Hippocampal Lesions of Pick's Disease

J. Constantinidis and R. Tissot

Psychiatric Clinic, University of Geneva, 1225 Chène-Bourg, Switzerland

Pick's disease is a degenerative dementia with onset in the presenile and senile age periods, characterized by moria, apragmatism, stereotyped gestures, bizarre behaviour, decreased speech leading to complete mutism, prefrontal signs and, in some cases, pyramidal and extrapyramidal signs. Morphologically, its most characteristic form consists of atrophy of the temporal and frontal lobes, with gliosis and demyelinisation. In addition, two types of pathological changes in the neuronal bodies are observed: argyrophilic inclusions (AI) and neuronal ballooning (4,16).

The lesions in Pick's disease begin in the hippocampus

The AI in Pick's disease are observed initially in the hippocampus, and subsequently extend to the temporal, insular and orbito-frontal cortex, and sometimes even to the parietal cortex. The AI in the hippocampus are first observed in the neurons of the granular layer of the gyrus dentatus and gliosis is first seen in the area of mossy fibres originating from these neurons (Fig. 1). Later, the AI are observed in the neurons of CA1, the subiculum and the entorhinal cortex, and gliosis in the molecular layer of the gyrus dentatus, the stratum radiatum and the stratum oriens of CA1 and of the subiculum. In contrast, there is no gliosis in the layers of neuronal bodies containing AI. It seems that gliosis occurs exclusively in the axodendritic synapses formed by the axons originating from neuronal bodies with AI (5).

We wondered whether these systematic hippocampal changes found in the beginning stage of Pick's disease are related to disorders involving the intrinsic neurotransmitters of the hippocampal systems.

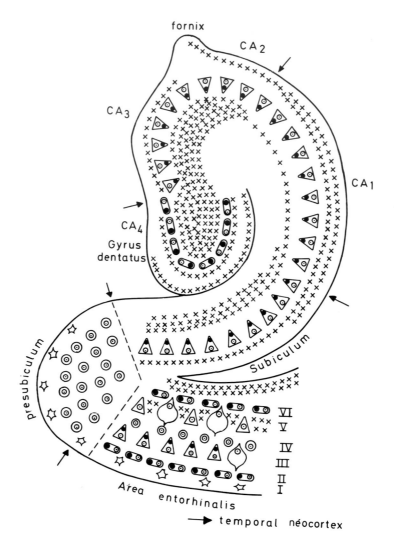

Fig 1. Topography of hippocampal lesions in Pick's disease:
x represent gliosis and full black circles are argyrophilic inclusions.

Glutamate is the intrinsic neurotransmitter of the hippocampus

It seems well established that the intrinsic system of the
neurons in the granular layer of the gyrus dentatus whose
axonal mossy fibres terminate in CA3 utilize glutamate (Glu)
as neurotransmitter (Fig.2). Neurons of CA3 project glutamin-

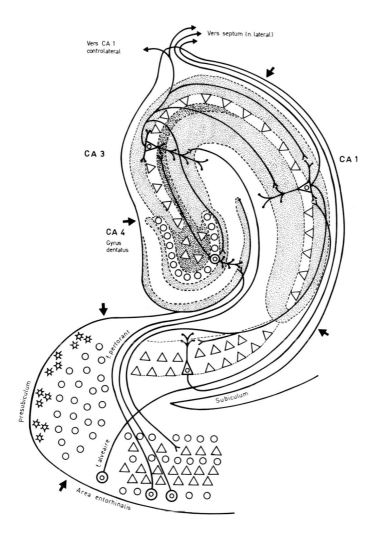

Fig.2. Neuronal organization of hippocampus according to Gastaut
and Lammers (6). Topography of the glutamate neurotransmitter expressed in dots according to Storm-Mathisen (14).

ergic axons to the dendrites of gyrus dentatus, and to the CA1
area bilaterally. CA1 neurons project axons utilizing Glu or
aspartate (Asp) as neurotransmitters to the lateral septal
nucleus, the subiculum and the entorhinal cortex. Lastly, the
entorhinal cortex projects the Glu mediated perforating pathway
to the dendrites of gyrus dentatus and CA3 (1,10,13,14, 18).
Thus intrahippocampal and interhippocampal connections and the

hippocampo-septal pathways are Glu or Asp mediated. Hippocampal afferences from the medial septal nucleus are mediated by acetylcholine (Ach) and form axosomatic synapses in gyrus dentatus, CA3 and CA1. Similarly, the Fleschig pathway, which originates in the cingulate gyrus and terminates in the pre-subiculum, is also Ach mediated. The GABAergic systems of the hippocampus are exclusively intrinsic and correspond to the basket cells of Cajal (14) which form inhibitory axosomatic and axodendritic synapses.

It should be noted that the hippocampus receives also afferent noradrenergic (NA) impulses from the locus coeruleus and serotoninergic (5-HT) impulses from the raphé.

It is clear that the AI-containing neurons in Pick's disease (gyrus dentatus, CA1, subiculum, entorhinal cortex) receive afferent impulses mediated by Ach, GABA, NA, 5-HT, but their efferent impulses and interconnections are mediated by Glu and Asp.

It seems to us justified to hypothesize that these latter neurotransmitters might be those initially involved when hippocampal changes occur in Pick's disease.

It is important to measure Glu levels in this illness. Post-mortem cerebral assays present certain problems which have now been resolved. We have begun to perform these assays in collaboration with Lloyd and Bartholini.

It will however require considerable time to accumulate sufficient data because of the rarity of this disease. In addition, since this amino acid intervenes in the Krebs cycle, problems are presented when one attempts to distinguish between Glu functioning as neurotransmitter and Glu participating in energy metabolism.

Topographic parallelism between neurotransmitter Glutamate and zinc

Therefore we proposed another approach to evaluating changes in neurotransmitter Glu. As demonstrated by the method of Timm (15,8) there exists a strict parallelism between the localization of Glu-containing synaptic buttons and the localisation of zinc. This correlation is particularly evident in the hippocampus (Fig. 3): the mossy fibres area, rich in Glu, is the part of the brain containing the highest zinc concentration; the same correlation between Glu and zinc exists in the proximal and distal parts of the molecular layer of the gyrus dentatus and the dendritic layers of CA1 and the subiculum. A parallelism between the distribution of Glu and zinc is also found in the lateral septal nucleus, in the neostriatum and the neocortical layers (2).

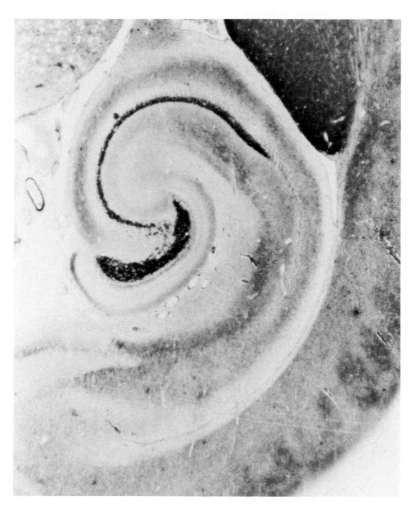

Fig.3. Topography of hippocampal zinc coloured by Timm's method.

Zinc is localized in the synaptic vesicles of the terminal buttons of the mossy fibres (7,9). Glu-dehydrogenase, one of the enzymes which metabolize this amino acid, is a zinc-containing metalloenzyme (17). Possibly, part of the zinc of the mossy fibres is incorporated in this enzyme; other correlations are also possible between zinc and neurotransmitter Glu. In any case, the zinc which is localized in the synaptic buttons of glutaminergic synapses may be considered as a marker of neurotransmitter Glu. Its topographical distribution and alterations can be taken to correspond to the topographical distribution and alterations of neurotransmitter Glu.

Zinc in Pick's disease

When several human hippocampi which had been rapidly removed post-mortem were stained with Timm's method which colors zinc, we observed deeper staining in Pick's disease than in Alzheimer's disease and in control brains of eldery subjects (5).

The hypothesis of an excess of zinc in patients with Pick's disease is supported by post-mortem hippocampal zinc measurements using atomic absorption spectrophotometry. Hippocampal zinc is higher in Pick's disease than in Alzheimer's disease or controls. Similarly, the blood cells and urine of patients with Pick's disease contain more zinc than those of patients with Alzheimer's disease or controls (Fig. 4).

Zinc chelators (Disulfiram, calcium EDTA) increase urinary excretion of zinc. This increase is greater in patients with Pick's disease than in patients with Alzheimer's disease (Fig.5).

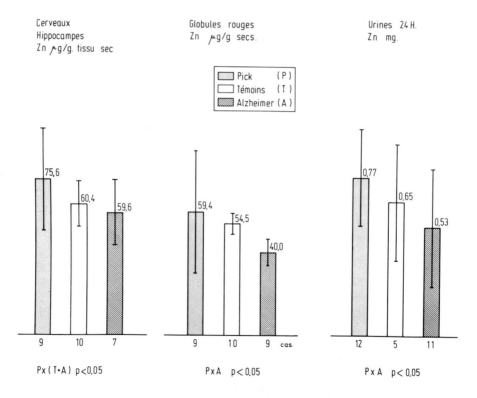

Fig.4. Zinc levels in hippocampus, blood cells and urines in Pick's disease, controls and Alzheimer's disease.

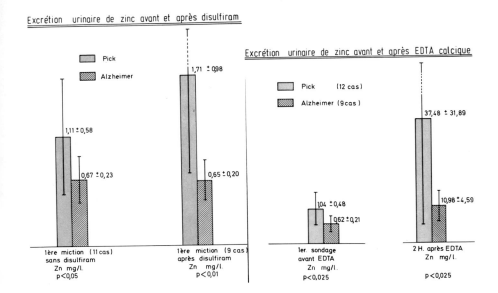

Excrétion urinaire de zinc avant et après disulfiram

Excrétion urinaire de zinc avant et après EDTA calcique

Fig.5. Zinc urinary excretion before and after administration of chelators (Disulfiram and calcium EDTA) in Pick's and Alzheimer's disease.

These results support the concept of a generalized excess of zinc in Pick's disease. Are there abnormalities of the metabolism and transport of this metal? Zinc is considered to be transported in blood by albumins and alpha globulins. We have found that patients with Pick's disease have less albumins and more alpha-1 globulins than those with Alzheimer's disease. We have found significant correlations between serum zinc and alpha-1 globulins in Pick's disease and between serum zinc and albumin levels in Alzheimer's disease (5).

We performed zinc assays on serum fractions after starch bloc electrophoresis (3). We found that concentrations of zinc in alpha globulins and in albumins are significantly higher in Pick's disease than in Alzheimer's disease and controls.

The increase in zinc concentration in Pick's disease is relatively more important in the alpha globulins than in the albumin fractions. In controls and in patients with Alzheimer's disease, there is 50% less zinc in the alpha globulins than in albumins, whereas in Pick's disease zinc levels are equally high in the alpha globulins and in albumins (Table 1). These results are consistent with the hypothesis of an excess of plasma transport of zinc in Pick's disease, involving particularly the alpha globulins.

Table 1. Zinc concentrations expressed in μ g/g protein, in seric β-globulins, α-globulins and albumins separated by starch block electrophoresis of 10ml serum.

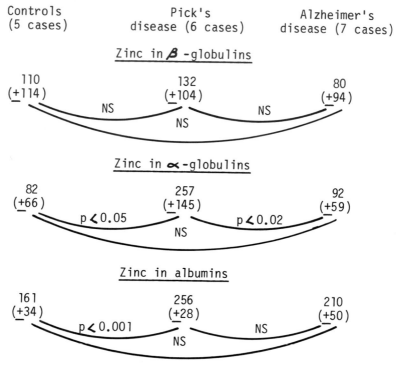

Controls (5 cases)   Pick's disease (6 cases)   Alzheimer's disease (7 cases)

Zinc in β-globulins

110 (+114)   132 (+104)   80 (+94)

NS   NS   NS

Zinc in α-globulins

82 (+66)   257 (+145)   92 (+59)

$p < 0.05$ $p < 0.02$ NS

Zinc in albumins

161 (+34)   256 (+28)   210 (+50)

$p < 0.001$ NS   NS

Pathogenic hypotheses

What pathogenic hypotheses can we formulate by synthetizing these data? In Pick's disease a generalized excess of zinc, probably related to changes in transport proteins, produces excess zinc deposits in areas which usually fix this metal. In the brain, this deposit is particularly abundant in the mossy fibres area of the hippocampus. Here, excess zinc might correspond to an excess of the metalloenzyme Glu-dehydrogenase. Activation of this Glu metabolizing enzyme could produce changes in the neurotransmitter Glu, synaptic dysfunction and gliosis. This could in turn produce a reaction of the neuronal cell bodies in the gyrus dentatus where the mossy fibres originate, thus producing AI.

The following observations can be made if the lesions in Pick's disease (gliosis and AI) are projected upon the hippocampal distribution of zinc and neurotransmitters. The gliosis/ AI pair is found in other systems in addition to the mossy

fibres/neurons of the gyrus dentatus. For example, gliosis in
the external molecular layer of the gyrus dentatus which is
rich in zinc and in Glu/AI in the entorhinal cortex; gliosis
in the dendritic layer of the subiculum/AI in CA1. It should
be noted that gliosis is absent in the layers of neuronal cell
bodies where no Glu mediated axons terminate, but where Ach
and GABA mediated axons synapse. The presubiculum which
is richly afferented by Ach (Fleschig's pathway) does not
show either gliosis or AI. In the neocortex where the process
extends from the hippocampus there is also a parallel between
the localization of the lesions and that of zinc, and probably
that of Glu as well. AI predominate in the neurons of superficial layers II and III and those of the VIth layer, the
majority of whose axons form homolateral or commissural
cortico-cortical association pathways. Gliosis is found in
layers III and V which are rich in zinc and probably also in
Glu, while layer IV which is unaffected in Pick's disease
contains little zinc.

Treatment of Pick's disease with a zinc chelator

The hypothesis that the primary defect in Pick's disease
is an excess of zinc led us to treat several patients with a
heavy metal chelator, calcium EDTA (11,12). In the 10 patients
treated for long periods, 6 showed transient or even long-term
improvement. Clinical improvement was shown in the following
areas: attention, contact, collaboration, initiative, communication, verbal fluency, comprehension; a decrease in persever-
ations, echolalia and verbal stereotypies has also been
observed. Prefrontal signs, when present, were more difficult
to demonstrate or even disappeared. In several patients, improvement in EEG records was observed. Clinical improvement
was seen in the least advanced cases and no improvement was
seen in those patients where one may suppose the most extensive cerebral lesions were present.

Conclusions

Because the lesions of Pick's disease are initially seen
in the hippocampus and because the intrinsic neurotransmitter
in this structure is glutamate, we hypothesized that glutamate
would be altered initially in this disease. The close topographical correlations between glutamate and zinc in the hippocampus and also in other cerebral structures, and the possible
role of zinc in glutamate metabolism (glutamate dehydrogenase
is a zinc metalloenzyme) led us to study this metal. We observed that zinc levels in the hippocampus, blood cells, urine,
serum-albumins and alpha globulins are higher in Pick's disease than in Alzheimer's disease and controls.
We formulated the following heuristic theory: Pick's
disease is related to generalized elevated zinc levels,

probably resulting from a defect in its transport by the plasma proteins. Zinc accumulates in various tissues including brain. This excess of cerebral zinc would produce neuronal lesions, either by direct action or mediated by metalloenzymes, particularly glutamate dehydrogenase. A disturbance of the neurotransmitter glutamate would occur, producing synaptic lesions (gliosis) and subsequently lesions of neuronal cell bodies (argyrophilic inclusions). This process would be initiated in the hippocampus with later extension to the neocortex.

Favorable clinical results were obtained in Pick's disease with a zinc chelator which probably normalizes cerebral glutamate by lowering zinc levels.

References

1. Bradford H.F.and Richards C.D.(1976): Brain Res.,105: 168-172.
2. Constantinidis J.(1980): In: Etats déficitaires cérébraux liés à l'âge. Métabolisme énergétique des acides aminés neurotransmetteurs, Masson, Paris (in press).
3. Constantinidis J., Richard J., Despont J.-P., Cruchaud A. and Tissot R.(1979): In: Biological psychiatry today, eds. J. Obiols, C. Ballus, E. Gonzales Monclus & J. Pujol, pp. 626-630. Elsevier/North-Holland, Biomedical Press.
4. Constantinidis J., Richard J. and Tissot R.(1974): Europ. Neurol. 11: 208-217.
5. Constantinidis J., Richard J. and Tissot R.(1977): Rev. neurol. (Paris) 133: 685-696.
6. Gastaut H. and Lammers H.J.(1961): Anatomie du rhinencéphale, Masson, Paris.
7. Haug F.-M.S.(1967): Histochemie, 8: 355-368.
8. Haug F.-M.S.(1974): Z. Anat. Entwickl.-Gesch., 145: 1-27.
9. Ibata Y. and Otsuka N. J.(1969): Histochem. Cytochem. 17: 171-175.
10. Nadler J.V., Vaca K.M., White W.F., Lynch G.S and Cotman C.W. (1976): Nature (Lond.), 260: 538-540.
11. Richard J., Constantinidis J. and Tissot R.(1978): Nouv. Presse méd. 7, No 15.
12. Richard J., Constantinidis J., Tissot R.(1979): In: Gérontopsychiatrie 7, eds. Ch. Muller & J. Wertheimer, pp. 83-88, Janssen Pharmaceutica, Switzerland.
13. Storm-Mathisen J.(1977): Prog. Neurobiol. 8: 119-181.
14. Storm-Mathisen J.(1978): In: Functions of the septohippocampal system, Ciba Foundation Symposium, 58: 49-79.
15. Timm F.(1958): Z. Zellforsch. 48: 548-555.
16. Tissot R., Constantinidis J.and Richard J.(1975): La maladie de Pick, Masson, Paris.
17. Vallée B.L.(1962): In: Mineral metabolism, eds. C.L. Comar, F. Bronner, Vol.2B: p. 463. Academic Press, New York.
18. White W.F., Nadler J.V., Hamberger A., Cotman C.W. and Cummins J.T.(1977): Nature (Lond.) 270: 356-357.

Glutamate as a Neurotransmitter,
edited by G. Di Chiara and G. L. Gessa
Raven Press, New York © 1981.

Neuroendocrine Effects of Excitotoxic Amino Acids

John W. Olney and Madelon T. Price

*Department of Psychiatry, Washington University School of Medicine,
St. Louis, Missouri 63110*

The ability of systemically administered glutamate (Glu), aspartate (Asp) and certain structural analogs of these putative excitatory neurotransmitters and known neurotoxins, to selectively
penetrate a specific region of the endocrine hypothalamus, the arcuate nucleus (AH), and either stimulate firing of AH neurons or
destroy them, makes these "excitotoxic" agents useful as either
provocative or ablative neuroendocrine investigational tools.
Here we will briefly review information obtained over the past decade in studies involving the ablative use of excitotoxins and
then will describe recent research in which these agents have been
used as provocative tools for studying the role of AH neurons in
the regulation of luteinizing hormone (LH) output.

ABLATION APPROACH

It was first demonstrated 10 years ago (4), and has subsequently been confirmed repeatedly (6, 7) that it is possible to delete
about 80% of the neurons of AH by treating rodents subcutaneously
(sc) in infancy with Glu (Fig. 1). Other excitatory analogues of
Glu reproduce the AH lesion but Glu itself has been the agent employed in most AH ablation studies. Glu-treated animals, including mice, rats, and hamsters, manifest a complex syndrome of endo-
crine-type disturbances, including normophagic obesity (Fig. 1),
skeletal stunting, impaired reproductive capacity, reduced mass
of the anterior pituitary (Fig. 1) and gonads, and reduced pituitary content of growth hormone (GH), prolactin (Prl) and luteinizing hormone (LH). Pulsatile amplitude of serum GH is markedly
reduced and basal serum levels of GH and LH also tend to be depressed. Responsiveness of hypothalamic Prl release mechanisms
are altered - Prl response to estrogenic stimulation is weakened
but to serotonergic stimuli is exaggerated. In Glu-treated rats,
serum triiodothyronine and free thyroxine indices are in the hypo-
thyroid range and serum corticosterone levels are strikingly elevated in Glu-treated mice. While the mechanism by which Glu-
treatment results in obesity remains uncertain, the AH lesion is

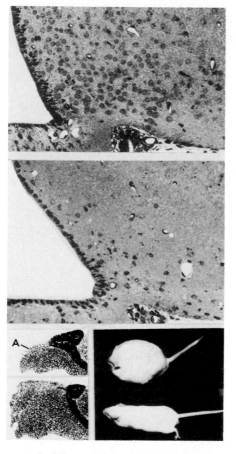

FIG. 1.   The normal arcuate hypothalamic nucleus (AH) of an infant mouse is shown at the top
with the same brain region of an
immature mouse 4 days following
sc Glu treatment depicted below.
In the AH of the Glu-treated animal, note the absence of neurons
(most of the cell bodies visible
are glia) and widening of the
ventricle in compensation for
the loss of neuronal mass.   A
short, fat adult mouse bearing
an AH lesion from neonatal Glu
treatment is depicted at the lower right with a normal litter-
mate control immediately below.
Directly across from each mouse
is his pituitary gland (½ of
each gland is shown).   In the absence of AH neurons, the adeno-
hypophysis (A) of the Glu-treated mouse has failed to develop
to the normal size.

probably responsible since treatment with other Glu analogues
that reproduce the AH lesion also cause obesity.   The Glu lesioned animal provides an interesting model for studying obesity,
since the adiposity develops despite normal or subnormal food in-
take.   It has been suggested that Glu lesioning may provide a
means of gaining insight into the role of the hypothalamus in
both obesity and diabetes since diabetes is unmasked by Glu treatment of inbred mouse strains that are genetically susceptible to
diabetes.

Analysis of the mediobasal hypothalamus following Glu treatment, suggests that, in terms of neurotransmitter content, the
deleted AH neurons are composed of at least two subpopulations -
dopaminergic (DA) and cholinergic (Ach).   In recent immunohistochemical studies, evidence has been presented that all or nearly
all β-endorphin-containing neuronal cell bodies in the brain are
located within the AH region and the same may be true for α-MSH-
containing neurons.   In apparent corroboration of this observation, the deletion of AH neurons by Glu treatment of rodents in
infancy reportedly results in a marked reduction of the

β-endorphin and α-MSH content in both the mediobasalar hypothalamus and in certain extra-hypothalamic brain regions where the fiber systems of these neurons are thought to terminate. A complete set of references to the information summarized above is contained in recent reviews (6, 7).

PROVOCATIVE APPROACH

If our proposal that an excitatory mechanism underlies the toxic action of Glu and related compounds on AH neurons is correct, it follows that subtoxic doses of these compounds - that is, doses that do not damage AH neurons - may excite them to fire at an accelerated rate, just as the application of tiny amounts of these compounds iontophoretically stimulates accelerated firing of neurons throughout many brain regions. Since bioelectric discharge may be the first step in the chain of events through which AH neurons influence pituitary hormonal outputs, increased AH discharge activity may give rise to altered hormonal outputs. Experiments recently undertaken to explore this proposal in relation to the hypothalamic regulation of LH output will be discussed. The serum LH determinations in all of the studies described were performed by radioimmunoassay using reagents supplied by Drs. A.F. Parlow, Gordon Niswender or Leo Reichert of the Rat Pituitary Hormone Distribution Program of NIAMDD.

Acute Effects of Glu or Potent Glu Analogs on Serum LH

When we administered Glu (5) and its potent excitatory analogs (9) kainic acid (KA), N-methyl DL-aspartic acid (NMA) and DL-homocysteic acid (HCA), in subtoxic doses to the weanling or adult male rat,we observed that it results in a rapid elevation of serum luteinizing hormone (LH) and that the order of potencies for the LH releasing activities of these compounds was proportional to the order of their excitatory or toxic potencies. We also evaluated the brain damaging potential of each compound on 25 day old male rats and found that the lowest doses of NMA and HCA effective in producing AH damage were 3-4 times higher than the lowest doses required to induce LH elevations. For KA, however, there was little or no practical margin between a brain damaging and LH-stimulating dose; more importantly, we found that KA tended to damage several extra hypothalamic regions of brain (hippocampus, olfactory cortex, amygdala, lateral septal nucleus and several thalamic nuclei) much more readily than it damaged AH (2, 6). Therefore, we judged KA relatively unsuitable for neuroendocrine investigational purposes and selected NMA - the next most potent excitant - as the agent of choice for exploring LH regulatory mechanisms. NMA, like other straight-chain excitatory amino acids, when administered systemically, exerts excitotoxic action only in select brain regions that lie outside blood brain barriers, the so-called circumventricular organs (CVO). Since one of the CVO, the arcuate hypothalamic nucleus (AH), is particularly

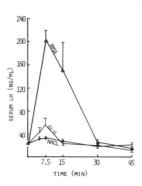

FIG. 2. The time curves of the LH response to non-toxic doses of Glu (1000 mg/kg) or NMA (25 mg/kg) administered sc to weanling male rats. Although the amplitude of the response to NMA is much greater, all other characteristics of the NMA and Glu curves are identical. The LH response, in either case, is rapid of onset and brief in duration with peak amplitude occurring at 7.5 minutes after sc injection of the excitant. (From Olney and Price, Ref. 7)

sensitive to the neurotoxic actions of these agents and is known to have neuroendocrine regulatory function, it is logical to as-cribe the acute effects of amino acid excitants on the LH axis to their interaction with AH neurons. Assuming lack of blood brain barriers is the basis for localization of NMA effects to the AH region, it is curious that systemically administered KA, although capable of destroying AH neurons (8), is relatively more toxic for various other neurons. We suspect that KA penetrates blood brain barriers diffusely to gain access to both CVO and non-CVO neurons and that CVO neurons, perhaps because they have primarily "Asp-preferring" receptors, are hyposensitive to KA excitotoxic-ity compared to certain non-CVO neurons.

Characteristics of the NMA-sensitive LH Release Pathway

Schainker and Cicero (13) and Price et al., (12) have inten-sively examined the LH-releasing activity of NMA and have demon-strated that when this agent is administered sc in non-toxic doses (15-40 mg/kg) to weanling or young adult male rats, it in-duces LH release by an action which is reversible, rapid of onset, brief in duration (Fig. 2), has a suprasellar locus of action and is dependent on AH neurons. The latter points were established by the finding that NMA does not induce release of LH from pitui-tary in vitro (13) and that the LH-releasing action of NMA is not demonstrable in vivo in rats whose AH neurons have been deleted by Glu treatment in infancy (7, 12). These observations, coupled with other related evidence, allowed a tentative characterization of the NMA sensitive LH release pathway in relatively specific terms, i.e., it is subject to stimulation by putative excitatory transmitters acting apparently at specific excitatory receptors on the dendrosomal surfaces of a particular group of hypothalamic neurons whose axons presumably terminate in the median eminence region. Efforts to manipulate this system pharmacologically to provide further insights into its mechanisms and component parts were therefore undertaken.

Not Mediated Through DA or Ach Neurons

Since some AH neurons are thought to be dopaminergic, whereas others may be cholinergic, we employed DA and Ach blocking agents to explore whether the NMA sensitive LH release pathway involves either of these AH neuronal subpopulations, the assumption being that if the AH neurons which effect release of LH in response to NMA stimulation do so by either a DA or Ach mechanism, DA or Ach receptors are presumably involved and antagonists of these receptors should block NMA-stimulated LH release. When the DA receptor blocking agents, pimozide and chlorpromazine were administered (11) 24, 14 and 2 hours prior to NMA challenge, and adequate doses for receptor blocking purposes were employed, the LH-releasing potential of NMA was totally unaffected. When cholinergic blocking agents (atropine, a muscarinic antagonist, and mecamylamine, a nicotinic antagonist) were administered sc to 25 day old male rats (7), these agents also failed to suppress NMA-stimulated LH release. It appears, therefore, that neither the DA nor Ach subpopulation of AH neurons is an integral part of the NMA sensitive LH-release pathway.

GABA and Taurine Block LH-Releasing But Not AH Neurotoxic Actions of NMA

In the early work of Curtis and Watkins (1), it was established that the neuroinhibitory amino acids GABA and taurine, when applied iontophoretically, are effective in blocking the excitatory responses of central neurons to Glu, Asp and their structural analogs. To explore the hypothesis that excitatory amino acids induce LH release by excitation of AH neurons, we administered NMA to 25 day old rats in a dose (25 mg/kg) known to be non-toxic but sufficient to assure a reliable LH response and attempted to block this response by simultaneous administration of GABA or taurine (11). Neither GABA nor taurine by itself influenced serum LH concentrations, but when given with NMA, either compound completely blocked the striking 5 to 10-fold LH elevation typically observed in rats $7\frac{1}{2}$ min after NMA treatment (Table 1). When bicuculline, a specific GABA antagonist, was administered together with GABA, it prevented GABA from blocking NMA-induced LH release (Table 1). This suggests that the inhibitory influence of GABA on the NMA-sensitive LH release pathway may be mediated through a GABAergic inhibitory synapse. Since bicuculline by itself did not alter serum LH levels, the NMA-sensitive LH release pathway is presumably not under tonic GABAergic inhibition. It may be assumed that the inhibitory action of GABA is exerted at a suprasellar rather than pituitary level, since addition of GABA in concentrations from 10^{-7} to 10^{-3} M does not suppress release of LH stimulated from pituitary in vitro by LHRH (10^{-8}M). (Price and Olney, unpublished).

If both the LH-releasing and neurotoxic actions of NMA are mediated by the excitatory actions of NMA and the LH-releasing

TABLE 1.   GABA and Taurine Block NMA-Induced LH Release*

Agents	n	Dose (mg/kg)	Serum LH (ng/ml $\pm$ SEM)
Saline	100		30.1 $\pm$ 1.6
GABA	10	1000	32.8 $\pm$ 5.4
Bicuculline	15	1	32.2 $\pm$ 4.6
Taurine	10	1000	36.6 $\pm$ 6.1
NMA	70	25	247.0 $\pm$ 13.1
NMA + Taurine	15	25 + 1000	27.6 $\pm$ 3.0
NMA + GABA	30	25 + 1000	26.6 $\pm$ 3.0
NMA + GABA	55	25 + 500	24.1 $\pm$ 1.7
NMA + GABA	10	25 + 300	43.0 $\pm$ 7.2
NMA + GABA	15	25 + 200	51.2 $\pm$ 7.5
NMA + GABA	10	25 + 100	196.7 $\pm$ 40.6
NMA + Bicuculline + GABA	20	25 + 1 + 500	187.4 $\pm$ 28.2

*When GABA, taurine or bicuculline are injected sc into 25 day old rats, basal serum LH levels are unaffected. Administering taurine or GABA, together with NMA, results in blockade of NMA-induced LH release. The lowest effective dose of GABA was 200 mg/kg. Adding bicuculline (1 mg/kg) to an effective blocking dose of GABA (500 mg/kg) rendered GABA ineffective in blocking NMA-induced LH release.

effect is blocked by antagonists (GABA or taurine) of NMA-induced excitations, is the neurotoxic action of NMA also subject to such antagonism? We recently conducted a series of experiments aimed at clarifying this question. GABA and taurine were administered simultaneously with NMA and with other excitotoxins, such as Glu itself, in various dose combinations and in both mice and rats at several ages spanning infancy to adulthood. The data in Table 2 are representative findings - in no instance were we able to block the neurotoxic manifestations of NMA or other excitotoxins with GABA or taurine. As discussed below, we believe that these findings can best be understood in terms of GABA and taurine exerting their blocking actions elsewhere than at the NMA excitatory receptor.

α-Aminoadipate Blocks Both the LH-Releasing and AH Neurotoxic Actions of NMA

From recent microelectrophoretic experiments (14) it appears that α-aminoadipate (αAA) is a relatively specific antagonist of the depolarizing action of NMA on central mammalian neurons. Therefore, it was of interest to determine whether this agent might antagonize either the LH-releasing or AH neurotoxic effects

TABLE 2. NMA Neurotoxicity Blocked by DL-αAA But Not
GABA or Taurine

Agent(s)	n	Dose (mg/g)	Lesion Severity[a]
NMA	36	0.075	100.0 ± 3.33
NMA + GABA	12	0.075 + 1.0	103.9 ± 6.70
NMA + Taurine	6	0.075 + 1.0	105.8 ± 6.36
NMA + αAA	22	0.075 + 1.0	43.8 ± 5.07[b]
NMA + Glu	8	0.075 + 2.0	174.4 ± 3.64[b]

(a) Test compounds were administered sc to 35-40 day old mice and
the mean (± SEM) number of acutely necrotic AH neurons/section at
point of maximal damage was determined. Control means (animals
receiving only NMA) were assigned a value of 100 and means for
combination treatments are given as percent ± SEM of the control.
DL-αAA effectively blocks the neurotoxicity of NMA but GABA and
taurine do not. Note that when neuroexcitants are administered
in combination (NMA + Glu), they add to one anothers neurotoxicity.
(b) p < 0.001

of NMA. As Tables 2 & 3 reveal, αAA effectively antagonizes both
the LH releasing and AH neurotoxic actions of NMA. We also have
noted that αAA less effectively, but to a statistically significant degree, antagonizes the AH neurotoxicity of Glu (Table 2).
According to the dual receptor hypothesis (3), some central synapses are "Glu-preferring" and others "Asp-preferring" and Glu
acts interchangeably at either receptor type but Asp may be optimally active only at Asp-preferring receptors. NMA and KA, potent excitotoxic analogs of Asp and Glu respectively, have been
proposed as probe molecules for distinguishing the two receptor
populations. The particular efficacy of NMA as both an AH neurotoxic and LH-releasing agent, the greater efficiency of αAA in
blocking the AH neurotoxic effects of NMA compared to those of Glu
and the peculiar failure of KA to destroy AH neurons as readily as
it destroys neurons in various other regions of brain all tend to
suggest that the majority of excitatory amino acid receptors on
the surfaces of AH neurons are of the Asp-preferring type.

Possible Roles of Excitatory and Inhibitory Amino Acids
In Neuroendocrine Regulation

For reasons just discussed, it appears that AH neurons may
have predominantly Asp-preferring receptors, which suggests the
possibility that physiologically they are innervated by an aspartergic fiber tract. Thus, one might postulate (Fig. 3) that AH
neurons are a major link in an LH release pathway that is driven
by aspartergic excitatory input to synaptic receptors on the

dendrosomal surfaces of AH neurons and is subject to GABAergic inhibition mediated at other receptors in the pathway. Since αAA is
thought to block NMA excitations specifically at the NMA excitatory receptor (14), αAA would be expected to block both the LH releasing and AH neurotoxic actions of NMA. Since GABA and taurine
are considered non-specific antagonists of NMA (they also block
cholinergic excitations), these agents probably exert their blocking action at some point other than either the NMA or cholinergic
receptor; they may exert blocking action, for example, at some
point along the course of the AH axon. Failure of GABA or taurine
to block at the dendrosomal excitatory receptor where the depolarizing action of NMA is translated into a neurotoxic reaction,
would explain why these inhibitory amino acids do not block the
AH neurotoxicity of NMA. If the locus of their inhibitory effect
is at some point along the AH axon, however, this would explain
their blocking action on LH release, i.e., by a presynaptic

TABLE 3.　DL-αAA Blocks NMA-Induced LH Release[*]

Agents	n	Dose (mg/kg)	Serum LH (ng/ml $\pm$ SEM)
Saline (5 cc/kg)	55	-	26.8 $\pm$ 2.1
αAA	20	2000	60.4 $\pm$ 12.9
NMA	25	25	183.3 $\pm$ 23.0
NMA + αAA	15	25 + 2000	54.9 $\pm$ 11.8
NMA + αAA	5	25 + 1500	56.3 $\pm$ 16.3
NMA + αAA	10	25 + 1000	59.3 $\pm$ 19.6
NMA + αAA	10	25 + 500	112.5 $\pm$ 30.6
NMA + αAA	5	25 + 250	223.0 $\pm$ 114.6

[*]DL-alpha aminoadipate (αAA), when administered sc to 25 day old
male rats in high dosage (2000 mg/kg), appears to be a weak sti-
mulant of LH release. The blockade of NMA-induced LH release is
dose dependent in the αAA dose range from 250-1000 mg/kg but no
greater antagonism is achieved by further increasing the αAA dose.
Possibly these findings reflect the fact that L-αAA is a weak
neuroexcitant and that D-αAA may be particularly effective in
blocking NMA-sensitive receptors and only partially effective in
blocking the excitatory receptors with which L-αAA interacts. We
suspect this is not the correct explanation, however, because we
recently found that L-αAA has significant neurotoxic and gliotoxic activity and that D-αAA fully blocks the former but not the
latter. The LH-releasing action of αAA, therefore, might conceivably reflect an interaction between αAA and AH glia. A role
for AH glia (tanycytes) as well as neurons in LH regulation has
long been postulated.

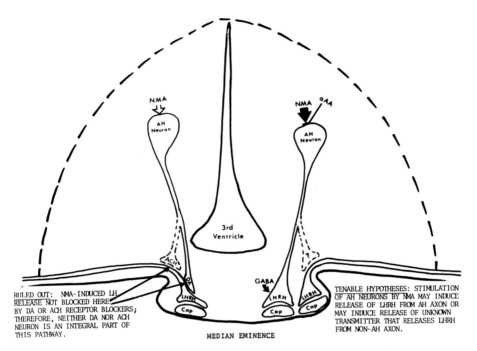

FIG. 3. This schematic depicts the arcuate nucleus-median eminence region of the hypothalamus and illustrates tenable (right) and untenable (left) hypotheses regarding the mechanisms and component parts of the NMA-sensitive LH release pathway. An aspartergic fiber tract may innervate the pathway at the NMA-sensitive excitatory receptor locus, which is also the putative locus of αAA blocking action. A GABAergic synapse at the axonal locus indicated (GABA, arrow) may abort the action potential and thereby prevent the aspartergic stimulus from resulting in secretion of LHRH into the portal capillary system.

inhibition mechanism, they may abort the action potential that presumably is necessary to effect secretion of LH-releasing hormone (LHRH) from either the AH axon or median eminence storage terminals with which it is in contact (Fig. 3).

CONCLUSIONS

We have presented information pertaining to the use of excitotoxic amino acids as neuroendocrine research tools and have focused particularly on recent studies suggesting that amino acid excitants, when administered sc in subtoxic doses, penetrate a specific region of the endocrine hypothalamus, the arcuate nucleus (AH), and by stimulating excitatory receptors on the dendrosomal surfaces of AH neurons, effect an acute release of luteinizing hormone (LH) from the pituitary. Our finding that α-aminoadipate blocks both the LH-releasing and AH neurotoxic actions of NMA, whereas GABA and taurine block only the LH-releasing action, when interpreted in light of other available evidence, suggests that AH neurons may be an integral part of an LH release pathway which is driven by aspartergic excitatory input and is inhibited by GABAergic (or taurinergic) input. The GABAergic influence over this pathway is subject to antagonism by bicuculline. We tentatively propose that this influence is exerted at some point between the AH neuronal cell body and the median eminence storage terminals that presumably secrete LH-releasing hormone (LHRH) in response to the excitatory signal from the AH neuron.

ACKNOWLEDGEMENTS

Supported in part by USPHS grants NS-09156, DA-00259, Career Research Scientist Award MH-38894 (JWO) and Wills Foundation grant.

REFERENCES

1. Curtis, D.R. and Watkins, J.C. (1969): J. Neurochem. 6: 117-141.
2. Fuller, T.A. and Olney, J.W. (1978): Life Sciences 24: 1793-1798.
3. Johnston, G.A.R., Curtis, D.R., Davies, J. and McCulloch, R. M. (1974): Nature 248: 804-805.
4. Olney, J.W. (1969): Science 164: 719-721.
5. Olney, J.W., Cicero, T.J., Meyer, E.R. and de Gubareff, T. (1976): Brain Res. 112: 420-424.
6. Olney, J.W. and Price, M.T. (1978): In: Kainic Acid As A Tool In Neurobiology, edited by E.G. McGeer, J.W. Olney and P.L. McGeer, pp. 239-264. Raven Press, New York.
7. Olney, J.W. and Price, M.T. (In press, 1980): Brain Res. Bull.
8. Olney, J.W., Rhee, V. and Ho, O.L. (1974): Brain Res. 77: 507-512.
9. Price, M.T., Olney, J.W. and Cicero, T.J. (1978): Neuroendocrinology 26: 352-358.
10. Price, M.T., Olney, J.W., Anglim, M. and Buchsbaum (1979): Brain Res. 176: 165-168.
11. Price, M.T., Olney, J.W., Mitchell, M.V., Fuller, T. and Cicero, T.J. (1978): Brain Res. 158: 461-465.
12. Price, M.T., Olney, J.W., Anglim, M., Mitchell, V. and Buchsbaum, S. (1979): Neurosci. Abstr. 5: 456.
13. Schainker, B.A. and Cicero, T.J. (1980): Brain Res. 184: 425-437.
14. Watkins, J.C. (1978): In: Kainic Acid As A Tool In Neurobiology, edited by E.G. McGeer, J.W. Olney and P.L. McGeer, pp. 37-69. Raven Press, New York.

Subject Index